Neuroimaging: An Issue of Radiologic Clinics

Neuroimaging: An Issue of Radiologic Clinics

Editor: Miles Scott

AMERICAN
MEDICAL PUBLISHERS
www.americanmedicalpublishers.com

AMERICAN
MEDICAL PUBLISHERS
www.americanmedicalpublishers.com

Cataloging-in-publication Data

Neuroimaging : an issue of radiologic clinics / edited by Miles Scott.
p. cm.
Includes bibliographical references and index.
ISBN 979-8-88740-309-0
1. Brain--Imaging. 2. Nervous system--Radiography. 3. Brain--Diseases--Imaging.
4. Nervous system--Imaging. 5. Brain--Diseases--Diagnosis. 6. Diagnostic imaging.
I. Scott, Miles.
RC386.6.D52 N483 2023
616.804 754--dc23

American Medical Publishers,
41 Flatbush Avenue,
1st Floor, New York,
NY 11217, USA

ISBN 979-8-88740-309-0 (Hardback)

Contents

Preface

Neuroimaging is a specialized field of medical imaging that uses a wide range of structural and functional imaging techniques to study the structure and function of the CNS and the brain. Neurology makes use of quantitative techniques. From large sectional anatomy to the subatomic level, structural neuroimaging encompasses all scales of anatomical imaging. The primary methods for structural neuroimaging are computerized tomography (CT) scans and magnetic resonance imaging (MRI). Radiology is a medical specialty that involves the use of medical imaging techniques to diagnose and treat diseases. Radiology, unlike neuroimaging, uses qualitative methods based on subjective impressions and substantial clinical training but it does occasionally employ quantitative tools. Functional brain imaging techniques like functional magnetic resonance imaging (fMRI) are standard in neuroimaging but uncommon in radiology. This book discusses the fundamental and modern approaches to neuroimaging. It includes some of the vital pieces of work being conducted worldwide on various topics related to neuroimaging and radiology. This book will serve as a source of comprehensive knowledge to the readers.

Various studies have approached the subject by analyzing it with a single perspective, but the present book provides diverse methodologies and techniques to address this field. This book contains theories and applications needed for understanding the subject from different perspectives. The aim is to keep the readers informed about the progresses in the field; therefore, the contributions were carefully examined to compile novel researches by specialists from across the globe.

Indeed, the job of the editor is the most crucial and challenging in compiling all chapters into a single book. In the end, I would extend my sincere thanks to the chapter authors for their profound work. I am also thankful for the support provided by my family and colleagues during the compilation of this book.

Editor

1

Functional MRI in Alzheimer's Disease

Julia Kivistö, Hilkka Soininen and Maija Pihlajamäki

1. Introduction

Alzheimer's disease (AD) is the most common form of dementia affecting millions of people worldwide. AD results in progressive brain atrophy, memory loss and widespread neurologic deterioration. The first AD-related neuropathological changes appear in the medial temporal lobe (MTL) memory structures already years prior to the manifestation of clinical dementia. Atrophy of the MTL structures as revealed by structural magnetic resonance imaging (MRI) is nowadays considered to be a valid diagnostic marker at the mild cognitive impairment stage, although structural imaging findings may be somewhat nonspecific. "Mild cognitive impairment" (MCI) is in fact one of the recent concepts to describe the possible prodromal state of AD, that is a stage between healthy aging and full-blown clinical AD, for example in terms of neuropathological, imaging and cognitive changes.

Despite extensive research, the fundamental neural basis of memory impairment characteristic to early AD is still largely unknown. Particularly, the relationship between β-amyloid (Aβ) pathology and alterations in memory function remains to be fully elucidated. During recent years, clinical functional MRI (fMRI) has provided tools to investigate the neural underpinnings of AD-related cognitive alterations and thus novel insights into the pathognomonic changes in the MTL structures and related whole-brain memory networks. The ultimate clinical goal of fMRI research is to develop means to reliably define alterations in brain function related to the earliest symptoms of AD before development of significant irreversible structural damage. Since the MTL memory structures are known to be the site of early neuropathological alterations (e.g., neurofibrillary tangles) in AD, previous fMRI studies have largely focused on investigating this particular region of the brain. FMRI during tasks probing episodic memory encoding, which is the cognitive function most characteristically impaired in early AD, is of particular interest.

In this chapter, we will summarize previous studies demonstrating changes in task-related fMRI activity, primarily focusing on memory tasks, as well as studies investigating resting state fMRI findings in clinical AD patients compared to healthy elderly individuals. In a nutshell, fMRI studies in AD patients have demonstrated hypoactivation of the MTL structures during memory task performance, whereas studies in elderly individuals with MCI have reported both increased and decreased MTL responses depending on the severity of the cognitive impairment and underlying structural atrophy. Additionally, recent fMRI findings in MCI and AD patients are beginning to reveal functional abnormalities between the MTL and posteromedial regions such as posterior cingulate and precuneal cortices. In addition to MCI and clinical AD, we will also review recent advances in our understanding of the neuroimaging correlates of cognitively intact elderly subjects at increased risk to develop AD in terms of carrying the apolipoprotein E ε4 (*APOE* ε4) allele.

The long asymptomatic or minimally symptomatic phase of AD provides a potential period for early therapeutic interventions to slow down – and perhaps ultimately prevent – the progression to clinical dementia. Large-scale worldwide multimodal imaging studies on reliable predictors of AD are on-going. There is great hope that imaging of the MTL memory structures and related whole-brain networks would facilitate early diagnosis of AD and other dementias as well as improve treatment options of these devastating diseases in the near future.

2. Alzheimer's disease

AD was originally described in 1907 by the German physician Alois Alzheimer (Alzheimer, 1907; Maurer et al., 1997). Today it is the most common form of dementia in the elderly (Bookmayer et al., 1998). AD is a progressive neurodegenerative syndrome which typically begins with insidious impairment of episodic memory (*i.e.*, memory for past personal experiences in a particular spatial and temporal context).

The most common form of AD is often termed sporadic or late-onset AD as opposed to the relatively rare early-onset forms of the disease (Tanzi & Bertram, 2001). For late-onset AD, the main known genetic risk factor is the *APOE* ε4 allele in chromosome 19 (Bertram et al., 2007; Saunders et al., 1993). Neuropathologically, the disease is characterized by the accumulation of extracellular deposits of Aβ plaques, intracellular neurofibrillary tangles (NFTs) consisting of hyperphosphorylated tau protein, and brain atrophy with regional synaptic, neuronal, and axonal loss (Braak & Braak, 1991). Interestingly, as opposed to the NFT pathology, at the early stages of the disease, Aβ accumulation is often modest within the MTL memory structures but more pronounced, for example, in the posteromedial cortices of the brain. Presentation and clinical course of the AD syndrome can, however, be very variable. Accordingly, AD can be heterogeneous in terms of genetic background (Bertram et al., 2007), response to treatment (Kaduszkiewicz et al., 2005) as well as neuropathological and neuroradiological patterns (Henry-Feugeas, 2007; Jagust et al., 2008; Jellinger, 2002).

The diagnosis of AD relies on clinical judgement. Perhaps the most widely used criteria for defining AD were developed by the National Institute of Neurological and Communicative Disorders and Stroke / Alzheimer's Disease and Related Disorders Association (NINCDS-ADRDA; McKhann et al., 1984). A recent proposal for new research criteria for AD suggests that various biomarkers could be used as supportive features in the diagnostics to improve the specific identification of AD as early as possible (Dubois et al., 2007; Dubois et al., 2010). According to this suggestion, the diagnosis of AD requires meeting the core criterion of significant episodic memory impairment together with at least one or more of the supportive biomarker criteria. Hippocampal atrophy as revealed by structural MRI is one of the most widely documented supportive biomarkers of AD, in addition to abnormal cerebrospinal fluid (CSF) Aβ and tau findings, and a specific pattern of temporoparietal hypometabolism as indicated by [^{18}F]fluorodeoxyglucose positron emission tomography (FDG-PET). Currently, a diagnosis of *definite* AD can, however, only be done by *post mortem* neuropathological evaluation.

The concept of MCI (mild cognitive impairment) refers to subjects with cognitive impairment beyond that expected for their age and education but who are not demented (Petersen et al., 1999; Petersen et al., 2001; Petersen et al., 2004; Petersen et al., 2009; Winblad et al., 2004). During recent years, MCI has had a number of definitions. Diagnostic criteria for the amnestic subtype of MCI widely used during recent years are as follows: 1) memory complaint, preferably corroborated by an informant; 2) objective memory impairment; 3) normal general cognitive function; 4) intact activities of daily living; and 5) not demented (Petersen et al., 2001). Persons who present with amnestic MCI have an increased risk of developing clinical AD with an annual conversion rate of 12 – 15 %, in contrast to 1 – 2 % risk of conversion in healthy elderly individuals (Petersen et al., 1999). Not all subjects with MCI progress to dementia / AD, but a high number of MCI subjects remain stable or may even revert back to normal during follow-up (Ganguli et al., 2004; Gauthier et al., 2006; Larrieu et al., 2002; Petersen, 2004). As noted above, however, a lively discussion on revisions of the MCI / AD diagnostic criteria is on-going among researchers and clinicians.

3. Methodological basis for fMRI in AD

During the past fifteen years, fMRI – together with complementary imaging modalities and sophisticated data analysis methods – has proved to be a very useful tool in investigating the neural basis of intact human memory and other higher cognitive functions. Activation of the hippocampal and parahippocampal regions of the MTL during successful memory encoding has been demonstrated in several fMRI studies in healthy young subjects (Brewer et al., 1998; Pihlajamäki et al., 2003; Sperling et al., 2003b; Stern et al., 1996; Wagner et al., 1998;). These human fMRI findings strongly support the notion that the MTL structures are critical for encoding new events into long-term memory (Eichenbaum, 2000; Mesulam, 1998; Squire & Zola-Morgan, 1991).

Clinical fMRI research into the pathophysiology of age-associated neurodegenerative diseases has become established more recently. Neuroimaging tools such as fMRI provide *in vivo* methods to investigate the integrity of the resting human brain as well as mapping neural networks supporting higher cognitive functions (*e.g.*, memory). fMRI is non-invasive, radiation-free and offers a combination of good spatial and reasonable temporal resolution. Nowadays, the most widely used fMRI technique to measure hemodynamic changes related to underlying cellular activity is based on imaging of the endogenous blood-oxygen-level-dependent (BOLD) contrast (Kwong et al., 1992; Ogawa et al., 1992). In a nutshell, the relative decrease in the amount of deoxygenated hemoglobin enhances the MRI signal locally in brain areas activated during a particular cognitive task. In addition to observed increases in BOLD signal in "activated" brain areas, it has recently been shown that negative BOLD responses are also related to underlying neural activity and originate in decreases in neuronal activity below spontaneous activity in "deactivated" brain regions (Logothetis et al., 2001; Shmuel et al., 2006).

Typically, fMRI experiments compare the BOLD signal during one cognitive condition (*e.g.*, encoding novel pictures) to a control task (*e.g.*, viewing familiar pictures) or to a passive baseline condition (*e.g.*, visual fixation on a cross-hair). This can be done in a "block design" paradigm, in which stimuli of each cognitive condition are grouped together in blocks lasting 20–40 s, or in "event-related" paradigms, in which single stimuli from several different conditions are interspersed.

In addition to functional activation studies, there has recently been considerable interest in studying the baseline activity, or the "default mode" activity, of the resting human brain using FDG-PET and various fMRI techniques (Buckner et al., 2005; Gusnard & Raichle, 2001). It is very interesting that the same brain areas which show high default mode activity and predilection for task-induced fMRI deactivation responses have also demonstrated the earliest hypometabolic changes in AD in previous FDG-PET studies as well as early accumulation of Aβ pathology in recent molecular PET studies using a tracer called [11C]Pittsburgh Combound B, or PIB (Buckner et al., 2005; Cavanna & Trimble, 2006; Klunk et al., 2004; Minoshima et al., 1997; Nestor et al., 2003).

Taken together, fMRI based on BOLD contrast offers a unique, safe and widely available technique for the study of intact human cognition as well as alterations in neuronal function related to healthy aging and dysfunction related to neurodegenerative diseases such as AD.

4. FMRI activation studies

4.1. FMRI activation studies in AD and MCI patients

The hallmark of early AD is the inability to form new enduring episodic memories. At the same time, mild AD patients typically present with neuropathological changes such as synaptic alterations, selective neuronal loss and neurofibrillary tangles in the MTL structures (Braak & Braak 1991; Gomez-Isla et al., 1997; Hyman et al., 1984; Kordower et al., 2001; Scheff et al., 2006; Scheff et al., 2007). In addition to the critical role of the MTL, successful memory formation is thought to require a carefully synchronized interplay between the

MTL and large-scale neural networks (Buckner et al., 2005; Eichenbaum, 2000; Lavenex & Amaral, 2000; Mesulam, 1998; Squire & Zola-Morgan, 1991; Suzuki, 2007; Tulving & Markowitsch, 1998).

Given the prominence of MTL pathology and structural atrophy in early AD, the pioneering fMRI studies on AD focused on investigating alterations in hippocampal activation during various episodic memory tasks (Kato et al., 2001; Machulda et al., 2003; Rombouts et al., 2000; Small et al., 1999; Sperling et al., 2003a). To date, there are several fMRI studies, which have consistently reported diminished or absent MTL activation in AD compared to healthy elderly controls (Fig. 1), during encoding numerous different types of novel stimuli such as faces, face-name pairs, line-drawings, scenes, and geometric shapes (Dickerson et al., 2005; Golby et al., 2005; Grön & Riepe, 2004; Hämäläinen et al., 2007; Kato et al., 2001; Machulda et al., 2003; Pariente et al., 2005; Remy et al., 2005; Rombouts et al., 2000; Small et al., 1999; Sperling et al., 2003a).

Subjects with amnestic MCI (Petersen et al., 2001; Petersen et al., 2009) are an important group to investigate, as they are at increased risk for developing dementia, AD in particular. Consonant with the notion of clinical heterogeneity, results of fMRI studies in MCI subjects relative to controls and AD patients have been variable, findings of hippocampal activation ranging from hyperactivation during encoding (Dickerson et al., 2004; Dickerson et al., 2005; Hämäläinen et al., 2007; Kircher et al., 2007; Woodard et al., 2009; Yassa et al., 2010) to hypoactivation both during encoding and retrieval tasks (Johnson et al., 2006a; Machulda et al., 2003; Mandzia et al., 2009; Petrella et al., 2006). In addition to the heterogeneity of the MCI population, some of the diversity of fMRI results in MCI subjects may be explained by differences in subject selection criteria and the level of clinical severity and underlying MTL atrophy, fMRI paradigms and their difficulty as well as functional imaging and data analysis methods. The mechanistic underpinnings of the observed MTL hyperactivation still remain unclear. In addition to pathological changes in cellular, synaptic or neurotransmitter activity, for example, multiple non-neural factors (such as resting hypoperfusion and metabolism) may also confound the interpretation of BOLD fMRI results in MCI and AD. Typically MCI subjects with significantly impaired memory have, however, similar to AD patients, shown decreased hippocampal activity compared with controls (Machulda et al., 2003; Petrella et al., 2006).

Interestingly, there is also evidence of increased MTL activity in AD patients during specific contrasts, primarily involving the brain response to repetitive stimuli. Golby et al. (2005) reported impaired fMRI repetition suppression paralleled by more MTL activation in AD patients than in older controls during processing of repeated scenes. Another recent study provided evidence that the normal suppression of MTL activity to repeated face-name pairs as compared to visual fixation is impaired in AD (Pihlajamäki et al., 2008). Similar findings have been reported in individuals with amnestic MCI (Johnson et al., 2004). Failure of the hippocampus and surrounding MTL cortices to discriminate familiar from novel information at encoding has also been related to both poor associative recognition memory and poor performance in neuropsychological tests of episodic memory across a range of age and cognitive impairment (Pihlajamäki et al., 2011).

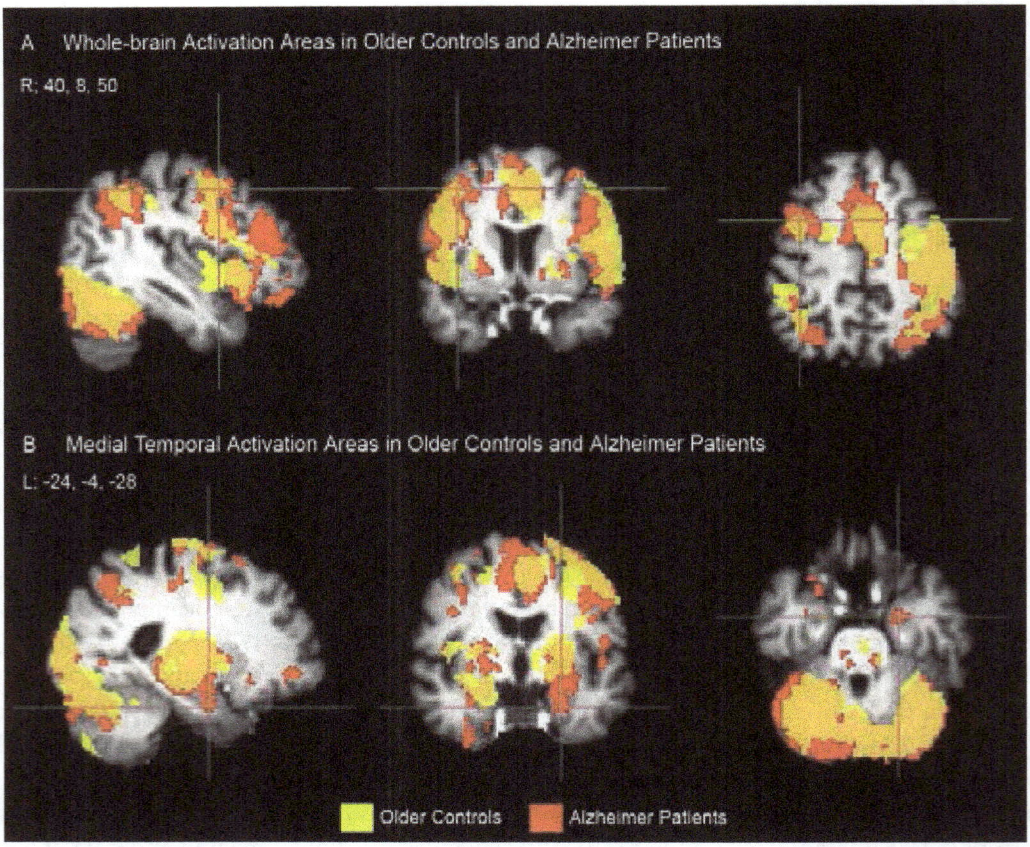

Figure 1. Increased fMRI activity in neocortical (A) and medial temporal (B) brain areas during processing of repeated face-name stimuli in patients with Alzheimer's disease (in red) relative to healthy older control subjects (in yellow). A: Crosshair is located in the right (R) prefrontal cortex, MNI coordinate: 40, 8, 50; B: Crosshair is located in the left (L) anterior hippocampus, MNI coordinate: -24, -4, -28.

As mentioned above, not only the hippocampus but also whole-brain neural networks interconnected with the MTL, are critical for higher cognitive functions such as episodic memory formation (Buckner et al., 2005; Eichenbaum, 2000; Mesulam, 1998). It can be hypothesized that – as opposed to focal changes in the MTL only – multiple nodes within these networks and their mutual interconnectivity are affected at the earliest stage of AD (Scheff et al., 2006; Selkoe, 2002). A recent meta-analysis (Schwindt & Black, 2009) of both fMRI and FDG-PET memory activation studies of AD identified several cortical regions as being more likely to show greater encoding-related activation in controls than in AD patients, including the ventrolateral prefrontal, precuneal, cingulate and lingual cortices. On the other hand, in addition to consistent findings of decreased MTL activation during novel encoding memory tasks, several groups have found evidence of increased fMRI or PET activation in neocortical brain regions, such as frontal and parietal cortices in mild AD patients compared to controls (Grady et al., 2003; Sperling et al., 2003a; Pariente et al., 2005; Celone et al., 2006). This may represent a compensatory process in the setting of MTL dysfunction.

In summary, previous fMRI studies in AD patients, compared to healthy elderly individuals, have reported decreased MTL activity during processing of novel versus repeated information (Dickerson et al., 2005; Golby et al., 2005; Rombouts et al., 2000; Sperling et al., 2003b). These findings of decreased hippocampal activity when comparing novel to repeated stimuli in AD or MCI patients are, in fact, likely to be explained at least to some degree by failure of hippocampal repetition suppression to repeatedly presented stimuli as reviewed above (Golby et al., 2005; Johnson et al., 2004; Pihlajamäki et al., 2008; Pihlajamäki et al., 2011). There is also converging evidence that AD patients show increases in brain activity to compensate for cognitive difficulties in brain regions such as frontal areas that are pathologically less affected than the MTL at the early stages of the disease (Braak & Braak, 1991; Johnson & Albert, 2000; Lehtovirta et al., 1996). Future studies combining multiple imaging modalities such as various structural and functional MRI techniques and PIB-PET imaging (Klunk et al., 2004) are likely to expand our knowledge of the relationships between cognitive impairment, neuropathological changes and alterations in functional imaging patterns.

4.2. FMRI activation studies in *APOE* ε4 carriers

Several experiments in cognitively intact elderly control subjects have demonstrated that elderly individuals are able to activate their hippocampus during successful associative encoding largely to the same degree as young subjects (Miller et al., 2008a; Rand-Giovannetti et al., 2006; Sperling et al., 2003a; Sperling et al., 2003b), although age-related alterations in fMRI activity during normal aging have also been reported (Cabeza et al., 2004; Daselaar et al., 2006a, Daselaar et al., 2006b; Dennis et al., 2007). It has been suggested that age-related changes in memory performance may primarily be due to alterations in cortical regions or in the connectivity between the MTL and neocortical regions.

Similarly to MCI subjects, results of fMRI studies comparing activation in *APOE* ε4 carriers at risk for AD versus their non-carrier counterparts have been diverse. Increased hippocampal and cortical activation has been reported during tasks such as encoding novel and repeated pictures or face-name pairs, encoding and retrieval of word-pairs, a letter fluency task, and an auditory verbal *n*-back working memory task, and has usually been interpreted to reflect compensatory neural mechanisms (Bondi et al., 2005; Bookheimer et al., 2000; Burggren et al., 2002; Dickerson et al., 2005; Fleisher et al., 2005; Han et al., 2007; Pihlajamäki & Sperling, 2009; Smith et al., 2002; Wishart et al., 2006). At the same time, several studies have demonstrated reduced functional brain activity in the MTL and other brain areas in cognitively normal ε4 carriers (Borghesani et al., 2007; Lind et al., 2006; Smith et al., 1999; Trivedi et al., 2006). Several of the above mentioned studies have carefully matched the study groups regarding age, gender and cognitive performance. It is difficult to draw firm conclusions of the ε4 effects on BOLD fMRI activation pattern. In the most recent large-scale fMRI studies, more complex patterns of alterations in brain activation differentially affected by *APOE* ε4 and family history of AD have been suggested (Bassett et al., 2006; Johnson et al., 2006). Longitudinal fMRI testing of subjects at genetic risk for AD would likely be informative, optimally in combination with metabolic FDG- and molecular PIB-PET imaging to improve our understanding of the temporal sequence of events early in the course of prodromal AD.

4.3. FMRI in prediction of cognitive decline

Since some of the MCI subjects will remain stable and some will progress to dementia over time, great interest has been focused on attempts to identify the features predicting future conversion from MCI to clinical AD. As reviewed above, previous cross-sectional fMRI studies in subjects with MCI / prodromal AD have reported variable results, ranging from MTL hypoactivation to hyperactivation compared to cognitively normal elderly individuals. It has been hypothesized that subjects in early phases of prodromal AD may present a short period of paradoxical hippocampal hyperactivation, which is then followed by loss of hippocampal activation along with progressive cognitive decline. FMRI studies with clinical follow-up data on MCI subjects have reported that increased MTL activity at baseline in MCI compared to elderly control subjects may indicate higher likelihood of subsequent cognitive decline (Dickerson et al., 2004; Miller et al., 2008b). Similar findings of a temporary period with abnormally enhanced MTL activity during a preclinical stage of AD have been reported in *APOE* ε4 carriers relative to non-carriers (Bookheimer et al., 2000).

Recently, one longitudinal fMRI study (O'Brien et al., 2010) demonstrated both the highest hippocampal activation at baseline and the greatest loss of hippocampal activation during follow-up in cognitively impaired subjects with the most rapid decline during the follow-up period. The authors concluded that cognitive decline is associated with loss of hippocampal activation and suggested that fMRI may prove valuable in tracking very early progression of brain dysfunction on the trajectory towards clinical AD but prior to the point of irreversible neuronal loss and significant macroscopic atrophy. Thus, it seems that there may be a temporary phase of abnormal MTL hyperactivity along the course of MCI to clinical AD, which may in turn be an indicator of compensatory neural mechanisms recruited in MCI subjects in order to keep memory performance close to the level of cognitively normal elderly subjects. Around the conversion from MCI to clinical AD, the ability to compensate for the MTL pathology is lost, which is then seen as poor task performance and disrupted hippocampal fMRI activity. In other words, hippocampal hyperactivity observed in some previous fMRI studies during the progression of MCI to clinical AD may be a compensatory phenomenon, but it may also be a harbinger of impending hippocampal failure.

5. FMRI resting state studies in AD, MCI and *APOE* ε4 carriers

In addition to task-related fMRI activation studies primarily focusing on the MTL function, recent functional imaging studies have demonstrated AD-related alterations in the so called brain "default mode", or resting state activity. The default mode of the human brain was originally identified by its consistent activity increases during passive task states as compared to a wide range of goal-directed activation tasks (Buckner et al., 2008; Gusnard & Raichle, 2001; Mazoyer et al., 2001; Raichle et al., 2001; Shulman et al., 1997). Regions of the default network show high resting glucose metabolism and blood flow relative to other brain regions as well as coordinated low frequency fluctuations in states of relative rest (Buckner et al., 2008; Minoshima et al., 1997; Raichle et al., 2001; Shulman et al., 1997). Anatomically, the key default mode regions consist of the posteromedial and lateral parietal regions as well as midline and lateral frontal regions. Interestingly, the same default mode regions which are upregulated at rest appear to be suppressed during various cognitive activities, including intentional encoding of new memories (Pihlajamäki et al., 2008; Rombouts et al., 2005a; Shulman et al., 1997). Deactivation of key nodes of the default mode network, in coordination with hippocampal activation, seems in fact to be a prerequisite for successful memory encoding (Daselaar et al., 2004; Miller et al., 2008a; Weissman et al., 2006).

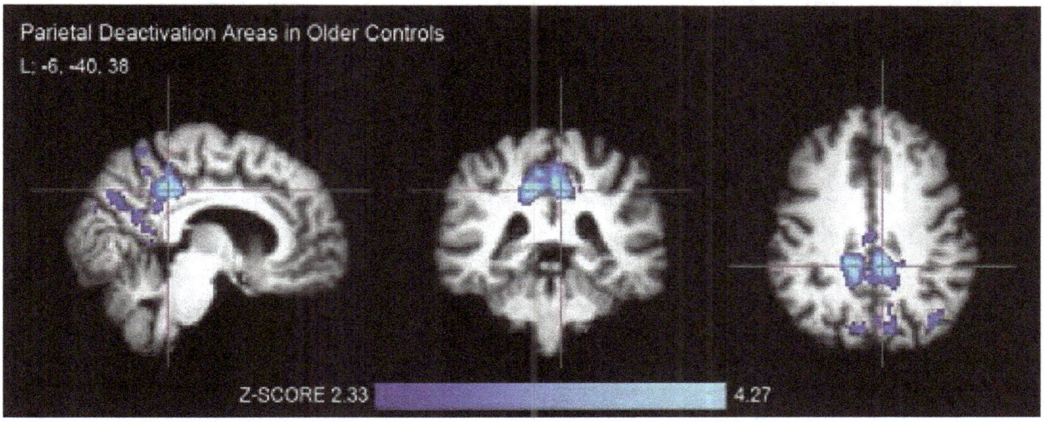

Figure 2. FMRI deactivation areas during processing of repeated face-name stimuli in healthy older subjects (in blue). Crosshair is located in the left (L) posterior cingulated cortex, MNI coordinate: -6, -40. 38.

Previous FDG-PET studies in clinical AD patients and older individuals at risk for AD have revealed hypometabolism of the posteromedial and other association cortical regions (Herholz et al. 2002; Minoshima et al. 1997; Mosconi et al. 2008b; Rapoport 1991; Reiman et al., 1996). In recent fMRI studies of AD, corresponding brain default mode regions have been found to demonstrate an abnormal fMRI task-induced deactivation pattern (Greicius et al., 2004; Lustig et al., 2003; Petrella et al., 2007a; Petrella et al., 2007b; Pihlajamäki et al., 2008; Rombouts et al., 2005a; Rombouts et al., 2005b). Predilection of the posteromedial core regions of the default network to demonstrate task-induced deactivation (*i.e.*, relative decreases in the BOLD fMRI signal) during paradigms requiring attention to external stimuli has been consistently demonstrated in both young and old healthy subjects (Fig. 2) using a multitude of cognitive stimuli and both fMRI and PET imaging modalities (Buckner et al., 2005, 2008; Cavanna & Trimble, 2006; Daselaar et al., 2004; Fransson & Marrelec, 2008; Gusnard et al., 2001; Mazoyer et al., 2001; Miller et al., 2008a; Otten & Rugg, 2001; Raichle et al., 2001; Shulman et al., 1997). In other words, the relative decreases in fMRI signal normally observed in the default mode regions in healthy subjects performing a cognitive task are not seen in AD patients, or may even be reversed to a paradoxical activation response (Grady et al., 2006; Lustig et al., 2003; Miller et al., 2008a; Otten & Rugg, 2001).

Recent fMRI studies have also revealed alterations in the deactivation pattern in elderly individuals at risk for AD by virtue of their *APOE* e4 genotype or evidence of MCI. The pattern of fMRI task-induced deactivation seems to be progressively disrupted along the continuum from normal aging to MCI and to clinical AD and more impaired in ε4 carriers than in non-carriers (Persson et al., 2008; Pihlajamäki et al., 2009). It is likely that the pathologically affected MCI or AD brain (Selkoe, 2002; Tanzi, 2005) is no longer capable of "turning off" the default mode activity during focused cognitive processing as it should in order to optimally recruit other networks – such as the hippocampal memory network or the frontoparietal attentional network – for task performance (Eichenbaum, 2000; Mesulam, 1998; Miller et al., 2008a; Weissman et al., 2006). This finding is consonant with recent studies in healthy young and elderly adults demonstrating that the ability to suspend default mode activity during goal-directed cognitive tasks, *i.e.* to reallocate neurocognitive resources to those brain regions optimal for the task performance, may be critical for successful cognitive performance (Daselaar et al., 2004; Grady et al., 2006; Miller et al., 2008a; Otten & Rugg, 2001; Weissman et al., 2006). Posteromedial cortical regions of the default mode network not only overlap topographically with the pattern of FDG-PET hypometabolism but also with the distribution of the fibrillar Aβ deposition in AD (Buckner et al., 2005). Recent PIB-PET studies, the tracer PIB labeling Aβ plaques (Edison et al., 2007; Klunk et al., 2004), have suggested that the posteromedial cortical areas of high default mode activity may in fact be among the earliest sites of Aβ pathology in AD (Mintun et al., 2006). Thus, functional (as well as structural) imaging studies focusing on this region are pathobiologically very relevant when searching for potential early markers of prodromal AD.

In MCI and AD patients, alterations observed in the fMRI deactivation pattern of the posteromedial cortices (Greicius et al., 2004; Lustig et al., 2003; Petrella et al., 2007a; Petrella et al., 2007b; Pihlajamäki et al., 2008; Rombouts et al., 2005a; Rombouts et al., 2005b) may also reflect remote effects of the MTL pathology and atrophy. The MTL, which is thought to be responsible for the episodic memory deficits observed in amnestic MCI and AD and is known to present the earliest neurofibrillary changes and neuronal and synapse loss, is strongly interconnected to the posteromedial nodes of the default network (Braak & Braak, 1991; Gomez-Isla et al., 1997; Hyman et al., 1984; Insausti et al., 1987; Kordower et al., 2001; Leichnetz, 2001; Suzuki & Amaral, 1994). It is also possible that local structural atrophy of the underlying posteromedial brain regions may explain some of the findings of altered fMRI deactivation (Greicius et al., 2004; Lustig et al., 2003; Petrella et al., 2007a; Petrella et al., 2007b; Pihlajamäki et al., 2008; Rombouts et al., 2005a; Rombouts et al., 2005b).

A more recent imaging approach, that is the functional connectivity MRI (fcMRI), identifies brain systems via intrinsic functional (activity) correlations (Damoiseaux et al., 2006; Fox & Raichle, 2007; Greicius et al., 2003; Greicius & Menon, 2004). Recent fcMRI studies in healthy young subjects have demonstrated the consistency of the resting state networks in the human brain and have also corroborated the findings of altered task-induced deactivation in MCI and AD relative to controls (Celone et al., 2006; Sorg et al., 2007; Supekar et al., 2008;

Wang et al., 2007; Zhou et al., 2008). As an example, functional connectivity between the posteromedial and MTL cortices has been reported to be impaired even in MCI subjects relative to healthy elderly controls (Sorg et al., 2007; Zhou et al., 2008). Resting state fcMRI between the MTL and posteromedial cortices has also been demonstrated to reflect underlying structural connectivity as revealed by diffusion tensor imaging. Future studies investigating the relations between, for example, the fMRI task-induced activation / deactivation, resting fcMRI and PIB-PET amyloid imaging findings will further expand our understanding of the role of the Aβ pathology and impaired default mode network function in the pathogenesis and cognitive symptomatology of AD.

6. Conclusions and future directions of fMRI in AD

There have been a number of promising clinically relevant imaging studies targeting brain functional alterations in AD, MCI and subjects at-risk for AD relative to normal aging. Functional imaging during memory paradigms has shown evidence of specific alterations in the MTL and related whole-brain memory networks that may be able to differentiate the process of very early AD from normal aging. The greatest potential of functional imaging most likely lies in the study of very early stages of dementias, at the point of emerging neuronal dysfunction without significant macroscopic brain atrophy. In the context of early diagnostics of AD, the most interesting and challenging target group to be investigated continues to be the elderly subjects with subtle memory impairment as these subjects would still have preserved brain function and thus scope for therapeutic interventions. Recent revisions of the criteria for AD and MCI strongly emphasize the use of imaging biomarkers in future clinical diagnostics of these disorders. Structural MRI evaluation of the hippocampus is already widely used as a supportive biomarker for AD diagnosis.

The past two decades have seen remarkable advances in our understanding of the pathophysiology of neurodegenerative dementias. As reviewed above, fMRI has many potential advantages in studying patients with cognitive impairment. FMRI can be acquired on a standard clinical magnet during the same session as structural imaging. Because it is non-invasive and subjects are not exposed to radiation, fMRI can be safely repeated many times over the course of longitudinal studies. Perhaps the greatest potential advantage of fMRI is that we can image patients with memory disorders while they are attempting to do the type of cognitive process that is causing them difficulty in their daily living. The use of event-related designs enables investigation of the hemodynamic correlates of specific behavioral events, such as successful long-term memory formation.

There are, however, several challenges in performing fMRI studies in patients with neurodegenerative dementias. It is likely that fMRI will remain quite problematic in examining patients with more severe cognitive impairment. High-field fMRI with optimized imaging parameters can offer spatial resolution as high as in the order of 1 mm, or even less. This is, however, currently not realistic with demented patients as the technique is sensitive to head motion. Inherently, the signal-to-noise ratio of BOLD signal changes between activation and baseline conditions is low, which necessitates repeated measurements and thus leads to relatively long scanning sessions. There is a need for continued technical advances, such as real-time motion correction and high-speed acquisition, to fully realize the potential of this technology in dementia research. Also, if the patients are not able to adequately perform the cognitive task, one of the major advantages of fMRI activation studies is lost. Differences in task performance between patient and control groups complicate data interpretation, as the ability to perform the task may greatly influence the pattern and degree of observed fMRI activity. Resting state fMRI can, however, be performed with less co-operative subjects and is thus better applicable to imaging more severely impaired patients.

It is important to remember that BOLD fMRI is an indirect measure of neuronal activity. The BOLD fMRI signal, and neurovascular coupling linking cellular activity to hemodynamic changes, is likely to undergo changes during healthy aging and during AD-related pathological processes. Some of the changes that may occur even in healthy elderly subjects include, for example, increased atherosclerosis. In AD, the presence of Aβ in the cerebral vasculature, together with altered neurotransmitter activity, impairs synaptic, neuronal and glial function, and may thus lead to attenuated BOLD response. Both increased and decreased BOLD fMRI responses have, however, been reported in MCI and AD and MCI compared to elderly controls, which does not support the view of attenuation of the BOLD signal solely due to vascular reasons (Golby et al., 2005; Grady et al., 2003; Sperling et al., 2003a). The alterations in BOLD activity reported in AD also appear to be quite regionally specific and dependent on the nature of the cognitive task, thus making it relatively unlikely that the changes observed in fMRI studies represent global pathophysiological alterations in neurovascular coupling.

In terms of using fMRI in longitudinal or pharmacological studies, it is critical to complete further validation experiments. The reproducibility of BOLD signal changes within young healthy individuals during memory encoding tasks across separate days is reported to be reasonable (Sperling et al., 2002; Harrington et al., 2006). However, reproducibility of task-related or resting state fMRI activity in older and cognitively impaired subjects has not yet been well established. More longitudinal functional imaging studies are needed to track the evolution of alterations in the fMRI activation / deactivation pattern over the course of the cognitive continuum from healthy aging to AD. It is also important to evaluate the contribution of structural atrophy to changes observed with functional imaging. A combination of structural MRI, fMRI and other functional and molecular imaging techniques such as PIB-PET may eventually serve as a valuable method for the *in vivo* detection of AD prior to clinical dementia, at the point when disease modifying therapies would likely be most efficacious.

In summary, despite technical challenges, there have been a number of promising fMRI studies in elderly individuals with prodromal AD. Neuroimaging, and in particular BOLD fMRI has produced invaluable information and will likely enable even deeper understanding of the human brain function both in health and disease in the future. Carefully designed future studies using multimodal imaging are hoped to yield us new tools that aid in the early identification of subjects likely to develop dementia. Further longitudinal studies are needed to track the evolution of brain functional alterations over the course of the cognitive continuum from healthy aging to clinical dementias such as AD, and perhaps also the pharmacological efficacy for novel disease-modifying therapies.

Acknowledgements

The original work from our laboratory described in this chapter was supported by Health Research Council of the Academy of Finland, grant #121038 (HS) and grants #108188 and #214050 (MP), and Kuopio University Hospital EVO grants #477311 and #5772720. We express special gratitude to the subjects who participated in this study.

Author details

Julia Kivistö[1], Hilkka Soininen[1,2] and Maija Pihlajamäki[1,2]

1 Department of Neurology, Kuopio University Hospital, Kuopio, Finland

2 Unit of Neurology, Institute of Clinical Medicine, School of Medicine, University of Eastern Finland, Kuopio, Finland

References

[1] Alzheimer, A. (1907). Über eine eigenartige Erkrankung der Hirnrinde. Allgem Z Psychiatr Psych-Gerisch Med, , 64, 146-148.

[2] Bassett, S. S., Yousem, D. M., Cristinzio, C., Kusevic, I., Yassa, M. A., Caffo, B. S., & Zeger, S. L. (2006). Familiar risk for Alzheimer's disease alters fMRI activation patterns. Brain, , 129, 1229-1239.

[3] Bertram, L., Mcqueen, M. B., Mullin, K., Blacker, D., & Tanzi, R. E. (2007). Systematic metaanalyses of Alzheimer's disease genetic association studies: the AlzGene database. Nat Genet, , 39, 17-23.

[4] Bondi, M. W., Houston, W. S., Eyler, L. T., & Brown, G. G. (2005). fMRI evidence of compensatory mechanisms in older adults at genetic risk for Alzheimer disease. *Neurology*, 64, 501-508.

[5] Bookheimer, S. Y., Strojwas, M. H., Cohen, M. S., Saunders, A. M., Pericak-vance, M. A., Mazziotta, J. C., & Small, G. W. (2000). Patterns of brain activation in people at risk for Alzheimer's disease. *N Engl J Med.*, 343, 450-456.

[6] Borghesani, P. R., Johnson, L. C., Shelton, A. L., Peskind, E. R., Aylward, E. H., Schellenberg, G. D., et al. (2007). Altered medial temporal lobe responses during visuospatial encoding in healty APOE*4 carriers. Neurobiol Aging, , 82, 239-259.

[7] Braak, H., & Braak, E. (1991). Neuropathological stageing of Alzheimer-related changes. *Acta Neuropathol (Berl),*, 82, 239-259.

[8] Brewer, J. B., Zhao, Z., Desmond, J. E., Glover, G. H., & Gabrieli, J. D. (1998). Making memories: brain activity that predicts how well visual experience will be remembered. *Science,* 281, 1185-1187.

[9] Brookmayer, R. Gray,.S & Kawas, C. ((1998). Projections of Alzheimer's disease in the United States and the public health impact of delaying disease onset. Am J Public Health, , 88, 1337-1342.

[10] Buckner, R. L. (2004). Memory and executive function in aging and AD: multiple factors that cause decline and reserve factors that compensate. *Neuron,* 44, 195-208.

[11] Buckner, R. L., Snyder, A. Z., & Shannon, B. J. LaRossa, G., Sachs, R., Fotenos, A. F., Sheline, Y.I., Klunk, W.E., Mathis, C.A., Morris, J.C. & Mintun, M.A. ((2005). Molecular, structural, and functional characterization of Alzheimer's disease: Evidence for a relationship between default activity, amyloid, and memory. Journal of Neuroscience, , 25, 7709-7717.

[12] Buckner, R. L., Andrews-hanna, J. R., & Schacter, D. L. (2008). The brain's default network: Anatomy, function and relevance to disease. *Annals of the New York Academy of Sciences,* 1124, 1-38.

[13] Burggren, A. C., Small, G. W., Sabb, F. W., & Bookheimer, S. Y. (2002). Specificity of brain activation patterns in people at genetic risk for Alzheimer disease. *Am J Geriatr Psychiatry,*, 10, 44-51.

[14] Cavanna, A. E., & Trimble, M. R. (2006). The precuneus: A review of its functional anatomy and behavioural correlates. *Brain,* 129, 564-583.

[15] Cabeza, R., Daselaar, S. M., Dolcos, F., Prince, S. E., Budde, M., & Nyberg, L. (2004). Task-independent and task-specific age effects on brain activity during working memory, visual attention and episodic retrieval. *Cereb Cortex,*, 14, 364-375.

[16] Celone, K. A., Calhoun, V. D., Dickerson, B. C., Atri, A., Chua, E. F., Miller, S., Depeau, K., Rentz, D. M., Selkoe, D. J., Blacker, D., Albert, M. S., & Sperling, R. A. (2006). Alterations in memory networks in mild cognitive impairment and Alzheimer's disease: an independent component analysis. *J. Neurosci.,* 26, 10222-10231.

[17] Damoiseaux, J. S., Rombouts, S. A., Barkhof, F., Scheltens, P., Stam, C. J., Smith, S. M., & Beckmann, C. F. (2006). Consistent resting-state networks across healthy subjects. *Proc Natl Acad Sci U S A,* 103, 13848-13853.

[18] Daselaar, S. M., Prince, S. E., & Cabeza, R. (2004). When less means more: deactivations during encoding that predict subsequent memory. *NeuroImage*, 23, 921-927.

[19] Daselaar, S. M., Fleck, M. S., Dobbins, I. G., Madden, D. J., & Cadeza, R. (2006a). Effects of healty aging on hippocampal and rhinal memory functions: an event-related study. Cereb Cortex, , 16, 1771-1782.

[20] Daselaar, S. M., Fleck, M. S., & Cebeza, R. (2006b). Triple dissociation in the medial temporal lobes: recollection, familiarity, and novelty. *J Neurophysiol,*, 96, 1902-1911.

[21] Dennis, N. A., Kim, H., & Cadeza, R. (2007). Effects of aging on true and false memory formation: an fMRI study. *Neuropsychologia*, 45, 74-79.

[22] Dickerson, B. C., Salat, D. H., Bates, J. F., Atiya, M., Killiany, R. J., Greve, D. N., et al. (2004). Medial temporal lobe function and structure in mild cognitive impairment. Ann Neurol, , 56, 27-35.

[23] Dickerson, B. C., Salat, D. H., Greve, D. N., Chua, E. F., Rand-giovannetti, E., Rentz, D. M., Bertram, L., Mullin, K., Tanzi, R. E., Blacker, D., Albert, M. S., & Sperling, R. A. (2005). Increased hippocampal activation in mild cognitive impairment compared to normal aging and AD. *Neurology*, 65, 404-411.

[24] Dubois, B., Feldman, H. H., Jacova, C., Dekosky, S. T., Barberger-gateau, P., Cummings, J., Delacourte, A., Galasko, D., Gauthier, S., Jicha, G., Meguro, K., Brien, O., Pasquier, J., Robert, F., Rossor, P., Salloway, M., Stern, S., Visser, Y., & Scheltens, P. J. P. ((2007). Research criteria for the diagnosis of Alzheimer's disease: revising the NINCDS-ADRDA criteria. Lancet Neurol, , 6, 734-746.

[25] Dubois, B., Feldman, H. H., Jacova, C., Cummings, J. L., Dekosky, S. T., Barberger-gateau, P., Delacourte, A., Frisoni, G., Fox, N. C., Galasko, D., Gauthier, S., Hampel, H., Jicha, G., Meguro, K., Brien, O., Pasquier, J., Robert, F., Rossor, P., Salloway, M., Sarazin, S., De Souza, M., Stern, L. C., Visser, Y., & Scheltens, P. J. P. ((2010). Revising the definition of Alzheimer's disease: a new lexicon. Lancet Neurol, , 9, 1118-1127.

[26] Edison, P. E., Archer, H. A., Hinz, R., Hammers, A., Pavese, N., Tai, Y., et al. (2007). Amyloid, hypometabolism, and cognition in Alzheimer disease: an [11C]PIB and [18F]FDG PET study, Neurology , 68, 501-508.

[27] Eichenbaum, H. system for declarative memory. Nat Neurosci , 1, 41-50.

[28] Fleisher, A. S., Houston, W. S., Eyler, L. T., Frye, S., Jenkins, C., Thal, L. J., & Bondi, M. W. (2005). Identification of Alzheimer disease risk by fMRI. Arch Neurol, , 62, 1881-1888.

[29] Fox, M. D., & Raichle, M. E. (2007). Spontaneous fluctuations in brain activity observed with functional magnetic resonance imaging,. *Nat Rev Neurosci*, 8, 700-711.

[30] Fransson, P., & Marrelec, G. (2008). The precuneus/posterior cingulate cortex plays a pivotal role in the default mode network: Evidence from a partial correlation network analysis. *Neuroimage*, 42, 1178-1184.

[31] Ganguli, M., Dodge, H. H., Shen, C., & Dekosky, S. T. (2004). Mild cognitive impairment amnestic type: an epidemiologic study. *Neurology*, 63, 115-121.

[32] Gauthier, S., Reisberg, B., Zaudig, M., Petersen, R. C., Ritchie, K., Broich, K., Belleville, S., Brodaty, H., Bennett, D., Chertkow, H., Cummings, J. L., De Leon, M., Feldman, H., Ganguli, M., Hampel, H., Scheltens, P., Tierney, M. C., Whitehouse, P., & Winblad, B. (2006). Mild cognitive impairment. Lancet, , 367, 1262-1270.

[33] Golby, A., Silverberg, G., Race, E., Gabrieli, S., Shea, O., Knierim, J., Stebbins, K., & Gabrieli, G. J. ((2005). Memory encoding in Alzheimer's disease: an fMRI study of explicit and implicit memory. Brain, 128, 773-787.

[34] Gomez IslaT., Hollister, R., West, H., Mui, S., Growdon, J.H., Petersen, R.C., Parisi, J.E. & Hyman, B.T. ((1997). Neuronal loss correlates with but exceeds neurofibrillary tangles in Alzheimer's disease. Ann Neurol, , 41, 17-24.

[35] Grady, C. L., Mcintosh, A. R., Beig, S., Keightley, M. L., Burian, H., & Black, S. E. (2003). Evidence from functional neuroimaging of a compensatory prefrontal network in Alzheimer's disease. *J Neurosci,*, 23, 986-993.

[36] Grady, C. L., Springer, M. V., Hongwanishkul, D., Mcintosh, A. R., & Winocur, G. (2006). Age related changes in brain activity across the adult lifespan. J Cogn Neurosci, , 18, 227-241.

[37] Greicius, M. D., Krasnow, B., Reiss, A. L., & Menon, V. (2003). Functional connectivity in the resting brain: a network analysis of the default mode hypothesis. Proc Natl Acad Sci U S A, , 100, 253-258.

[38] Greicius, M. D., & Menon, V. (2004). Default-mode activity during a passive sensory task: uncoupled from deactivation but impacting activation,. J Cogn Neurosci, , 16, 1484-1492.

[39] Greicius, M. D., Srivastava, G., Reiss, A. L., & Menon, V. (2004). Default-mode network activity distinguishes Alzheimer's disease from healthy aging: Evidence from functional MRI. Proc Natl Acad Sci USA, , 101, 4637-4642.

[40] Grön, G., & Riepe, M. W. (2004). Neural basis for the cognitive continuum in episodic memory from health to Alzheimer's disease. Am J Geriatr Psychiatry, , 12, 648-652.

[41] Gusnard, D. A., & Raichle, M. E. (2001). Searching for a baseline: Functional imaging and the resting human brain. Nat Rev Neurosci, , 2, 685-694.

[42] Harrington, G. S. Tomaszewski Farias, S., Buonocore, M. H., & Yonelinas, A. The intersubject and intrasubject reproducibility of FMRI activation during three encoding tasks: Implications for clinical applications. Neuroradiology, 2006.

[43] Henry-feugeas, M. C. (2007). MRI of the `Alzheimer syndrome`. *J Neuroradiol,*, 34, 220-227.

[44] Hyman, B. T., Van Hoesen, G. W., Damasio, A. R., & Barnes, C. L. (1984). Alzheimer's disease: cell-specific pathology isolates the hippocampal formation. Science, 225, 1168-1170.

[45] Hämäläinen, A., Pihlajamäki, M., Tanila, H., Hänninen, T., Niskanen, E., Tervo, S., et al. (2007). Increased fMRI responses during encoding in mild cognitive impairment. *Neurobiol Aging,*, 28, 1889-1903.

[46] Insausti, R., Amaral, D. G., & Cowan, W. M. (1987). The entorhinal cortex of the monkey: II. Cortical afferents,. J Comp Neurol, , 264, 356-395.

[47] Jagust, W. J., Zheng, L., Harvey, D. J., Mack, W. J., Vinters, H. V., Weiner, M. W., Ellis, W. G., Zarow, C., Mungas, D., Reed, B. R., Kramer, J. H., Schuff, N., Decarli, C., & Chui, H. C. (2008). Neuropathological basis of magnetic resonance images in aging and dementia. *Ann Neurol,*, 63, 72-80.

[48] Jellinger, K. A. (2002). Alzheimer disease and cerebrovascular pathology: an update. *J Neural Transm,*, 109, 813-836.

[49] Johnson, K. A., & Albert, M. S. (2000). Perfusion abnormalities in prodromal AD. *Neurobiol Aging,*, 21, 289-299.

[50] Johnson, S. C., Baxter, L. C., Susskind-wilder, L., Connor, D. J., Sabbagh, M. N., & Caselli, R. J. (2004). Hippocampal adaptation to face repetition in healthy elderly and mild cognitive impairment. *Neuropsychologia,* 42, 980-989.

[51] Johnson, S. C., Schmitz, T. W., Trivedi, M. A., Ries, M. L., Torgerson, B. M., Carlsson, C. M., et al. (2006). The influence of Alzheimer disease family history and apolipoprotein E epsilon4 on mesial temporal lobe activation. *J Neurosci,*, 26, 6069-6076.

[52] Kaduszkiewicz, H., Zimmermann, T., & Beck-bornholdt, H. P. Van Den Bussche, H. (2005). Cholinesterase inhibitors for patients with Alzheimer's disease: systematic review of randomised clinical trials. BMJ, , 331, 321-327.

[53] Kato, T., Knopman, D., & Liu, H. (2001). Dissociation of regional activation in mild AD during visual encoding: a functional MRI study. *Neurology,* 57, 812-816.

[54] Kircher, T. T., Weis, S., Freyman, K., Erb, M., Jessen, F., Grodd, W., Heun, R., & Leube, D. T. (2007). Hippocampal activation in MCI patients is necessary for successful memory encoding. J Neurol Neurosurgery Psychiatry, , 78, 812-818.

[55] Klunk, W. E., Engler, H., Nordberg, A., Wang, Y., Blomqvist, G., Holt, D. P., Bergström, M., Savitcheva, I., Huang, G. F., Estrada, S., Ausén, B., Debnath, M. L., Barletta, J., Price, J. C., Sandell, J., Lopresti, B. J., Wall, A., Koivisto, P., Antoni, G., Mathis, C. A., & Långström, B. (2004). Imaging brain amyloid in Alzheimer's disease with Pittsburgh Compound-B. Ann Neurol, , 55, 306-319.

[56] Kordower, J. H., Chu, Y., Stebbins, G. T., Dekosky, S. T., Cochran, E. J., Bennett, D., & Mufson, E. J. (2001). Loss and atrophy of layer II entorhinal cortex neurons in elderly people with mild cognitive impairment. Ann Neurol, , 49, 202-213.

[57] Kwong, K. K., Belliveau, J. W., Chesler, D. A., Goldberg, I. E., Weisskoff, R. M., Poncelet, B. P., Kennedy, D. N., Hoppel, B. E., Cohen, M. S., Turner, R., et al. (1992). Dynamic magnetic resonance imaging of human brain activity during primary sensory stimulation. Proc Natl Acad Sci USA, , 89, 5675-5679.

[58] Larrieu, S., Letenneur, L., Orgogozo, J. M., Fabrigoule, C., & Amieva, H. Le Carret, N., Barberger-Gateau, P. & Dartigues, J.F. ((2002). Incidence and outcome of mild cognitive impairment in a population-based prospective cohort. Neurology, 59, 1594-1599.

[59] Lavenex, P., & Amaral, D. G. (2000). Hippocampal-neocortical interaction: a hierarchy of associativity. *Hippocampus*, 10, 420-430.

[60] Lind, J., Persson, J., Ingvar, M., Larsson, A., Curts, M., Van Broeckhoven, C., Adolfsson, R., Bäckman, L., Nilsson, L. G., Petersson, K. M., & Nyberg, L. (2006). Reduced functional brain activity response in cognitively intact apolipoprotein E epsilon 4 carriers. Brain, , 129, 1240-1248.

[61] Lehtovirta, M., Soininen, H., Laakso, M. P., Partanen, K., Helisalmi, S., Mannermaa, A., Ryynänen, M., Kuikka, J., Hartikainen, P., & Riekkinen, P. J. Sr. ((1996). SPECT and MRI analysis in Alzheimer's disease: relation to apolipoprotein E epsilon 4 allele. J Neurol Neurosurg Psychiatry, , 60, 644-649.

[62] Leichnetz, G. R. (2001). Connections of the medial posterior parietal cortex (area 7m) in the monkey,. Anat Rec, , 263, 215-236.

[63] Logothetis, N. K., Pauls, J., Augath, M., Trinath, T., & Oeltermann, A. (2001). Neurophysiological investigation of the basis of the fMRI signal. *Nature*, 412, 150-157.

[64] Lustig, C., Snyder, A. Z., Bhakta, M., Brien, O., Mcavoy, K. C., Raichle, M., Morris, M. E., & Buckner, J. C. R.L. ((2003). Functional deactivations: change with age and dementia of the Alzheimer type. Proc Natl Acad Sci USA, , 100, 14504-14509.

[65] Machulda, M. M., Ward, H. A., Borowski, B., Gunter, J. L., Cha, R. H., Brien, O., Petersen, P. C., Boeve, R. C., Knopman, B. F., Tang-wai, D., Ivnik, D. F., Smith, R. J., Tangalos, G. E., Jack, E. G., & Jr, C. R. (2003). Comparison of memory fMRI response among normal, MCI and Alzheimer's patients. *Neurology*, 61, 500-506.

[66] Mandzia, J. L., Mcandrews, M. P., Grady, C. L., Graham, S. J., & Black, S. E. (2009). Neural correlates of incidental memory in mild cognitive impairment: an fMRI study. *Neurobiol Aging,*, 30, 717-730.

[67] Maurer, K., Volk, S., & Gerbaldo, H. and Alzheimer's disease. Lancet, , 349, 1546-1549.

[68] Mazoyer, B., Zago, L., Mellet, E., Bricogne, S., Etard, O., Houde, O., Crivello, F., Joliot, M., Petit, L., & Tzourio-mazoyer, N. (2001). Cortical networks for working memory and executive functions sustain the conscious resting state in man. Brain Res Bull, , 54, 287-298.

[69] Mckhann, G., Drachman, D., Folstein, M., Katzman, R., Price, D., & Stadlan, E. M. (1984). Clinical diagnosis of Alzheimer's disease: report of the NINCDS-ADRDA Work Group under the auspices of Department of Health and Human Services Task Force on Alzheimer's Disease. *Neurology,* 34, 939-944.

[70] Mesulam, M. M. (1998). From Sensation to cognition. *Brain,,* 121, 1013-1052.

[71] Miller, S. L., Celone, K., Depeau, K., Diamond, E., Dickerson, B. C., Rentz, D., Pihlajamäki, M., & Sperling, R. A. memory impairment associated with loss of parietal deactivation but preserved hippocampal activation. Proc Natl Acad Sci USA, , 105, 2181-2186.

[72] Miller, S. L., Fenstermacher, E., Bates, J., Blacker, D., Sperling, R., & Dickerson, B. C. (2008b). Hippocampal activation in adults with mild cognitive impairment predicts subsequent cognitive decline. *J Neurol Neurosurg Psychiatry,,* 79, 630-635.

[73] Minoshima, S., Giordani, B., Berent, S., Frey, K. A., Foster, N. L., & Kuhl, D. E. (1997). Metabolic reduction in the posterior cingulate cortex in very early Alzheimer's disease. *Ann Neurol,,* 42, 85-94.

[74] Mintun, M. A., Larossa, G. N., Sheline, Y. I., Dence, C. S., Lee, S. Y., Mach, R. H., et al. (2006). [11C]PIB in a nondemented population: potential antecedent marker of Alzheimer disease. *Neurology,* 67, 446-452.

[75] Nestor, P. J., Fryer, T. D., Smielewski, P., & Hodges, J. R. (2003). Limbic hypometabolism in Alzheimer's disease and mild cognitive impairment. *Ann Neurol,,* 54, 343-351.

[76] Brien, O, Keefe, J.L., O, & La, K.M. . & Sperling, R.A. (2010). Longitudinal fMRI study in elderly reveals loss of hippocampal activation with clinical decline. Neurology, Vol. 71, pp. 1969-76.

[77] Otten, L. J., & Rugg, M. D. (2001). When more means less: neural activity related to unsuccessful memory encoding. Curr Biol, , 11, 1528-1530.

[78] Ogawa, S., Tank, D. W., Menon, R., Ellermann, J. M., Kim, S. G., Merkle, H., & Ugurbil, K. (1992). Intrinsic signal changes accompanying sensory stimulation: Functional brain mapping with magnetic resonance imaging. Proc Natl Acad Sci USA, , 89, 5951-5955.

[79] Pariente, J., Cole, S., Henson, R., Clare, L., Kennedy, A., Rossor, M., Cipoloti, L., Puel, M., Demonet, J. F., Chollet, F., & Frackowiak, R. S. (2005). Alzheimer's patients engage an alternative network during a memory task. Ann Neurol, , 58, 870-879.

[80] Persson, J., Lind, J., Larsson, A., Ingvar, M., Sleegers, K., Van Broeckhoven, C., Adolfsson, R., Nilsson, L. G., & Nyberg, L. (2008). Altered deactivation in individuals with genetic risk for Alzheimer's disease. *Neuropsychologia*, 46, 1679-1687.

[81] Petersen, R. C., Smith, G. E., Waring, S. C., Ivnik, R. J., Tangalos, E. G., & Kokmen, E. (1999). Mild cognitive impairment: clinical characterization and outcome. *Arch Neurol,*, 56, 303-308.

[82] Petersen, R. C., Doody, R., Kurz, A., Mohs, R. C., Morris, J. C., Rabins, P. V., Ritchie, K., Rossor, M., Thal, L., & Winblad, B. (2001). Current concepts in mild cognitive impairment. *Arch Neurol,*, 58, 1985-1992.

[83] Petersen, R. C. (2004). Mild cognitive impairment as a diagnostic entity. *J Intern Med,*, 256, 183-194.

[84] Petersen, R. C., Roberts, R. O., Knopman, D. S., Boeve, B. F., Geda, Y. E., Ivnik, R. J., Smith, G. E., & Jack, C. R. Jr. ((2009). Mild Cognitive impairment: Ten years later. Arch Neurol, , 66, 1447-1455.

[85] Petrella, J. R., Krishnan, S., Slavian, M. J., Tran, T. T., Murty, L., & Doraiswamy, P. M. (2006). Mild cognitive impairment: evaluation with 4-T functional MR imaging. *Radiology*, 240, 177-186.

[86] Petrella, J. R., Prince, S. E., Wang, L., Hellegers, C., & Doraiswamy, P. M. (2007a). Prognostic value of posteromedial cortex deactivation in mild cognitive impairment. PLoS ONE, e1104., 2

[87] Petrella, J. R., Wang, L., Krishnan, S., Slavin, M. J., Prince, S. E., Tran, T. T., & Doraiswamy, P. M. (2007b). Cortical deactivation in mild cognitive impairment: high-field-strength functional MR imaging. *Radiology*, 245, 224-235.

[88] Pihlajamäki, M., Tanila, H., Hänninen, T., Könönen, M., Mikkonen, M., Jalkanen, V., Partanen, K., Aronen, H. J., & Soininen, H. (2003). Encoding of novel picture pairs activates the perirhinal cortex: an fMRI study. *Hippocampus*, 13, 67-80.

[89] Pihlajamäki, M., Depeau, K. M., Blacker, D., & Sperling, R. A. (2008). Impaired medial temporal repetition suppression is related to failure of parietal deactivation in Alzheimer's disease. Am J Geriatr Psychiatry, , 16, 283-292.

[90] Pihlajamäki, M., Keefe, O., Bertram, K., Tanzi, L., Dickerson, R. E., Blacker, B. C., Albert, D., & Sperling, M. S. R.A. ((2010). Evidence of altered posteromedial cortical fMRI activity in subjects at risk for Alzheimer disease. Alzheimer Disease and Associated Disorders, 24, 28-36.

[91] Pihlajamäki, M., & Sperling, R. A. (2009). Functional MRI assessment of task-induced deactivation of the default mode network in Alzheimer's disease and at-risk older individuals. Behavioral Neurology, , 21, 77-91.

[92] Pihlajamäki, M., Keefe, O., Brien, K. , O., Blacker, J., & Sperling, D. R.A. ((2011). Failure of repetition suppression and memory encoding in aging and Alzheimer's disease. Brain Imaging Behav, , 5, 36-44.

[93] Raichle, M. E. MacLeod, A.M., Snyder, A.Z., Powers, W.J. Gusnard, D.A. & Shulman, G.I. ((2001). A default mode of brain function. Proc Natl Acad Sci U S A , 98, 676-682.

[94] Remy, F., Mirrashed, F., Cambell, B., & Richter, W. (2005). Verbal episodic memory impairment in Alzheimer's disease: a combined structural and functional MRI study. *Neuroimage*, 25, 253-266.

[95] Rombouts, S. A., Barkhof, F., Veltman, D. J., Machielsen, W. C., Witter, M. P., Bierlaagh, M. A., Lazeron, R. H., Valk, J., & Scheltens, P. (2000). Functional MR imaging in Alzheimer's disease during memory encoding. *Am J Neuroradiol,*, 21, 1869-1875.

[96] Rombouts, S. A., Barkhof, F., Goekoop, R., Stam, C. J., & Scheltens, P. (2005a). Altered resting state networks in mild cognitive impairment and mild Alzheimer's disease: An fMRI study. Hum Brain Mapp, , 26, 231-239.

[97] Rombouts, S. A., Goekoop, R., Stam, C. J., Barkhof, F., & Scheltens, P. (2005b). Delayed rather than decreased BOLD response as a marker for early Alzheimer's disease. *Neuroimage*, 26, 1078-1085.

[98] Saunders, A. M., Strittmatter, W. J., Schmechel, D., George-hyslop, P. H., Pericakvance, M. A., Joo, S. H., Rosi, B. L., & Gusella, J. F. Crapper-MacLachlan, D.R., Alberts, M.J., et al. ((1993). Association of apolipoprotein E allele epsilon 4 with late-onset familial and sporadic Alzheimer's disease. Neurology, 43, 1467-1472.

[99] Scheff, S. W., Price, D. A., Schmitt, F. A., & Mufson, E. J. (2006). Hippocampal synaptic loss in early Alzheimer's disease and mild cognitive impairment. Neurobiol Aging, , 27, 1372-1384.

[100] Scheff, S. W., Price, D. A., Schmitt, F. A., Dekosky, S. T., & Mufson, E. J. (2007). Synaptic alterations in CA1 in mild Alzheimer disease and mild cognitive impairment. *Neurology*, 68, 1501-1508.

[101] Schwindt, G. C., & Black, S. E. (2009). Functional imaging studies of episodic memory in Alzheimer's disease: A quantative meta-analysis. Neuroimage, , 45, 181-190.

[102] Selkoe, D. J. (2002). Alzheimer's disease is a synaptic failure, Science, 298, 789-791.

[103] Shmuel, A., Augath, M., Oeltermann, A., & Logothetis, N. K. (2006). Negative functional MRI response correlates with decreases in neuronal activity in monkey visual area V1. *Nat Neurosci,*, 9, 569-577.

[104] Shulman, G., Fiez, J. A., Corbetta, M., Buckner, R. L., Miezin, F. M., & Raichle, M. E. (1997). Common blood flow changes across visual tasks: II. Decreases in cerebral cortex. J Cogn Neurosci, , 9, 648-663.

[105] Small, S. A., & Perera, G. M. DeLaPaz, R., Mayeux, R. & Stern, Y. ((1999). Differential regional dysfunction of the hippocampal formation among elderly with memory decline and Alzheimer's disease. Ann Neurol, , 45, 466-472.

[106] Smith, C. D., Andersen, A. H., Kryscio, R. J., Schmitt, F. A., Kindy, M. S., Blonder, L. X., & Acison, M. J. (1999). Altered brain activation in cognitively intact individuals at high risk for Alzheimer's disease. *Neurology*, 53, 1391-1396.

[107] Smith, C. D., Andersen, A. H., Kryscio, R. J., Schmitt, F. A., Kindy, M. S., Blonder, L. X., & Acison, M. J. (2002). Women at risk for AD show increased parietal actication during a fluent task. Neurology, , 58, 1197-1202.

[108] Sorg, C., Riedl, V., Muhlau, M., Calhoun, V. D., Eichele, T., Läer, L., Drzezga, A., Förstl, H., Kurz, A., Zimmer, C., & Wohlschläger, A. M. (2007). Selective changes of resting-state networks in individuals at risk for Alzheimer's disease. *Proc Natl Acad Sci USA*,, 104, 18760-18765.

[109] Sperling, R., Greve, D., Dale, A., Killiany, R., Holmes, J., Rosas, H. D., Cocchiarella, A., Firth, P., Rosen, B., Lake, S., Lange, N., Routledge, C., & Albert, M. (2002). Functional MRI detection of pharmacologically induced memory impairment. *Proc Natl Acad Sci USA.*, 99, 455-460.

[110] Sperling, R., Bates, J., Chua, E., Cocchiarella, A., Schacter, D. L., Rosen, B., Schacter, D. L., & Albert, M. S. (2003a). fMRI studies of associative encoding in young and elderly controls and mild AD patients. J Neurol Neurosurg Psychiatry, , 74, 44-50.

[111] Sperling, R., Chua, E., Cocchiarella, A., Rand-giovannetti, E., & Poldrack, R. Schacter, D.L & Albert, M. ((2003b). Putting names to faces: successful encoding of associative memories activates the anterior hippocampal formation. Neuroimage, 20, 1400-1410.

[112] Squire, L. R., & Zola-morgan, S. (1991). The medial temporal lobe memo. ry system. Science, , 11, 1380-1386.

[113] Stern, C. E., Corkin, S., Gonzalez, R. G., Guimaraes, A. G., Baker, J. R., Jennings, P. J., Carr, C. A., Sugiura, R. M., Vedantham, V., & Rosen, B. R. (1996). The hippocampal formation participates in novel picture encoding: evidence from functional magnetic resonance imaging. *Proc Natl Acad Sci USA*,, 93, 8660-8665.

[114] Supekar, K., Menon, V., Rubin, D., Musen, M., & Greicius, M. D. (2008). Network analysis of intrinsic functional brain connectivity in Alzheimer's disease. PLoS Comput Biol, e1000100., 4

[115] Suzuki, W. A., & Amaral, D. G. (1994). Perirhinal and parahippocampal cortices of the macaque monkey: cortical afferents. J Comp Neurol, , 350, 497-533.

[116] Suzuki, W. A. (2007). Making new memories: The role of the hippocampus in new associative learning. *Ann N Y Acad Sci*,, 1097, 1-11.

[117] Tanzi, R. E., & Bertram, L. (2001). New frontiers in Alzheimer's disease genetics. *Neuron,* 32, 181-184.

[118] Trivedi, M. A., Schmitz, T. W., Ries, M. L., Torgerson, B. M., Sager, M. A., Hermann, B. P., Asthana, S., & Johnson, S. C. (2006). Reduced hippocampal activation during episodic encoding in middle-aged individuals at genetic risk of Alzheimer's disease: a cross-sectional study. *BMC Med,,* 4, 1 EOF.

[119] Tulving, E., & Markowitsch, H. J. (1998). Episodic and declarative memory: role of the hippocampus. *Tulving, E. & Markowitsch, H.J. (1998). Episodic and declarative memory: role of the hippocampus. Hippocampus, Vol. 8, pp. 198-204.,* 8, 198-204.

[120] Wagner, A. D., Schacter, D. L., Rotte, M., Koutstaal, W., Maril, A., Dale, A. M., Rosen, B. R., & Buckner, R. L. (1998). Building memories: remembering and forgetting of verbal experiences as predicted by brain activity. *Science,* 281, 1188-1191.

[121] Wang, K., Liang, M., Wang, L., Tian, L., Zhang, X., Li, K., & Jiang, T. (2007). Altered functional connectivity in early Alzheimer's disease: A resting-state fMRI study. Hum Brain Mapp, , 28, 967-978.

[122] Weissman, D. H., Roberts, K. C., Visscher, K. M., & Woldorff, M. G. (2006). The neural bases of momentary lapses in attention. Nat Neurosci, , 9, 971-978.

[123] Winblad, B., Palmer, K., Kivipelto, M., Jelic, V., Fratiglioni, L., Wahlund, L. O., Nordberg, A., Bäckman, L., Albert, M., Almkvist, O., Arai, H., Basun, H., Blennow, K., De Leon, M., Decarli, C., Erkinjuntti, T., Giacobini, E., Graff, C., Hardy, J., Jack, C., Jorm, A., Ritchie, K., Van Duijn, C., Visser, P., & Petersen, R. C. (2004). Mild cognitive impairment--beyond controversies, towards a consensus: report of the International Working Group on Mild Cognitive Impairment. J Intern Med, , 256, 240-246.

[124] Wishart, H. A., Saykin, A. J., Rabin, L. A., Santulli, R. B., Flashman, L. A., Guerin, S. J., Mamourian, A. C., Belloni, D. R., Rhodes, C. H., & Mcallister, T. W. (2006). Increased brain activation during working memory in cognitively intact adults with the APOE epsilon4 allele. *Am J Psychiatry,,* 163, 1603-1610.

[125] Woodard, J. L., Seidenberg, M., Nielson, K. A., Antuono, P., Guidotti, L., Durgerian, S., Zhang, Q., Lancaster, M., Hantke, N., Butts, A., & Rao, S. M. (2009). Semantic memory activation in amnestic mild cognitive impairment. Brain, , 132, 2068-2078.

[126] Yassa, M. A., Stark, S. M., Bakker, A., Albert, M. S., Gallagher, M., & Stark, C. E. (2010). High-resolution structural and functional MRI of hippocampal CA3 and dentate gyrus in patients with amnestic Mild Cognitive Impairment. *Neuroimage,* 51, 1242-1252.

[127] Zhou, Z. Dougherty, Jr. J.H, Hubner, K.F., Bai, B., Cannon R.L. & Hutson R.K. ((2008). Abnormal connectivity in the posterior cingulate and hippocampus in early Alzheimer's disease and mild cognitive impairment. Alzheimers Dement, , 4, 265-270.

2

The Neurofunctional Architecture of Motor Imagery

Aymeric Guillot, Franck Di Rienzo and Christian Collet

1. Introduction

The remarkable ability of the human brain to mentally simulate sensations and actions has become a major focus of research during the last two decades. Such mental simulation process is called mental imagery and resembles perception, but without the immediate actual corresponding sensory input. Typically, mental imagery is often referred to as the experience of seeing with the mind's eye, hearing with the mind's ear. In other words, mental images can be generated from any sensorial system. Imagery experience is usually understood as evocation, copy, or reconstruction of actual perceptual experience from the long term memory systems, which is first recalled and then internally reproduced within working memory. At other times, participants may also anticipate possible or forthcoming events through imagery as a consequence of what they are expecting. A key feature of this simulation process is that it gives the ability to mentally rehearse motor acts without overt body movement, which is known as the motor imagery (MI) experience. Practically, MI is more often used when the whole human body or body segments are involved, hence requiring participants to imagine the body as the generator of acting forces and not only the effects of these forces on the external world. In this latter case, the information from the body is mainly used to build the mental image of the movement, e.g. tactile or any kind of proprioceptive data, from the muscles, the joints or the inner ear. In the wealth of motor learning literature, it is now well-established that MI is a valuable complement to physical practice to enhance cognitive and motor performance (Driskell et al., 1994; Guillot and Collet, 2008), as well as to promote motor recovery (Sharma, Pomeroy, and Baron, 2006; de Vries and Mulder, 2007). Interestingly, different types of MI can be described and easily combined. While people commonly report using visual imagery (either through a first-person or third-person perspective), auditory imagery, and kinaesthetic imagery (Kosslyn et al., 1990), each perceptual modality can be accompanied by imagery. On the other hand, and with reference to perception, mental imagery combines several cues from different sensorial systems, making the imagery a global sensory-motor experience. Investigating and assessing MI remains difficult due to its concealed nature.

Early on, MI has attracted attention from cognitive neuroscientists. In particular, understanding the neural correlates of goal-directed action, whether executed or imagined, has been an important purpose of cognitive brain research since the advent of neuroimaging techniques such as functional Magnetic Resonance Imaging (fMRI). Providing physiological recordings that correlate to the MI experience was therefore a major issue of the past two decades. In short, but not only, neuroimaging research demonstrated that MI engages motor systems, and that the cerebral plasticity due to actual practice also occurred during MI as well. These findings help to explain why MI can improve actual performance, and further contribute to motor memory consolidation. The present chapter was designed to provide an overview of the neural correlates of MI, with a threefold aim: *i)* to explain why recording human brain functioning with fMRI during MI is of particular interest and provides an objective measurement of imagery processes, *ii)* to give a clear picture of the neural networks mediating MI and actual execution of the same movement, while considering the issue of brain plasticity in the light of individual differences in imagery ability, motor expertise, the different forms of imagery, and the level of motor learning, and *iii)* to consider the recent fMRI methodological advances, e.g. using real-time fMRI, as well as recording changes in functional and effective connectivity in the neural networks activated during MI.

2. Using fMRI to assess brain activity during motor imagery

The most common aim of fMRI data analysis is to investigate the neural processes mediating higher cognitive functions, and detect correlations between brain activations and the task the participants have to perform during the scan. Since the early 1980s, fMRI has come to dominate the MI-related brain mapping research. During typical fMRI image acquisitions, participants are asked to alternatively perform a movement, either physically or mentally. These experimental conditions are also compared with a rest/control condition.

There are two main types of experimental design in fMRI: the block design and the event-related design. The block design paradigm consists of several epochs representing experimental conditions, during which stimuli are presented and actual execution or MI are required from participants, which are interleaved with time blocks of rest. Event-related designs rather associate brain processes with discrete events, with stimulus events being randomly presented one at a time, and being separated by an inter-stimulus interval of a pre-determined length. Habituation effects can be reduced, and stimuli are usually presented either tens of seconds apart or at a faster rate (e.g., every second). It could be noted that event-related designs are more sensitive to the details of the hemodynamic response model use. Figure 1 provides a schematic illustration of these two experimental designs when comparing the neural networks mediating MI and actual execution of the same movement.

There is not a universal procedure yet to acquire and process functional data and many researchers independently developed their methods and analyses, using different software. Practically, the most commonly technique used to map brain activity is based on the Blood Oxygenation Level Dependent (BOLD) effect, measuring regional differences in hemoglobin oxygenation. Therefore, a considerable amount of experimental studies investigated BOLD changes during MI. They primarily aimed at comparing the neuronal activations recorded during MI and actual practice of the same movement. For example, Grèzes and Decety (2001) provided evidence of a functional equivalence between intending, simulating, observing, and performing an action, as shown by the great deal of overlap among the corresponding neural substrates. Interestingly, brain activations recorded during MI do however not exactly match those of actual movement execution (Lotze and Halsband, 2006). Some differences also appear when comparing different types of MI or with regard to the individual features of the sample of participants. Put simply, fMRI allows the measurement of different neuronal activity in participants with high vs. low MI ability (Guillot et al., 2008), as well as differences in the patterns of cerebral activity related to the degree of expertise of the participants with the motor task (Lotze et al., 2003; Ross et al., 2003; Milton et al., 2007, 2008). Based on such evidence, fMRI offers a way to evidence the MI experience (Guillot et al., 2008). Finally, recent fMRI data suggested that different types of imagery elicit different patterns of neural activation (Solodkin et al., 2004; Jackson et al., 2006; Guillot et al., 2009; Lorey et al., 2009), while others nicely demonstrated, through positron emission tomography (PET), that the cerebral plasticity occurring after physical practice was reflected during MI (Lafleur et al., 2002; Jackson et al., 2003), hence reinforcing the principle of functional equivalence between MI and physical performance of the same task. Before we consider these issues and review the main related findings in the next section, an important methodological question remains to be addressed. Specifically, what are the additional benefits provided by fMRI to the study of MI compared to other neuroimaging and electrophysiological techniques, and, in turn, what are the limitations of fMRI recordings?

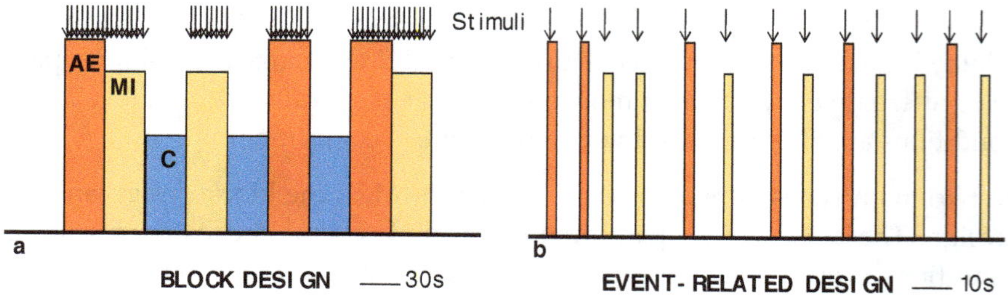

Figure 1. Schematic representation of a block design (a) and an event-related design (b) fMRI paradigm. In the block design paradigm, sustained periods of 20–30s are used for actual execution (AE), motor imagery (MI), and control (C) conditions during which several trials are performed successively (vertical arrows). Before each block of practice, brief periods of time (2-3s) are necessary to provide participants some instructions related to the forthcoming condition. Brief 'rest' periods can also be included. In the event-related design, each experimental condition is presented at random (orange and red vertical bars and vertical arrows).

A first advantage of fMRI, compared to PET, is its non-invasive nature. There is no radiation exposure, and no need for injection of radioactive materials with fMRI. Another strength is its high spatial resolution allowing the measurement of brain activity from deep structures. Unlike electrophysiological techniques such as electroencephalography (EEG) or even magnetoencephalography (MEG) which are somewhat biased towards the cortical surface, fMRI records signal from all regions of the brain, including subcortical structures. This is of particular importance when pinpointing the neural correlates of MI as activation of cerebellum and basal ganglia is commonly reported. As every technique, however, fMRI has also some methodological disadvantages or weaknesses for the study of MI (e.g., Dietrich, 2008). A first limit is related to the causality between brain activation and the task the participants perform in the scanner. Although the baseline activity is subtracted from that recorded during the task and the result is averaged for all participants, the causality between activated structures and characteristics of the task is not straightforward. In other words, some brain structures could remain activated although this activity is not directly related to the task. Such argument for the causality however also holds for other brain imaging techniques. Second, the temporal resolution, of about several seconds must also be considered, as fMRI cannot track the rapid temporal dynamics of the functioning brain compared to high temporal resolution methods, e.g. EEG or MEG. Neuromodulatory effects of some cognitive functions such as attention and memory are also likely to affect the spatiotemporal resolution of the signal as they can affect large masses of cells, and potentially induce larger changes in the fMRI signal than the sensory signals themselves (Logothetis, 2008). Fourth, regarding data interpretation, advanced statistical methods are required to identify active voxels, while modifications of the brain activity might be due either to an excitatory or inhibitory influence. Finally, the position in the scanner and the limitation of body movements make it difficult to investigate complex motor skills. Indeed, the participant is lying in supine position in the scanner, and then performs both actual execution and mental representation of the same movement. However, in such situation, only simple movement of fingers, hands, feet, or tongue, or more complex movements of limited amplitude can actually be studied.

As reported by Logothetis (2008), and despite the shortcomings mentioned above, fMRI remains probably the best current available technique for providing insights into brain function and formulating interesting testable hypotheses. Logothetis also stated that some limitations of fMRI are directly due to inappropriate experimental protocols that ignore the circuitry and complex functional organization of the human brain. This is a critical aspect that must be considered before drawing general conclusions and when comparing results across experimental studies. In particular, a specific attention should be paid to the control condition from which MI-related brain activity is reported. In fMRI data analyses, images of activity from experimental and control conditions are subtracted to determine significant peaks of activation. Hence, a difference which does not reach the significant threshold does not necessarily reflect a lack of activity, but can also be due to similar brain activations during both experimental and control tasks. In other words, if the control task is not thoroughly determined, the remaining activity of some brain regions might bias the pattern of activity observed during the experimental condition, i.e. MI. Inspection of the MI literature reveals great differences across studies. Among others, participants were asked either to listen for auditory stimuli without engaging in MI (perceptual control condition), having rest, projecting into a restful state, fixating a static stimulus on a screen, or even imagining a 'neutral' static motor task. Obviously, such differences might significantly influence the pattern of activity recorded when contrasting the experimental and the control conditions. This is likely to render the functional brain map, hence hindering the conclusions that one can reach. Another example is the fact that MI can be performed either with open or closed eyes. Marx et al. (2003) suggested that eye closure is likely to improve imagination, but in some circumstances, MI paradigms might require participants to open their eyes to fixate a screen and/or wait for instructions. As some activation or deactivation of cortical regions could be undetected with eyes open, however, MI could ideally be performed with closed eyes as it was asked for the rest condition (Marx et al., 2004).

3. Neural correlates of motor imagery

MI research provided convincing evidence that there is a functional equivalence between MI and motor performance (e.g., Jeannerod, 1994; Grèzes and Decety, 2001; Holmes and Collins, 2001). It is therefore not surprising that movement execution and MI reveal a high overlap of active brain regions, i.e. imagery draws on almost the same neural network that is used in actual perception and motor control (Murphy et al., 2008). Considerable evidence in support of the functional equivalence theory comes from fMRI studies which demonstrated that both cortical and subcortical brain areas are activated during MI. All studies showed that secondary motor areas are recruited during MI, but that the primary motor cortex might also be part of the network involved in imagined actions. Cerebellar and basal ganglia activations are also consistently reported during MI (Gerardin et al., 2000; Munzert et al., 2009). Finally, apart from motor-related areas, other regions such as parietal lobules are activated during mental simulation of actions (Gao et al., 2011). Taken together, these data support that MI and motor performance share the same neural substrate (Figure 2), but interestingly there are also some differences within the pattern of activity in these areas, as well as with regards to the characteristics of the participants or the content of the MI task.

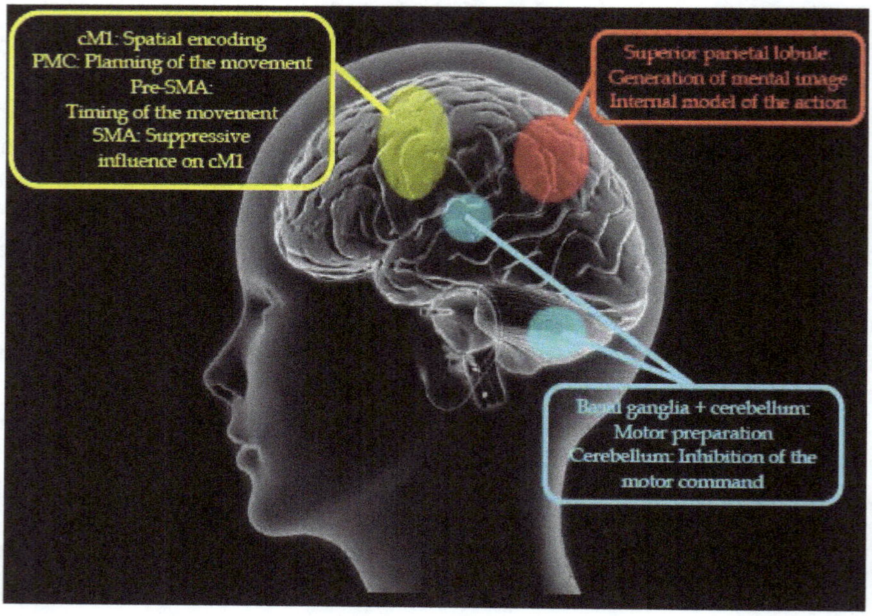

Figure 2. Schematization of brain activity during MI and possible roles of motor-related regions.

3.1. Contribution of the primary motor cortex

Since the pioneering PET study by Roland et al. (1980), who did not find a significant activation of the contralateral primary motor cortex (cM1) during MI, the question of the contribution of cM1 during imagined actions has attracted considerable attention and remains controversial (for reviews, see Lotze and Halsband, 2006; Sharma et al., 2008; Munzert et al., 2009; Lotze and Zentgraf, 2010). For example, Binkofski et al. (2000), Gerardin et al. (2000), Kuhtz-Bushbeck et al. (2003) and Hanakawa et al. (2003, 2008) failed to find peaks of activation in cM1, while Dechent et al. (2004) reported fleeting involvement. In contrast, several studies reported significant activation in cM1 during MI (Leonardo et al., 1995; Sabbah et al., 1995; Porro et al. 1996, 2000; Roth et al., 1996; Lotze et al., 1999; Ehrsson et al. 2003; Nair et al., 2003; Solodkin et al. 2004; Guillot et al., 2008, 2009). In a seminal paper, Ehrsson et al. (2003) even showed that the content of MI was reflected in the pattern of motor cortical activation. Accordingly, they found that MI of hand, foot and tongue movements specifically activated the corresponding hand, foot and tongue sections of cM1. Transcranial magnetic studies also revealed cM1 activation during MI (for review, see Stinear et al., 2010). Finally, and as previously reviewed by Munzert et al. (2009), similar cM1 activation was found during MI of movements with the impaired limb to that during motor execution with the unimpaired limb in amputees (Ersland et al., 1996). The same result was found in healthy controls during motor execution of the same movement and in patients with spinal cord injury (Alkadhi et al., 2005; Cramer et al., 2005). The fact that these patients do not need to inhibit the movement might have influenced the nature of the MI process (Munzert et al., 2009). A recent MEG study however revealed similar patterns of activity in cM1 during MI and actual practice of the same movement in a patient with spinal cord injury, while a loss of power was observed in the matched healthy control participant (Di Rienzo et al., 2011). These latter data support fMRI findings and further confirm both the contribution of cM1 during MI and the weakened inhibitory processes during MI in patients with spinal cord injury. Cerebral activations governing the inhibition of action during MI have not been yet fully explored. This would probably offer fruitful fMRI investigations in the future.

With regards to cM1 activation, Sharma et al. (2006) suggested that discrepancies in results may be due, at least partially, to methodological differences and difficulties in monitoring compliance with MI instructions. Definitely, the advent of fMRI techniques to investigate the contribution of cM1 during MI brought significant data into the debate. Furthermore, Sharma and colleagues argued that previous experimental studies did not specifically address whether the subdivisions of cM1 were differentially involved during MI. Furthermore, the primary motor cortex can be subdivided into an anterior component, thought to be executive in nature, while its posterior part would be involved in cognitive tasks or non-executive functions (Sanes and Donoghue, 2000). Accordingly, Sharma et al. (2008) reported that the cluster distribution in the anterior part of cM1 was significantly reduced during MI compared to the physical execution, while that of the posterior part was similar. Therefore, they proposed that the role of cM1 and its subdivisions may be related to spatial encoding. Despite these results, determining how MI participates to the activation of cM1 remains difficult. Typically, cM1 activation during MI is usually smaller compared to that during overt motor execution, and is not systematically observed in all participants (Munzert et al., 2009). It was also demonstrated that cM1 was increasingly involved along with the complexity of movements (Kuhtz-Buschbeck et al., 2003). As well, activation of cM1 might be differentially influenced by MI instructions, MI ability and motor expertise (Lotze and Zentgraf, 2010).

Taken together, and despite some controversial data, fMRI studies support that cM1 is actually activated during MI but more weakly than during actual movement. Such activation is not essential for imagery and the neurons are not in the same location than those active during movement execution (Lotze and Halsband, 2006). Moreover, cM1 might not only have an execution function for the motor system (Lotze and Zentgraf, 2010), and it is particularly preparation for MI that may impact significantly cM1 activation (Johnson et al., 2002; Zang et al., 2003; Munzert et al., 2009).

3.2. Activation of the other motor-related regions

Unlike the contribution of cM1, there is a general consensus regarding the activation of secondary motor areas of the cerebral cortex during MI. Accordingly, fMRI studies provided strong evidence that motor-related areas such as the ventral and dorsal parts of the premotor cortex (PMC), the supplementary motor area (SMA) and the pre-SMA, are active during MI of both simple and complex movements as well as subcortical areas such as the cerebellum and the putamen. Overall, it was shown that MI might activate a subset of the areas required for movement execution, albeit to a lesser extent (e.g., Macuga and Frey, 2011). Conversely, other activations could also be more robust in MI than during motor execution (e.g., Gerardin et al., 2000) thus leading to a partial overlapping of the networks mediating MI and actual execution of the same movement.

The activation of the SMA is now well-established during MI (Guillot et al., 2008; 2009; Hanakawa et al., 2003; Lotze et al., 1999; Munzert et al., 2009; Olsson et al., 2008; Solodkin et al., 2004). As neurons in the SMA are integrated in the functional loop controlling motor actions planning, it is therefore quite reasonable that similar preparatory aspects of the movement are engaged during MI. Kasess et al. (2008) further demonstrated that the SMA may inhibit activity of cM1 to prevent movement execution during MI. Interestingly, some authors also reported that the overlap of SMA activity during MI and motor execution is partial, and that the pre-SMA might rather play a specific role during imagined movements. Hence, the pattern of activity in this region could be higher during MI than during actual practice of the same task (Gerardin et al., 2000). Pre-SMA is known as being involved in acquiring new sequences, planning spatio-temporal actions, and updating motor plans for subsequent temporally ordered movements. As suggested by Malouin et al. (2003), the pre-SMA might thus be activated during MI to provide proper movement sequencing and timing. Taken together, MI would activate both the SMA and pre-SMA, not only for the preparation of the movement, but also for its suppressive influence on cM1 thus preventing movement execution.

Overlapping activity during MI and motor execution was also found in the premotor cortex (PMC-Guillot et al., 2008; Lotze and Halsband, 2006; Munzert et al., 2009), with potential more robust activity in the ventral part of the PMC during MI (Gerardin et al., 2000). The dorsal part of the PMC is involved in the preparation and control of movement, while the ventral part may play a crucial role in the planning of movements. Neurons with mirror properties which are active during action imitation and recognition were found in this region neighbouring Brodmann areas 44/45 (Rizzolatti et al., 1998). This may partially explain why more robust activity was reported in this area during MI than during motor execution.

Several studies also reported that MI and motor execution activate subcortical regions such as the basal ganglia and the cerebellum (e.g., Gerardin et al., 2000; Guillot et al., 2008; Lotze and Halsband, 2006; Munzert et al., 2009; Nair et al., 2003). These structures are known to strongly contribute to motor learning and motor preparation, and are closely connected to cortical motor-related areas. More specifically, the cerebellum contributes to predict movement outcomes as well as to correct the movement on the basis of sensori-motor feedback. Evidence that the cerebellum participates in the internal representation of movement, and therefore to MI, also comes from studies showing that cerebellar stroke disrupts MI (Battaglia et al., 2006; Gonzalez et al., 2005). In a seminal paper, Lotze et al. (1999) even postulated that the posterior cerebellum might play a crucial role in the inhibition of the motor command during MI (see also Lotze and Halsband, 2006). Likewise, basal ganglia play a substantial role in the storage of learned motor sequences, as well as in motor preparation (Alexander and Crutcher, 1990). While there is a general consensus regarding the activation of the basal ganglia during MI, few studies were devised to determine the specific role of this region. Li (2004) demonstrated that lesion of the putamen is likely to impair MI. More generally, however, studies on the effect of basal ganglia dysfunction on MI revealed inconsistent results (Heremans et al., 2011), with possible, but not systematic, MI impairment in patients with Parkinson's disease. Taken together, and even if experimental studies still have to understand in greater details how the cerebellum and the basal ganglia specifically contribute to the MI process, there is no doubt about their activation during imagined movements. Interestingly, distinct contributions of the cortico-striatal and cortico-cerebellar anatomical systems have been proposed in the motor learning literature (Doyon and Ungerleider, 2002; Doyon and Benali, 2005). Although functional interactions between these anatomical systems are essential at the beginning of the learning process, there is ample evidence that the cerebellum plays a weaker role when the sequence is well learned and has reached asymptotic performance (for review, see Doyon and Benali, 2005), while basal ganglia remain active during the later stages of motor learning. By comparing the pattern of cerebral activations in 13 skilled and 15 unskilled imagers during both physical execution and MI sequence of finger movements, Guillot et al. (2008) showed that poor imagers not only need to recruit the cortico-striatal system, but also activate the cortico-cerebellar system as well. Findings also suggested that compared to poor imagers, good imagers would have a more efficient recruitment of movement engrams. Although this remains a working hypothesis awaiting experimental investigation, the authors concluded that the pattern of cerebral activation recorded during MI in poor imagers might improve and evolve close to that observed in good imagers after MI training. This might suggest that the expected changes in subcortical brain activations during MI would reflect those elicited by the process of actual motor learning (see also Lafleur et al., 2002; Jackson et al., 2003).

3.3. Activation of parietal regions

Activation of parietal areas including possibly the somatosensory cortex, but more certainly the inferior and superior parietal lobules and the precuneus, is frequently reported during MI (Binkofski et al., 2000; Gerardin et al., 2000; Guillot et al., 2009; Hanakawa et al., 2003; Lotze et al., 1999; Munzert et al., 2009; Nair et al., 2003). More importantly, the parietal cortex, and perhaps predominantly the left parietal cortex, could play a critical role in the formation of mental images. Experimental studies in patients with lesions located in the superior region of the parietal cortex showed that the temporal congruence between actual and MI times, known as being a reliable measure of MI quality (Guillot and Collet, 2005; Guillot et al., 2011; Malouin et al., 2008), was affected (Malouin et al., 2004; Sabate et al., 2007; Sirigu et al., 1996). Sirigu et al. (1996) postulated that the parietal cortex might set up an internal model of the forthcoming movement making the participants to predict the expected movement outcome. After parietal damage, coding for the spatial properties of the movement to be imagined and predicting the temporal feature of the movement might therefore be more difficult, hence reflecting the critical role of the posterior parietal cortex in the use of MI.

Interestingly, bilateral parietal lesions resulted in a complete unawareness of movement execution during imagery (Schwoebel et al., 2002). In fact, the patient exhibited hand movements during MI of the same body segments, but explicitly denied that they occurred. These data strongly support that parietal areas are critically involved in the generation and guidance of imagined movements. More importantly, they further suggest that the patient failed to inhibit the motor consequences of MI, and therefore, that parietal areas may also play a critical role in the inhibitory processes of the motor command during MI. Finally, and in conjunction with previous fMRI data (Gerardin et al., 2000), these findings suggest a functional dissociation between cortical areas underlying MI and motor execution. The primary sensory area would be more activated during motor execution, due to sensory feedback processes, whereas MI might elicit greater activity both in the inferior and superior parietal cortices, especially in the left hemisphere.

3.4. The effect of motor imagery content

A limited number of fMRI studies examined the influence of MI content on brain activations, and most specifically whether visual imagery and kinaesthetic imagery recruit different neural networks. In a first study looking at this issue, Binkofski et al. (2000) reported that the anterior part of the intraparietal sulcus was more active during kinaesthetic imagery of finger movements, while visual imagery yielded stronger activation in the posterior part. Bilateral activations were also reported during kinaesthetic imagery in the opercular portion of the ventral PMC. In a seminal paper, Solodkin et al. (2004) later investigated the neural networks mediating physical execution, visual imagery and kinaesthetic imagery of hand movements. Although these two types of imagery shared similar neural substrates, including the connection from the superior parietal lobule to the SMA, the main difference was found in the inputs from the superior parietal lobule and the SMA to cM1, which were opposite to those observed during motor execution. In the same line of research, Guillot et al. (2009) examined whether the same group of participants with high imagery abilities recruited similar or distinct brain activations during visual imagery and kinaesthetic imagery of complex hand movements. Visual activated predominantly the visual pathways including the occipital regions and the precuneus, whereas the pattern of kinaesthetic imagery involved mainly motor-associated structures and the inferior parietal lobule (Figure 3). These data support the hypothesis that visual imagery of a motor sequence refers to the visual properties of visual perception, while kinaesthetic imagery includes in greater extent motor simulation processes related to the form and timing of actual movements (Michelon et al. 2006). Although visual and kinaesthetic imagery shared common brain structures, these data provide strong evidence that the patterns of neural activity mediating the ability to perform a specific MI type are partially different. Practically, it might suggest that participants are able to favor one sensory modality to form mental images, although MI is a multimodal and multidimensional construct.

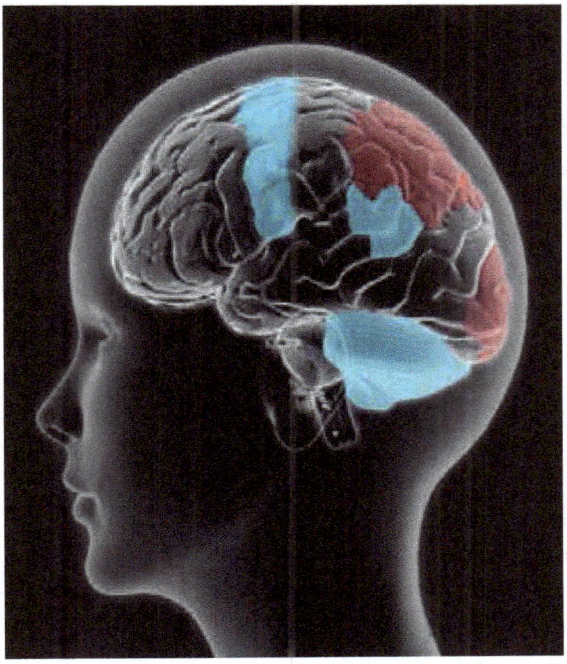

Figure 3. Schematization of brain activations during visual and kinaesthetic imagery. During kinaesthetic imagery (blue), the pattern of activity involves motor-related regions mainly, including cM1, PMC, SMA, cerebellum and basal ganglia (hidden from the view), as well as the inferior parietal cortex. In contrast, more activity is observed during visual imagery (red) in occipital regions and superior parietal lobule, including the precuneus.

Similar data have been reported in regards to the visual imagery perspectives, that is, by comparing first and third person imagery perspectives. The first study looking at this issue, was conducted by Ruby and Decety (2001) with PET scan. They investigated the neural networks mediating MI when the participants were asked either to mentally simulate an action or to imagine someone else (*i.e.,* the experimenter) performing the same movement. They found that the inferior parietal lobule and the somatosensory cortex were more activated during the first-person than the third-person perspective, while increased activity was observed in the precuneus and during the third-person perspective. Then, fMRI experiments were designed to examine in greater details whether using either the first or third-person imagery perspective lead to motor-areas-related changes. Jackson et al. (2006) explored the neural circuits involved in imitation and perspective-taking, and showed that first-person perspective was more tightly coupled to the sensory-motor system than the third-person perspective, which requires additional visuospatial transformation. More recently, Lorey et al. (2009) also found stronger activation of motor and motor-related brain structures, like the inferior parietal lobe, when imagining a movement through a first-person compared to a third-person perspective. They argued that proprioceptive information on actual body posture would be more relevant for internal visual imagery users, which reveals that bodily information is mainly integrated into the image of one's own body movement.

More generally, these results provide clear evidence that both imagery types (e.g. visual vs. kinaesthetic imagery) and perspectives (first-person vs. third-person imagery) are partially mediated through separate neural systems, which may therefore contribute differently during the process of motor learning and neurological rehabilitation. This assumption is supported by a remarkable fMRI study demonstrating that MI engages systematically the organized sections of cM1 in a somatotopic manner, i.e. that the content of the mental images is reflected in the pattern of motor cortical activation (Ehrsson et al., 2003).

3.5. Neural mechanisms for motor expertise

The fact that MI efficacy depends on the individual ability to form accurate mental images is now well-established. Although not systematic, this capacity to mentally simulate forthcoming actions may be influenced by the individual level of expertise in the corresponding motor task. While the concepts of motor expertise and MI ability measurements have been considered early on, researchers are able, for a short time, to assess the content of MI objectively using thorough procedures, in particular since the advent of functional brain mapping studies (Guillot et al., 2010). Taken overall, fMRI data strongly support the existence of distinct neural mechanisms of expertise in MI, as a function of the individual skill level. For instance, lower cortical activation was recorded in professional violinists as compared to amateurs (Lotze et al., 2003). Similar differences were observed in the neural networks mediating MI in novice and expert athletes (Milton et al., 2008). By comparing brain activations of six golfers of various handicaps during MI of a golf swing, Ross et al. (2003) found decreased activations of the SMA and cerebellum as a function of golf skill level, i.e. an inverse relationship between brain activity and skill level. Also, golf swing MI yielded few peaks of activation in the basal ganglia and cingulate gyri across all skill levels. Milton et al. (2007) finally reported that the posterior cingulate, the amygdala-forebrain complex, and the basal ganglia were activated in novices but not in elite golfers during motor planning of a golf swing movement, hence confirming that the neural networks controlling both motor planning and MI are influenced by the individual skill level. As a whole, changes in cerebral activations confirmed previous investigations showing that levels of expertise during the motor learning process are supported by different neural networks (Doyon and Benali, 2005).

Analogously, researchers investigated the neural networks mediating musical experience, training onset, and training stages. Langheim et al. (2002) first showed in participants who imagined playing a musical selection with their instrument that an associative network including the superior parietal lobule, the inferior frontal gyrus and the bilateral lateral cerebellum was activated. This network would be particularly activated during the coordination of the complex spatial and timing components of musical performance. As mentioned above, Lotze et al. (2003) compared the patterns of brain activation during auditory imagery in experienced and novice musicians, with the professionals reporting frequent use of imagery with high vividness. Interestingly, experienced musicians recruited very few cerebral areas, while amateurs manifested a widely distributed activation map. In the professional group, however, more activation was observed in the SMA, the PMC, the superior parietal lobule and the cerebellum. Finally, Kleber et al. (2007) reported an increased activation in the fronto-parietal regions during imagined singing, suggesting increased involvement of working memory processes during imagery.

To summarize, fMRI data provided strong evidence that partially separate neural networks are activated during MI of both motor and musical performance in regards to the individual differences in the level of expertise. These findings therefore strongly support the hypothesis of distinct neural mechanisms for expertise in imagery, independently of the imagery type, with the network integrating the superior parietal lobule mediating the imagery activity of highly experienced people.

4. fMRI advances in the study of motor imagery

Going beyond the usual comparison of brain activation patterns that are associated with MI and motor execution of the same movement is the next step in this field of research. To do so, researchers may take advantage of the recent methodological fMRI developments. Both the use of real time fMRI and the recording of changes in functional and effective connectivity in the neural networks activated during MI are of particular interest. Also, reporting more systematically negative BOLD responses might contribute to expand our knowledge on neuronal inhibition during MI.

It is now possible to image human brain functioning in real time with fMRI (Esposito et al., 2003; Weiskopf et al., 2003; for an extensive review, see deCharms, 2008). This technique provides a reconstruction of the raw data obtained with the brain scan, while the scan is going on. There are several exciting research perspectives for considering the contribution of real time fMRI dedicated to MI study. This technique may first be useful during the MI learning process, especially when the pattern of activation during mental simulation is not the one expected. Indeed, real time images are expected to provide participants some objective information related to the vividness of MI, since they have been educated to gain some familiarity with the neuroanatomy before neurofeedback fMRI sessions. Receiving a feedback from brain activation in predetermined regions of interest seems possible. An average 2-5s time lapse usually remains necessary, due to the physiological delay of the Hemodynamic response (a more simple feedback can also be used, e.g. a simple score using a Likert-type scale). A well-known study supporting the use of real time fMRI was published by Yoo and Jolesz (2002), who used visual feedback of brain activation to guide participants to adjust their motor task performance and to achieve the desired modulation of cortical activity. For example, during simple hand movements, participants spontaneously involved more muscle groups and increased tapping frequency along fMRI sessions. The biofeedback given to participants with regard to the activated neural network helped them to modulate their cortical activation. A significant illustration of the strength of this methodology in the field of MI was offered by deCharms et al. (2004) during imagery of a manual action task. In this study, participants received feedback about the activation level in the somatomotor cortex with a simple virtual reality interface. The results showed that they enhanced the fMRI level of activation driven by MI in the somatomotor cortex through the course of training. Moreover, the activation of this region after MI training was as robust as that recorded during actual practice. In a more recent study, Yoo et al. (2008) showed that real time fMRI might help individuals to learn how to increase region-specific cortical activity associated with a MI task. Practically, the level of increased activation in motor areas was consolidated after the 2-week self-practice period. Regarding the method for presentation of neurofeedback (intermittent presentation or continuous presentation) and the nature of the neurofeedback being presented to participants during a MI task (true or false neurofeedback regarding brain activations), Johnson et al. (2010) further reported that the intermittent presentation of feedback was more effective than the continuous presentation in promoting self-modulation of brain activity. Accordingly, regular interruptions in neurofeedback presentation allowed central processing and integration of the information conveyed in the feedback regarding brain activations. The authors also reported that false feedback resulted in irrelevant brain activations with regards to the regions of interest targeted by experimental instructions. Finally, Xie et al. (2011) supported the effectiveness of delivering neurofeedback during MI using real time fMRI, and further provided evidence that the SMA was controllable by participants. These data strongly support that real time fMRI is a valuable technique to investigate whether participants are able to use a cognitive strategy to control a target brain region in real time. In the field of neurorehabilitation, for example, a similar approach could be used to learn how controlling pain by learning to control the brain regions that mediate pain perception (deCharms et al., 2005). Indeed, there are multiple therapeutic applications of real time fMRI but it is too early to predict success or failure and new experimental results are awaited.

Real time fMRI might also be particularly useful in developing brain-computer interfaces (deCharms, 2008). A brain-computer interface is a novel communication system that translates human thoughts or intentions into a control signal without using any muscle activity (for review, see Pfurtscheller and Neuper, 2010). To date, many brain-computer interface systems have used MI tasks to modulate sensorimotor EEG activity taken to operate and control an external device. Pfurtscheller and Neuper (2010) nicely demonstrated how brain-computer interface systems using MI can contribute to help patients with various motor impairments and paralysis. Despite the temporal limitations of fMRI, using fMRI data for brain-computer interface remains plausible as many cognitive processes change slowly, over seconds or minutes (deCharms, 2008). Practically, the method is appealing although future experimental studies are necessary to determine its feasibility and effectiveness, such as during motor recovery of patients with motor impairment. Real time fMRI might also be used to explore the state of consciousness and communicate with patients in a persistent vegetative state. Accordingly, Owen et al. (2006) detected awareness in such a patient following instructions to mentally imagine moving around a house and playing tennis. Brain activations were observed in the parahippocampal gyrus, the posterior parietal lobe and the lateral PMC during MI of walking, and in the SMA when imagining playing tennis. These data provide evidence that real time fMRI might be used along with MI to actually communicate with people and/or patient who are physically or conventionally unable to interact with their environment (deCharms, 2008).

Creating functional connectivity maps of distinct spatial distributions of temporally correlated brain regions is another methodological advanced tool offered by fMRI. Functional and effective connectivity can be used to examine interactions among brain regions. Practically, these techniques go beyond the usual activation maps obtained through peak-detection methods, by looking respectively at temporal correlation between the time course of activation of two regions, and the influence of one neuronal population over another (Doyon and Benali, 2005; Friston and Büchel, 2003; Friston et al., 1995). Multiple innovative data-driven methods have been proposed to investigate the changes observed in cerebral networks over time, or to study functional and effective connectivity. Some reliable examples are the structural equation modeling and the dynamic causal modeling. In the field of MI, few researchers examined the inter-relationships among brain areas selectively activated along different experimental conditions, that is, the effective connectivity between network components. Solodkin et al. (2004) explored the effective connectivity of the neural networks mediating motor execution, visual imagery, and kinaesthetic imagery of a finger to thumb opposition task. Their results provided evidence that the networks underlying these behaviors were almost different, despite the extensive overlap between motor execution and kinaesthetic imagery. In particular, inputs from SMA and lateral PMC to cM1, which were facilitated during motor execution, exhibited the opposite activity during kinaesthetic imagery, suggesting a physiological mechanism whereby the system prevents overt movements. A second study looking at the effective connectivity between SMA and cM1 suggested that the lack of activation in cM1 during MI might result from a suppressive influence of the SMA (Kasess et al., 2008). More recently, Gao et al. (2008) and Chen et al. (2009) reported that, in right-handed participants, more brain regions showed effective connections to the SMA during right-hand MI than during left-hand MI, but that the strength of the casual influence was stronger during left-hand MI. Furthermore, they found forward and backward effective connectivity between the SMA and the bilateral dorsal PMC, the contralateral primary and somatosensory cortex, and cM1. A last study by the same group of researchers confirmed these findings, and further showed that motor execution has some increased causal connections because of additional processes for the overt behavior stage (Gao et al., 2011). Taken together, these experimental studies highlight the advantages of studying functional and/or effective connectivity through fMRI to expand our understanding of the neural underpinnings of MI.

Reporting an elevation in the fMRI BOLD signal, namely positive BOLD, has become a common routine for mapping neural activity in the human brain. Aside from positive BOLD signal changes, several studies have also observed negative BOLD responses. The negative BOLD signal is a physiological process correlated with a corresponding decrease in cerebral blood flow, oxygen consumption, and neuronal activity (for review, see Shmuel et al., 2002). Practically, negative BOLD signal might reflect less activation for a given task as compared to a baseline condition. The negative BOLD response might be caused by a reduction in cerebral blood flow and is associated with decrease in the rate of oxygen consumption. From a functional viewpoint, the negative BOLD response is further considered to carry information content that is stimulus-specific (Bressler et al., 2007). Its neurobiological mechanisms are yet not well understood, and much of the debate has centered on whether its source is primarily vascular or neuronal. The neuronal origin might reflect a suppression of the local neuronal activity and/or a reduction in the afferent input, whereas the vascular origin refers to a reduction in cerebral blood flow to the less demanding regions due to the increase in flow to the demanding areas, without a necessary decrease in neuronal activity in the negative regions (Schmuel et al., 2002). Until recently, very few experimental studies were designed to analyze negative BOLD responses during either visual or MI tasks. An interesting and innovative paper by Amedi et al. (2005) investigated the pattern of brain deactivation during visual imagery and compared it to the neural correlates of visual perception. While they found that visual imagery and visual perception share similar neural substrate, these two conditions yielded different brain-deactivation profiles as shown by negative BOLD responses. Of particular interest is that the authors reported a robust deactivation in early auditory areas as well as a selective deactivation in the somatosensory cortex during visual imagery, hence supporting that visual imagery is associated with deactivation of non-visual sensory processing. Based on these data, they stated that what they named 'pure visual imagery' might be characterized by an isolated activation of visual cortical areas with concurrent deactivation of sensory inputs that may potentially disrupt the image created by the mind's eye. They also considered that deactivation could be the consequence of filtering out irrelevant stimuli. The correlation between the level of deactivation and the vividness of visual imagery might support the hypothesis that participants with high imagery ability are able to shut down or disconnect the 'useless' cortices. To the best of our knowledge, unfortunately, there are no experimental studies specifically designed to look for similar results in MI paradigms *per se,* since most experimental work looking at the negative BOLD signal primarily focused on stimulus-based sensorial tasks rather than cognitive processes such as MI. Interestingly, it has been suggested that the prolonged negative BOLD signal reflects an inhibition or suppression of neuronal firing patterns (Raichle, 1998; Kastrup et al., 2008). Looking more systematically for negative BOLD responses might therefore be of particular interest to investigate the inhibitory processes of the motor command during imagined movements. Indeed, motor command inhibition mechanisms during MI remains rather unclear since no direct fMRI brain signal is known to characterize neural inhibitory processes, and inhibition during MI has been primarily studied from brain activation signals. The negative BOLD response might therefore be an interesting methodological complement to extend our knowledge of motor inhibition.

5. Conclusion

The data reviewed in this chapter strongly support that recording human brain functioning with fMRI during MI provides an objective measurement of the neural networks underlying MI processes. Although they are not totally overlapping, it is now well-established that the neural substrates mediating MI and actual execution of the same task are quite similar. Spurred by recent fMRI methodological advances, the next step of MI research will certainly contribute to understand in greater details the neural correlates of imagined movements, as well as the inhibition of the motor command. MI studies could therefore benefit from the use of real time fMRI, effective connectivity, and also negative BOLD. This latter technique might be of particular interest in investigating the inhibitory processes of the motor command during MI. Cerebral regions which are inhibited during mental operations or human behavior are certainly of the same scientific interest than those which are activated.

Author details

Aymeric Guillot*, Franck Di Rienzo and Christian Collet

Centre de Recherche et d'Innovation sur le Sport, Performance Motrice, Mentale et du Matériel (P3M), Université de Lyon, Université Claude Bernard Lyon1, France

References

[1] Alexander, G.E., and Crutcher, M.D. (1990). Functional architecture of basal ganglia circuits: neural substrates of parallel processing. *Trends in Neuroscience, 13,* 266-271.

[2] Alkadhi, H., Brugger, P., Boendermaker, S.H., Crelier, G., Curt, A., Hepp-Reymond, M.-C., and Kollias, S.S. (2005). What disconnection tells about motor imagery: evidence from paraplegic patients. *Cerebral Cortex, 15,* 131–140.

[3] Amedi, A., Malach, R., and Pascual-Leone, A. (2005). Negative BOLD Differentiates Visual Imagery and Perception. *Neuron, 48,* 859-872.

[4] Battaglia, F., Quartarone, A., Ghilardi, M.F., Dattola, R., Bagnato, S., Rizzo, V., Morgante, L., and Girlanda, P. (2006). Unilateral cerebellar stroke disrupts movement preparation and motor imagery. *Clinical Neurophysiology, 117,* 1009–1016.

[5] Bressler, D., Spotswood, N., and Whitney, D. (2007). Negative BOLD fMRI Response in the Visual Cortex Carries Precise Stimulus-Specific Information. *Plos One, 2,* e410.

[6] Binkofski, F., Amunts, K., Stephan, K.M., Posse, S., Schormann, T., Freund, H.J., Zilles, K., and Seitz, R.J. (2000). Broca's region subserves imagery of motion: a combined cytoarchitectonic and fMRI study. *Human Brain Mapping, 11,* 273-285.

[7] Chen, H., Yang, Q., Liao, W., Gong, Q., and Shen, S. (2009). Evaluation of the effective connectivity of supplementary motor areas during motor imagery using Granger causality mapping. *NeuroImage, 47,* 1844-1853.

[8] Cramer, S.C., Lastra, L., Lacourse, M., and Cohen, M.J. (2005). Brain motor system function after chronic, complete spinal cord injury. *Brain, 128,* 2941–2950.

[9] De Vries, S., and Mulder, T. (2007). Motor imagery and stroke rehabilitation: a critical discussion. *Journal of Rehabilitation Medicine, 39,* 5–13.

[10] deCharms, R.C. (2008). Applications of real-time fMRI. *Nature Review Neuroscience, 9,* 720-729.

[11] deCharms, R.C., Christoff, K., Glover, G.H., Pauly, J.M., Whitfield, S., and Gabrieli J.D. (2004). Learned regulation of spatially localized brain activation using real-time fMRI. *NeuroImage, 21,* 436-443.

[12] deCharms, R.C., Maeda, F., Glover, G.H., Ludlow, D., Pauly, J.M., Soneji, D., Gabrieli, J.D., and Mackey, S.C. (2005). Control over brain activation and pain learned by using real-time functional MRI. *PNAS, 102,* 18626-18631.

[13] Dechent, P., Merboldt, K.D., and Frahm, J. (2004). is the human primary motor cortex involved in motor imagery? *Cognitive Brain Research, 19,* 138-144.

[14] Dietrich, A. (2008). Imaging the imagination: the trouble with motor imagery. *Methods, 45,* 319-324.

[15] Di Rienzo, F., Guillot, A., Delpuech, C., Rode, G., Grangeon, M., and Collet C. (2011). Inhibition of the motor command during motor imagery: a MEG study with a tetraplegic patient. 17th Annual Meeting of the Organization on Human Brain Mapping, June 26-30, Quebec City, Canada, p. 40.

[16] Doyon, J., and Benali, H. (2005). Reorganization and plasticity in the adult brain during learning of motor skills. *Current Opinion in Neurobiology, 25,* 161-167,.

[17] Doyon, J., and Ungerleider, L.G. (2002). Functional anatomy of motor skill learning. In: *Neuropsychology of Memory,* Squire L.R and Schacter D.L. (Ed.), pp. 225-38, Guilford Press.

[18] Driskell, J. E., Copper, C., and Moran, A. (1994). Does mental practice enhance performance? *Journal of Applied Psychology, 79,* 481–492.

[19] Ehrsson, H.H., Geyer, S., and Naito, E. (2003). Imagery of voluntary movement of fingers, toes and tongue activates corresponding body-part-specific motor representations. *Journal of Neurophysiology, 90,* 3304-3316.

[20] Ersland, L., Rosen, G., Lundervold, A., Smievoll, A.I., Tillung, T., Sundberg, H., and Hugdahl, K. (1996). Phantom limb imaginary fingertapping causes primary motor cortex activation: an fMRI study. *Neuroreport,8,* 207–210.

[21] Esposito, F., Seifritz, E., Formisano, E., Morrone, R., Scarabino, T., Tedeschi, G., Cirillo, S., Goebel, R., and Di Salle, F. (2003). Real-time independent component analysis of fMRI time-series. *NeuroImage, 20,* 2209-2224.

[22] Friston, K.J., and Buchel, C. (2003). Functional connectivity. In: *Human Brain Function,* Frackowiak, R.S.J. et al., Eds), Academic Press (2nd Ed.).

[23] Friston, K., Ungerleider, L., Jezzard, P., and Turner, R., (1995). Characterizing modulatory interactions between V1 and V2 in human cortex with fMRI. *Human Brain Mapping, 2,* 211-224.

[24] Gao, Q., Chen, H., and Gong, Q. (2008). Evaluation of the effective connectivity of the dominant primary motor cortex during bimanual movement using Granger causality. *Neuroscience Letters, 443,* 1-6.

[25] Gao, Q., Duan, X., and Chen, H. (2011). Evaluation of effective connectivity of motor areas during motor imagery and execution using conditional Granger causality. *NeuroImage, 54,* 1280-1288.

[26] Gerardin, E., Sirigu, A., Lehericy, S., Poline, J.B., Gaymard, B., Marsault, C., Agid, Y., and Le Bihan, D. (2000). Partially overlapping neural networks for real and imagined hand movements. *Cerebral Cortex, 10,* 1093-1104.

[27] Gonzáles, B., Rodríguez, M., Ramirez, C., and Sabaté, M. (2005). Disturbance of motor imagery after cerebellar stroke. *Behavioral Neuroscience, 119,* 622–626.

[28] Grezes, J., and Decety, J. (2001). Functional anatomy of execution, mental simulation, observation, and verb generation of actions: a meta-analysis. *Human Brain Mapping, 12,* 1-19.

[29] Guillot, A., and Collet, C. (2005). Duration of mentally simulated movement: a review. *Journal of Motor Behavior, 37,* 10-20.

[30] Guillot, A., and Collet, C. (2008). Construction of the motor imagery integrative model in sport: a review and theoretical investigation of motor imagery use. *International Review of Sport and Exercice Psychology, 1,* 31–44.

[31] Guillot, A., Collet, C., Nguyen, V.A., Malouin, F., Richards, C., and Doyon, J. (2008). Functional neuroanatomical networks associated with expertise in motor imagery ability. *NeuroImage, 41,* 1471-1483.

[32] Guillot A., Collet C., Nguyen VA., Malouin F., Richards C., and Doyon J. (2009). Brain activity during visual versus kinesthetic imagery: an fMRI study. *Human Brain Mapping, 30,* 2157-2172.

[33] Guillot A., Louis M., and Collet C. (2010). Neurophysiological substrates of motor imagery ability. In: *The neurophysiological foundations of mental and motor imagery,* Guillot A. and Collet C. (Eds.) pp. 109-124, Oxford University Press.

[34] Guillot, A., Hoyek, N., Louis, M., and Collet, C. (2011). Understanding the timing of motor imagery: recent findings and future directions. *International Review of Sport and Exercice Psychology, in press.*

[35] Hanakawa, T., Immisch, I., Toma, K., Dimyan, M.A., Van Gelderen, P., and Hallett, M. (2003). Functional properties of brain areas associated with motor execution and imagery. *Journal of Neurophysiology, 89,* 989-1002.

[36] Hanakawa, T., Dimyan, M.A., and Hallett, M. (2008). Motor planning, imagery, and execution in the distributed motor network: a time-course study with functional MRI. *Cerebral Cortex, 18,* 2775–2788.

[37] Heremans, E., Feys, P., Nieuwboer, A., Vercruysse, S., Vandenberghe, W., Sharma, N., Helsen, W. (2011). Motor imagery ability in patients with early-and mid-stage Parkinson disease. *Neurorehabilitation and Neural Repair, 25,* 168-177.

[38] Holmes, P.S., and Collins, D.J. (2001). The PETTLEP approach to motor imagery: A functional equivalence model for sport psychologists. *Journal of Applied Sport Psychology, 13,* 60-83.

[39] Jackson, P.L., Meltzoff, A.L., and Decety, J. (2006). Neural circuits involved in imitation and perspective-taking. *NeuroImage, 31,* 429-439.

[40] Jackson, P.L., Lafleur, M.F., Malouin, F., Richards, C.L., and Doyon, J. (2003). Functional cerebral reorganization following motor sequence learning through mental practice with motor imagery. *NeuroImage, 20,* 1171-1180.

[41] Jeannerod, M. (1994). The representing brain: neural correlates of motor intention and imagery. *Behavioral and Brain Sciences, 17,* 187-202, 1994.

[42] Johnson, S.H., Rotte,M., Grafton, S.T., Hinrichs, H., Gazzaniga,M.S., and Heinze, H.J. (2002). Selective activation of a parietofrontal circuit during implicitly imagined prehension. *NeuroImage, 17,* 1693–1704.

[43] Johnson, K.A., Hartwell, K., Lematty, T., Borckardt, J., Morgan, P.S., Govindarajan, K., Brady, K., and George, M.S. (2010). Intermittent "Real-time" fMRI Feedback Is Superior to Continuous Presentation for a Motor Imagery Task: A Pilot Study. *Journal of Neuroimaging, in press,* doi: 10.1111/j.1552-6569.2010.00529.

[44] Kasess, C.H., Windischberger, C., Cunnington, R., Lanzenberger, R., Pezawas, L., and Moser, E. (2008). The suppressive influence of SMA on M1 in motor imagery revealed by fMRI and dynamic causal modeling. *NeuroImage, 40,* 828-837.

[45] Kastrup, A., Baudewig, J., Schnaudigel, S., Huonker, R., Becker, L., Sohns, J.M., Dechent, P., Klingner, C., and Wittec, O.W. (2008). Behavioral correlates of negative BOLD signal changes in the primary somatosensory cortex. *Neuroimage, 41,* 1341-1371.

[46] Kleber, B., Birbaumer, N., Veit, R., Trevorrow, T., and Lotze, M. (2007). Overt and imagined singing of an Italian aria. *NeuroImage,* 36, 889-900.

[47] Kosslyn, S.M., Segar, C., Pani, J., and Hillger, L.A. (1990). When is imagery used in everyday life? A diary study. *Journal of Mental Imagery, 14,* 131–52.

[48] Kuhtz-Buschbeck, J.P., Mahnkopf, C., Holzknecht, C., Siebner, H., Ulmer, S., and Jansen, O. (2003). Effector-independent representations of simple and complex imagined finger movements: a combined fMRI and TMS study. *European Journal of Neuroscience, 18,* 3375-3387.

[49] Lafleur, M.F., Jackson, P.L., Malouin, F., Richards, C.L., Evans, A.C., and Doyon, J. (2002). Motor learning produces parallel dynamic functional changes during the execution and imagination of sequential foot movements. *NeuroImage, 2,* 142-57.

[50] Langheim, F.J.P., Callicott, J.H., Mattay, V.S., Duyn, J.H., and Weinberger, D.R. (2002). Cortical systems associated with covert music rehearsal. *NeuroImage, 16,* 901-908, 2002.

[51] Leonardo, M., Fieldman, J., Sadato, N., Campbell, G., Ibanez, V., Cohen, L., Deiber, M.-P., Jezzard, P., Pons, T., Turner, R., Le Bihan, D., and Hallett, M. (1995). A functional magnetic resonance imaging study of cortical regions associated with motor task execution and motor ideation in humans. *Human Brain Mapping, 3,* 83–92.

[52] Li, C.R. (2000). Impairment of motor imagery in putamen lesions in humans. *Neuroscience Letters,* 287, 13-16.

[53] Logothetis, N. K. (2008). What we can do and what we cannot do with fMRI. *Nature,* 453, 869-878.

[54] Lorey, B., Bischoff, M., Pilgramm, S., Stark, R., Munzert, J., and Zentgraf, K. (2009). The embodied nature of motor imagery: the influence of posture and perspective. *Experimental Brain Research, 194,* 233-243.

[55] Lotze, M., and Halsband, U. (2006). Motor imagery. *Journal of Physiology (Paris),* 99, 386-395.

[56] Lotze, L., Montoya, P., Erb, M., Hulsmann, E., Flor, H., Klause, U., Birbaumer, N., and Grodd, W. (1999). Activation of cortical and cerebellar motor areas during executed and imagined hand movements: an fMRI study. *Journal of Cognitive Neuroscience, 11,* 491-501.

[57] Lotze, M., Scheler, G., Tan, H.R.M., Braun, C., and Birbaumer, N. (2003). The musician's brain: functional imaging of amateurs and professionals during performance and imagery. *NeuroImage, 20,* 1817-1829, 2003.

[58] Lotze, M. and Zentgraf, K. (2010). Contribution of the primary motor cortex to motor imagery. In: *The neurophysiological foundations of mental and motor imagery,* Guillot A. and Collet C. (Eds.), pp. 31-46, Oxford University Press.

[59] Macuga, K.L., and Frey, S.H. (2011). Neural representations involved in observed, imagined, and imitated actions are dissociable and hierarchically organized. *NeuroImage, in press.*

[60] Malouin, F., Belleville, S., Richards, C. L., Desrosiers, J., and Doyon, J. (2004). Working memory and mental practice outcomes after stroke. *Archives of Physical Medicine and Rehabilitation, 85,* 177–183.

[61] Malouin, F., Richards, C., Durand, A., and Doyon, J. (2008). Reliability of mental chronometry for assessing motor imagery ability after stroke. *Archives of Physical Medicine and Rehabilitation, 89,* 311-319.

[62] Malouin, F., Richards, C.L., Jackson, P.L., Dumas, F., and Doyon, J. (2003). Brain activations during motor imagery of locomotor-related tasks: a PET study. *Human Brain Mapping, 19,* 47–62.

[63] Marx, E., Deutschländer, A., Stephan, T., Dieterich, M., Wiesmann, M., and Brandt, T. (2004). Eyes open and eyes closed as rest conditions: Impact on brain activation patterns. *NeuroImage, 21,* 1818-1824.

[64] Marx, E., Stephan, T., Nolte, A., Deutschländer, A., Seelos, K.C., Dieterich, M., and Brandt, T. (2003). Eye closure in darkness animates sensory systems. *NeuroImage, 19,* 924–934.

[65] Michelon, P., Vettel, J.M., and Zacks, J.M. (2006). Lateral somatotopic organization during imagined and prepared movements. *Journal of Neurophysiology, 95,* 811-822.

[66] Milton, J., Solodkin, A., Hlustîk, P., and Small, S.L. (2007).The mind of expert motor performance is cool and focused. *NeuroImage, 35,* 804-813.

[67] Milton, J., Small, S.L., and Solodkin, A. (2008). Imaging motor imagery: methodological issues related to expertise. *Methods, 45,* 336-341.

[68] Munzert, J., Lorey, B., and Zentraf, K. (2009). Cognitive motor processes: The role of motor imagery in the study of motor representations. *Brain Research Reviews, 60,* 306-326.

[69] Murphy, S., Nordin, S.M., and Cumming, J. (2008). Imagery in sport, exercise and dance. In: *Advances in sport psychology,* Horn T.S. (Eds.), pp. 306–315, Champagne, IL: Human Kinetics.

[70] Nair, D.G., Purcott, K.L., Fuchs, A., Steinberg, F., and Kelso, J.A.K. (2003). Cortical and cerebellar activity of the human brain during imagined and executed unimanual and bimanual action sequences: a functional MRI study. *Cognitive Brain Research, 15,* 250-260.

[71] Olsson, C.J., Jonsson, B., and Nyberg, L. (2008). Internal imagery training in active high jumpers. *Scandinavian Journal of Psychology, 49,* 133–140.

[72] Owen, A.M., Coleman, M.R., Boly, M., Davis, M.H., Laureys, S., and Pickard, J.D. (2006). Detecting Awareness in the Vegetative State. *Science, 313,* 1402.

[73] Pfurtscheller, G., and Neuper, K. (2010). EEG-based brain–computer communication. In: *The neurophysiological foundations of mental and motor imagery,* Guillot A. and Collet C. (Eds.), pp. 203-212, Oxford University Press.

[74] Porro, C.A., Francescato, M.P., Cettolo, V., Diamond, M.E., Baraldi, P., Zuiani, C., Bazzocchi, M., and Di Prampero, P.E. (1996). Primary motor and sensory cortex activation during motor performance and motor imagery: a functional magnetic resonance imaging study. *Journal of Neuroscience, 16*, 7688-7698.

[75] Porro, C.A., Cettolo, V., Francescato, M.P., and Baraldi, P. (2000). Ipsilateral involvement of primary motor cortex during motor imagery. *European Journal of Neuroscience, 12*, 3059-3063.

[76] Raichle, M.E. (1998). Behind the scenes of functional brain imaging: a historical and physiological perspective. *Proceedings of the National Academy of Sciences (USA), 95*, 765–772.

[77] Rizzolatti, G., Luppino, G., and Matelli, M. (1998). The organization of the cortical motor system: new concepts. *Electroencephalographic and Clinical Neurophysiology, 106*, 283–296.

[78] Roland, P.E., Larsen, B., Lassen, N.A., and Skinhoj, E. (1980). Supplementary motor area and other cortical areas in organisation of voluntary movements in man. *Journal of Neurophysiology, 43*,118-136.

[79] Ross, J.S., Tkach, J., Ruggieri, P.M., Lieber, M., and Lapresto, E. (2003). The mind's eye: Functional MR imaging of golf motor imagery. *American Journal of Neuroradiology, 24*, 1036-1044.

[80] Roth, M., Decety, J., Raybaudi, M., Massarelli, R., Delon-Martin, C., Segebarth, C.M., Morand, S., Gemignani, A., Decorps, M., and Jeannerod, M. (1996). Possible involvement of primary motor cortex in mentally simulated movement: A functional magnetic resonance imagery study. *Neuroreport, 7*, 1280-1284.

[81] Ruby, P., and Decety, J. (2001). Effect of subjective perspective taking during simulation of action: a PET investigation of agency. *Nature Neuroscience, 4*, 546-50.

[82] Sabate, M., Gonzalez, B., and Rodriguez, M. (2007). Adapting movement planning to motor impairments: The motor-scanning system. *Neuropsychologia, 45*, 378-386.

[83] Sabbah, P., Simond, G., Levrier, O., Habib M, Trabaud V, Murayama N, Mazoyer BM, Briant JF, Raybaud C, and Salamon G. (1995). Functional magnetic resonance imaging at 1.5T during sensory motor and cognitive tasks. *European Neurology, 35*, 131–135.

[84] Sanes, J.N., and Donoghue, J.P. (2000). Plasticity and primary motor cortex. *Annual Review of Neuroscience, 23*, 393-415.

[85] Schmuel, A., Yacoub, E., Pfeuffer, J., Van de Moortele, P.F., Adriany, G., Hu, X., and Ugurbil, K. (2002). Sustained negative BOLD, blood flow and oxygen consumption response and its coupling to the positive response in the human brain. *Neuron, 36*, 1195-1210.

[86] Schwoebel, J., Boronat, C.B., and Coslett, H.B. (2002). The man who executed "imagined" movements: evidence for dissociable components of the body schema. *Brain and Cognition, 50,* 1–16.

[87] Sharma, M., Pomeroy, V.M., and Baron, J.C. (2006). Motor imagery: a backdoor to the motor system after stroke? *Stroke, 37,* 1941–1952.

[88] Sharma, M., Jones, P.S., Carpenter, T.A., and Baron, J.C. (2008). Mapping the involvement of BA 4a and 4p during motor imagery. *NeuroImage, 41,* 92–99.

[89] Sirigu, A., Duhamel, J.R., Cohen, L., Pillon, B., Dubois, B., and Agid, Y. (1996). The mental representation of hand movements after parietal cortex damage. *Science, 273,* 1564-1568.

[90] Solodkin, A., Hlustik, P., Chen, E.E., and Small, S.L. (2004). Fine modulation in network activation during motor execution and motor imagery. *Cerebral Cortex, 14,* 1246-1255.

[91] Stinear, C.M. (2010). Corticospinal facilitation during motor imagery. In: *The neurophysiological foundations of mental and motor imagery,* Guillot A. and Collet C. (Eds.), pp. 47-61, Oxford University Press.

[92] Weiskopf, N., Veit, R., Erb, M., Mathiak, K., Grodd, W., Goebel, R., and Birbaumer, N. (2003). Physiological self-regulation of regional brain activity using real-time functional magnetic resonance imaging (fMRI): methodology and exemplary data. *NeuroImage, 19,* 577-86.

[93] Xie, B., Ma, X., Yao, L., Long, Z., and Zhao, X. (2011). Real time fMRI data analysis using region of interest selection based on fast ICA. *Progress in Biomedical Optics and Imaging – Proceedings of SPIE, 7965,* article 79651s.

[94] Yoo, S.S, and Jolesz, F.A. (2002). Functional MRI for neurofeedback: feasability study on a hand motor task. *Neuroreport, 13,* 1377-81.

[95] Yoo, S.S., Lee, J.H., O'Leary, H., Panych, L.P., and Jolesz, F.A. (2008). Neurofeedback fMRI-mediated learning and consolidation of regional brain activation during motor imagery. *International Journal of Imaging Systems and Tecnhology, 18,* 69-78.

[96] Zang, Y., Jia, F., Weng, X., Li, E., Cui, S., Wang, Y., Hazeltine, E., and Ivry, R. (2003). Functional organization of the primary motor cortex characterized by event-related fMRI during movement preparation and execution. *Neuroscience Letters, 337,* 69–72.

3

Using fMRI to Examine Central Auditory Plasticity

Deborah A. Hall, Cornelis P. Lanting and Douglas E.H. Hartley

1. Introduction

During the last two decades or so, auditory neuroscience has made significant progress in understanding the functional organization of the auditory system in both normal-hearing listeners, patients with sensorineural hearing impairments and/or tinnitus, and following cochlear implantation. Modern brain imaging techniques have made an enormous contribution to that progress by enabling the *in vivo* study of human central auditory function. Since its introduction, magnetic resonance imaging (MRI) has evolved to become one of the most influential methods for investigating non-invasive human brain structure and function. Functional MRI (fMRI) has become the tool of choice for addressing many research questions concerning central auditory plasticity. First, fMRI has good spatial sensitivity and specificity and so can be used to map auditory responses with reasonably fine topographic detail (Logothetis et al., 2001). Second, fMRI is suitable for research use with children, as well as adults. Third, since multiple observations can be made on the same individual, fMRI permits the investigation of longer-term dynamic processes, such as functional plasticity after disease, damage, retraining or therapy. Finally, the need for averaging data across individuals is reduced, further improving the accuracy with which activations can be mapped onto subject-specific brain structure (e.g. Talavage et al., 2004). Despite these advantages, there are significant issues using this technique in certain clinical populations, such as individuals with a cochlear implant (CI). Subsequently, to investigate the effects of CIs on brain reorganization, it is necessary to consider alternative functional imaging methods, such as electroencephalography (e.g. Debener et al., 2008). Moreover, the high level of the scanner acoustic noise can have detrimental effects on central auditory function, patient anxiety and verbal communication between patient and scanner operator (Mechefske et al., 2002). In terms of central auditory function, the scanner acoustic noise can induce increases in the fMRI response of the auditory cortex as well as interfere with the perception of externally presented sound stimuli (Edmister et al., 1999; Hall et al., 1999).

Although- functional imaging of the central auditory pathway has not been widely used in Ear, Nose and Throat or Audiology clinics, there is a growing literature on its potential application. Using insights gained from functional imaging research with normal-hearing subjects, we can now transfer the most efficient protocols to study patients with hearing problems. For example, a choice of methods is available for noise reduction and a range of scanning parameters have been optimised to enhance the detection of brain activity.

This chapter discusses some of the theoretical and technical challenges of auditory fMRI and several of the major themes within this field, notably cortical reorganization underpinning tinnitus and deafness. Also we will consider the effect of CIs on the auditory brain, the difficulties associated with the use of conventional imaging methods in CI populations, and potential application of novel techniques, such as near infrared spectroscopy. Sections not only highlight evidence for neuroplasticity within the central auditory system, but also review what is currently known about the involvement and integration of information from other sensory modalities.

2. Challenges and limitations of auditory fMRI

Rather than directly measuring the stimulus- and task-related electrical activity of neurons, fMRI measures indirect changes in the magnetic properties of the blood. Most common methods make use of the blood-oxygen-level-dependent (BOLD) contrast. This technique is based on the increase in signal intensity caused by an increase in oxygen concentration of blood (Ogawa et al., 1990). The functional image represents the spatial distribution of blood oxygenation levels in the brain and the small fluctuations in these levels over time are correlated with the stimulus input or cognitive task.

To detect the magnetic properties of brain tissue, MR scanners operate using three different types of electromagnetic fields: a very high static field generated by a superconducting magnet, time-varying gradient magnetic fields and pulsed radiofrequency (RF) fields. The latter two fields are much weaker than the first, but all pose a number of unique and considerable technical challenges for conducting auditory fMRI research within this hostile environment.

In the first place, the static and time-varying magnetic fields preclude the use of many types of electronic sound presentation equipment, as well as preventing the safe scanning of patients who are wearing listening devices such as hearing aids or implants. Despite the restriction on the materials that can be used in a scanner, a number of different MR-compatible active headphone driving units have been produced for sound delivery. Several audio systems use electrostatic transducers to ensure high performance. Electrostatic headphones generate sound using a conductive diaphragm placed next to a fixed conducting panel. A high voltage polarises the fixed panel and the audio signal passing through the diaphragm rapidly switches between a positive and a negative signal, attracting or repelling it to the fixed panel and thus vibrating the air. Induced currents in the electronics, caused directly by the time-varying gradient magnetic fields or the RF pulses, are an additional hazard to the electronic devices themselves. Some materials can also absorb the RF energy causing local tissue heating and even burns if in contact with soft tissue. Hence, the digital audio source, electronics and power supply that drive the sound system are housed outside the RF screened scanner room to avoid electromagnetic interference with MRI. The electrical signal is then transferred from the audio source to the headphones in the RF screened scanner room using either filters through a filter panel or fibre-optic cable through the waveguide. For the same safety reasons, there are restrictions on scanning people who have electronic listening devices. These include hearing aids, cochlear implants and brainstem implants. Official approval for the manufacture of implant devices requires rigorous testing for susceptibility to electromagnetic fields, radiated electromagnetic fields and electrical safety testing (including susceptibility to electrical discharge). Typically however standard listening devices do not meet the more stringent criteria for compatibility with MR scanning. For the patient, risks include movement of the device and localised heating of brain tissue, whereas, for the device, the electronic components may be damaged. Some implant designs *have* been proven to be MR compatible (e.g. Shellock et al., 1993), but they are not routinely supplied in clinical practice. Given that implanted devices cannot be removed without surgical intervention, clinical imaging research of implantees has generally used other brain imaging methods, namely positron emission tomography (Giraud et al., 2001).

The high levels of scanner noise generated by the flexing of the gradient coils in the static magnetic field can reduce audibility and increase listening effort. Scanner noise increases nonlinearly with static magnetic field strength. For example, comparing scanners from 1 to 3 Tesla indicates a difference in sound level of about 10 dB SPL (Price et al., 2001). The sound level measured in the bore of the scanner is typically 99 dB SPL (98 dB(A)). Clearly, exposure to such an intense sound levels without protection is likely to cause a temporary threshold shift in hearing and tinnitus, and could be permanently damaging over a prolonged stay inside the bore of the scanner (Foster et al., 2000). The simplest way to treat the intense noise is to use ear protection in the form of ear defenders and/or ear plugs. Foam ear plugs can compromise the acoustic quality of the experimental sounds delivered to the subject and so circumaural headsets are preferable. Typically transducers are fitted into sound attenuating earmuffs to reduce the ambient noise level at the subject's ears. Considerable attenuation can be achieved in this manner (e.g., 25 dB of attenuation at 600 Hz rising to 40 dB at 4 kHz, Hall et al., 2009). Even with hearing protection, whenever the scanner noise coincides with the presented sound stimulus it produces changes in task performance and increases the attentional demands of the listening task. The frequency range of the scanner noise overlaps with the range that is crucial for speech intelligibility and so speech experiments can be particularly compromised in the noisy environment. For example, Blackman and Hall (2011) reported that speech intelligibility (measured as the proportion of keywords reported correctly) dropped by about 50% for words that were masked by the scanner noise compared to those that were not masked by the noise.

The high levels of ambient scanner noise can interfere with the patterns of brain activity measured during fMRI. The noise not only activates parts of the auditory brain, but also interacts with the patterns of activity evoked by experimental stimuli. Two novel methods have been developed by the Nottingham group to deal with these problems; sparse temporal sampling (Hall et al., 1999) and active noise reduction (Hall et al., 2009). In sparse sampling, a clustered acquisition of brain slices is combined with a long and fixed (e.g. 10 s) inter-scan interval and the scan acquisition is temporally offset from the presentation of the stimulus of interest (typically by 8-10 s). Although the scanner noise resulting from the acquisition still evokes an auditory BOLD response, it does not extend across time to the subsequent scan. Work in the mid-90s demonstrated that when the onset of the scan acquisition is synchronized to the offset of an epoch of the stimulus presentation in a sparse sampling paradigm, the activation associated with the experimental sound can be effectively separated from the activation associated with the scanner sound (Hall et al., 1999). Furthermore, because the scanner sound is temporally offset, it does not produce acoustical masking and does not distract the listener. Sparse sampling is often the scanning protocol of choice for identifying auditory cortical evoked responses in the absence of scanner noise. Active noise reduction achieves significant attenuation of the acoustic energy received at the ears. The system reduces the perceived level of the background noise by producing an output ('cancellation') signal that destructively interferes with the scanner sound (i.e. the incident sound wave) at each ear. Precise control over the frequency and phase of acoustic signals presented to participants is achieved through a digital-signal processing system that delivers sound stimuli via a high-fidelity electrostatic headset. Blackman and Hall (2011) evaluated the benefit of active noise reduction by asking whether sound reduction provided sufficient gains in both audibility and sensitivity to sound-related activity to remove the need for sparse temporal sampling. While both sparse sampling and cancellation were found to improve listening quality, these factors did not provide equivalent benefits for auditory fMRI experiments. Cancellation offered small improvements for spatially specific analyses within Heschl's gyrus and planum polare '(regions that are engaged in auditory perception and speech comprehension)' and for reducing some of the extra-auditory activity associated with the effort required for perceptual discrimination in a noisy environment. Nevertheless, sparse acquisition remained the more robust method for detecting auditory cortical activity by providing proper quiet intervals for stimulus presentation.

3. Central auditory processing: Beyond 3 Tesla fMRI

Brain imaging studies in humans are revealing parallels with the functional organization of the auditory brain discovered in electrophysiological studies in animals: sound-level dependencies as well as topographical mapping of stimulus frequencies are observed. This section provides a foundation to the remaining sections in this chapter by describing the BOLD effect and highlighting experiments that investigate the spatial specificity of this effect as a function of the external magnetic field strength and the parameters of the imaging sequence. We consequently describe fMRI experiments that focus on the functional organization of the auditory system. Specifically, we report an experiment on the topographical mapping of sound frequencies in human auditory cortex and discuss common findings and interpretations.

3.1. Characterizing BOLD signal changes at various field strengths

Research systems typically operate at 3 Tesla, but nowadays MRI systems that operate at magnetic field strengths exceeding this field strength are becoming more widely available.

Nottingham University is the home of the first ultra-high field 7 Tesla MRI scanner for human brain imaging in the UK. The key factor for the development of such high field MRI systems is the improvement in intrinsic signal-to-noise ratio and contrast-to-noise ratio with increasing field strength. A simple motor task, for example, elicits a signal change of approximately 1%, 2.5% and 5% for field strengths of respectively 1.5 Tesla, 3 Tesla and 7 Tesla (Van der Zwaag et al., 2009). Figure 1 shows the results for one of our typical auditory tasks acquired at a magnetic field strength of 7 Tesla. In this short experiment, a sound was alternated with silence in a block design. The signal change was 5.2% indicating that the obtained percent signal change is comparable to that obtained in the above motor task. The resulting increased BOLD effect is of great benefit for fMRI basic research studies and also for clinically focussed studies. It can be exploited to improve the spatial resolution and reduces the number of trials required to demonstrate significant levels of activation. An additional effect is the increased spatial specificity of the BOLD effect with increasing field strength. At higher field strengths the T2*time of blood is relatively short causing its signal, originating mainly from the vasculature, to be attenuated relative to that of tissue at the echo times used for BOLD fMRI (Yacoub et al., 2001). The contribution of venous signal to the BOLD effect is therefore reduced at high field strengths, increasing the spatial specificity of the BOLD effect.

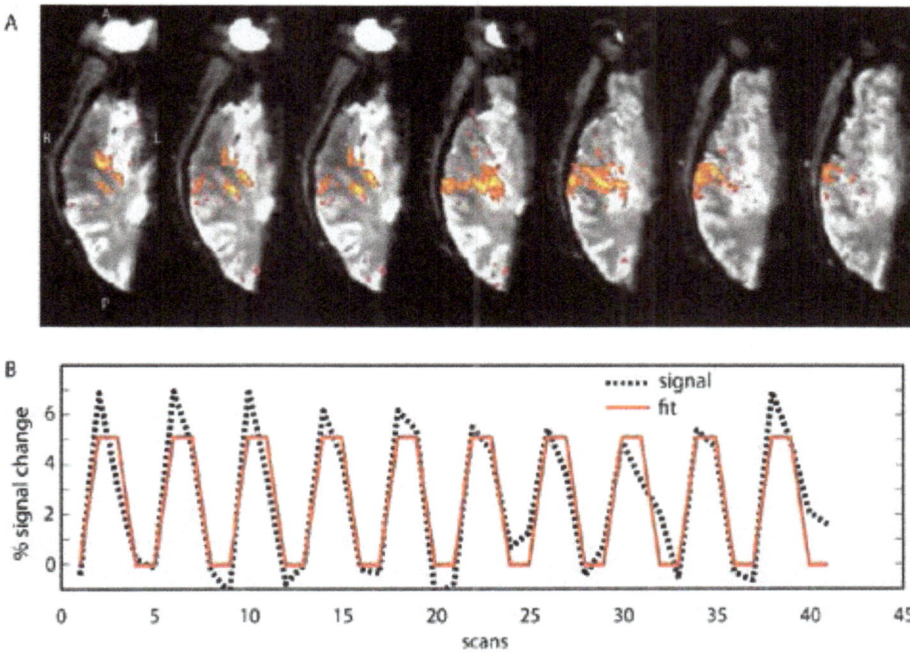

Figure 1. A) Sound-evoked activation maps obtained at 7 Tesla as overlaid on the average EPI image of one subject. The results show the primary auditory cortex, demarcated by the anterior Heschl's sulcus and the posterior Heschl's sulcus, as well as the secondary auditory cortex and higher order areas in the right hemisphere. B) shows the averaged time-course (black) and a linear fit (red) of all the active voxels following a simple block design where blocks of sound were alternated with silence. Abbreviation: A: anterior; P: posterior; R: right, L: left.

3.2. Characterizing the spatial resolution of the BOLD effect

The spatial resolution of the BOLD effect is, compared to most MRI imaging techniques, quite poor. T1-weighted anatomical images can, for example, be easily obtained with an isotropic resolution of well below 1 mm. In contrast, the spatial resolution of the BOLD effect is mostly determined by physiological sources, in the sense that the vascular response to neural activity extends over several millimetres (Logothetis et al., 2001). The BOLD signal originating from small capillaries and surrounding areas is thought to provide good spatial localization for neuronal activation. However, at low and intermediate field strengths, the gradient echo (GE) BOLD effects from large draining veins often contaminate the signal, causing inaccurate localization of the activity and also cause a widening of the point spread function of the BOLD response. GE BOLD is sensitive to extravascular effects around the large vessels while spin-echo (SE) sequences are relatively insensitive to these effects (Duong et al., 2003; Weisskoff et al., 1994). The 180° rephasing pulse in an SE sequence compensates for the constant field heterogeneities to obtain an echo that is weighted in T2 and not in T2*. Spin-echo sequences are therefore more closely related to neuronal activity than GE sequences, although there is still a large contribution of intravascular signal arising from blood. The benefit of high fields (i.e. at field strengths of 3 Tesla and higher) compared to a lower field strength is the reduced T_2 and T_2^* of blood relative to that of tissue, reducing the intravascular component even more (Yacoub et al., 2001). However, a major disadvantage with T_2-weighted SE sequences is linked to long inter-scan intervals, resulting in potentially prohibitive acquisition times.

The point spread function describes the response of the MRI scanning to a point source within the brain. Measurements of the point spread function have revealed a full-width at half-maximum (FWHM) of around 2.3 mm tangential to cortical surface of the visual cortex using GE BOLD at 7 Tesla (Shmuel et al., 2007). The FWHM of the point spread function at 7 Tesla is therefore narrower than at 1.5 Tesla (reported at 3.5 mm, Engel et al., 1997) and at 3 Tesla (reported at 3.9 mm, Parkes et al., 2005). Recently, Polimeni et al. (2010) measured the spatial spread of the BOLD response tangential to the cortical surface as a function of cortical depth. Sampling near the pial surface provided the highest signal strength, but it also introduced the most spatial error due to extravascular BOLD effects. Avoiding the surface laminae improved spatial localization considerably, at the cost of sensitivity, implying that optimal spatial resolution in fMRI of the cortex can be achieved using anatomically informed spatial sampling to avoid large pial vessels.

When comparing the point spread function of GE and SE BOLD sequences there is a 13% reduction of the FWHM of the SE sequence, but at a cost of at least 3-fold reduction in contrast to noise ratio (Parkes et al., 2005). fMRI suffers from susceptibility artifacts that are caused by the proximity of air-cavities like the ear canal and nasal cavity causing signal loss and distortion of the images (Ojemann et al., 1997). Many strategies have been proposed to overcome these effects which include the usage of shorter echo times, parallel imaging methods and improved shimming methods. Since static susceptibility artifacts can –at least partly- be refocused using SE techniques, it is less affected by susceptibility artifacts than GE methods and may increase the sensitivity in affected areas (Goense et al., 2008) such as auditory regions in the temporal lobe.

In conclusion, although there is a trade-off between sensitivity and specificity, and the fact that there are still some technical considerations that need to be assessed, most recent imaging literature agree on the advantages of ultra-high field fMRI (i.e. ≥ 7 Tesla), that is, the increased signal-to-noise ratio. This evolution is of special importance for the clinical field in general and the field of auditory research specifically. The next section discusses the application of fMRI to study the functional organization of the auditory cortex.

3.3. Tonotopic organization in the human auditory cortex revealed using fMRI

Many studies have elucidated the functional specialization and hierarchical organization of multiple areas of the auditory cortex in non-human primates using invasive neurophysiological recordings which are obviously not applicable to human studies. A method to map frequency mapping using noninvasive BOLD fMRI in primates is in its early infancy (Petkov, personal communication). At present, there are many applications of BOLD fMRI in experiments on the human auditory system, ranging from the characterization of the effects of sound intensity (Bilecen et al., 2002; Hart et al., 2003), the effects of the side of presentation (Jäncke et al., 2002) to more complex phenomena such as the interaction of scanner noise and sound-evoked responses (Gaab et al., 2007; Hall et al. 1999; Talavage & Edmister 2004) and feature sensitivity and attention modulation (Paltoglou et al., 2011). Mapping one of the most fundamental properties of the auditory system, that of frequency coding, remains elusive and only a few studies have demonstrated a clear topographical arrangement of the response to sound frequency in the auditory pathway. This organization, referred to as 'tonotopy', mirrors the distribution of receptors in the cochlea, with neurons at the base of the cochlea preferentially responding to high frequencies and neurons at the apex responding best to low frequencies (Ehret, 1978). Tonotopy is conveyed up to the level of auditory cortex by fibres in the lemniscal pathway (Figure 3). In the auditory cortex of nonhuman primates, the primary core cortex, consisting of A1, R and RT, exhibit tonotopic gradients that are mirror symmetric to each other (Hackett et al., 2001; Kaas & Hackett 2000; Morel et al., 1993).

Tonotopic organization has been identified in human auditory cortex using a variety of imaging techniques including positron emission tomography (PET) and fMRI. The majority of early studies were based on just two different stimulus frequencies (Bilecen et al., 1998; Lauter et al., 1985; Lockwood et al. 1999; Talavage et al., 2000; Wessinger et al., 1997). From the results a general pattern emerges where high frequencies are represented at the medial end of auditory cortex and low frequencies in the anterior and lateral part of Heschl's gyrus and surrounding areas, mostly as a single low-to-high frequency gradient. More recent studies used more frequencies allowing the identification of more fine-grained frequency gradients. However, the results and interpretations of these studies vary considerably. For example, Langers et al. (2007) reported a single high-to-low gradient extending from posterior medial to anterior lateral auditory areas, similar to earlier studies. Mapping of the left hemisphere at 7 Tesla using surface coils and sparse image acquisition revealed two mirror-symmetric tonotopic maps encompassing three linear gradients of frequency-sensitive BOLD responses in six subjects: (i) one connecting a high-frequency region in Heschl's sulcus with a low-frequency region halfway Heschl's gyrus and (ii) a second connected the same low-frequency region with a high-frequency region near the lateral junction of Heschl's gyrus and the superior temporal gyrus (Formisano et al., 2003). These results suggest that human auditory cortex conforms to the primate model with two mirror-symmetric tonotopic maps in primary auditory core and belt areas that are joined at a common low-frequency boundary (Petkov et al., 2006). Talavage and colleagues reported three consistent gradients, none of which clearly followed the long (medial-to-lateral) axis of Heschl's gyrus (Talavage et al., 2004). Schönwiesner et al. (2002) argued that the observed frequency selectivity does not necessarily represent frequency gradients but instead represent different functional regions within the auditory cortex (Schönwiesner et al., 2002). Based on this assumption, in combination with the models by Kaas et al. (2000), three recent studies investigated tonotopic mapping and related their findings to anatomical models.

Humphries reported two major mirror-symmetric frequency gradients, oriented roughly perpendicular to Heschl's gyrus, rather than parallel as previously assumed (Humphries et al., 2010). They found a single low-frequency area centered on Heschl's gyrus, bordered anteriorly and posteriorly by two high-frequency areas (planum temporale). This seems very similar to previous findings (Woods et al., 2009). Based on the observed mirror-symmetric frequency gradients, both sets of authors proposed boundaries of regions in human auditory cortex homologous to A1 and R regions in non-human primate cortex. Figure 2 shows the schematic outline of auditory fields as based on electrophysiology in primates and the original group data of both Woods et al. (2009) and Humphries et al. (2010) indicating similar tonotopic maps and a close correspondence between these maps and proposed boundaries as compared to primate data.

A different approach was taken by Striem-Amit et al. (2011), who used phase-encoding (travelling wave) fMRI, a technique previously used to map the visual field onto the visual cortex (Engel et al., 1997; Warnking, 2002). They found up to six mirror-symmetric frequency gradients covering most of Heschl's gyrus and extending to the superior temporal gyrus and superior temporal sulcus (Striem-Amit et al., 2011), beyond the areas previously reported by Woods et al. (2009) and Humphries et al. (2010). Such cochleotopic organization was identified in both left and right hemispheres. The maps of Striem-Amit et al. (2011) demonstrate that tonotopy persists well beyond the auditory core and belt.

The discovery of the tonotopic maps and proposed boundaries between auditory cortical fields might help our understanding of these fields and contributes in defining possible connectivity patterns between these fields. These advances ultimately help us understand the functional consequences of e.g., hearing loss and tinnitus which may affect the function or organization of the auditory cortex (Eggermont, 2006; Komiya & Eggermont, 2000). Both conditions are good examples of auditory disorders with an increasing prevalence due to an aging population.

4. Functional magnetic resonance imaging of tinnitus

4.1. A phantom sound?

Tinnitus is an auditory sensation without the presence of an external acoustic stimulus. In 6-20% of the adult population, tinnitus is a chronic condition and severely disrupts quality of life in 1-3%. Tinnitus is more prevalent in men than in women and its prevalence increases with advancing age (Axelsson & Ringdahl, 1989). Subjective tinnitus is the most common form of the disorder, but its neural origins remain rather elusive. Like any external acoustic percept, tinnitus is associated with neural activity in the central auditory system. Tinnitus-related activity may arise from abnormal cellular mechanisms in neurons of the central auditory system, or may result from aberrant input from the cochlea or non-auditory structures. Subjective tinnitus is often associated with peripheral hearing loss (Eggermont & Roberts, 2004; Nicolas-Puel et al., 2006) and many patients describe tinnitus as a sound in one or both ears. Therefore, it has been thought for many years that the tinnitus-related neural activity must also originate from the cochlea. Clinical observations however indicate the importance of central mechanisms. In patients that underwent sectioning of the eighth cranial nerve as part of retro-cochlear tumor surgery, tinnitus actually arose in 34% of the cases (Berliner et al., 1992). Surgically severing the connections between the cochlea and the brain has also been applied to provide relief of the tinnitus. This procedure was however not successful in 38-85% of cases (Kaltenbach et al., 2005).

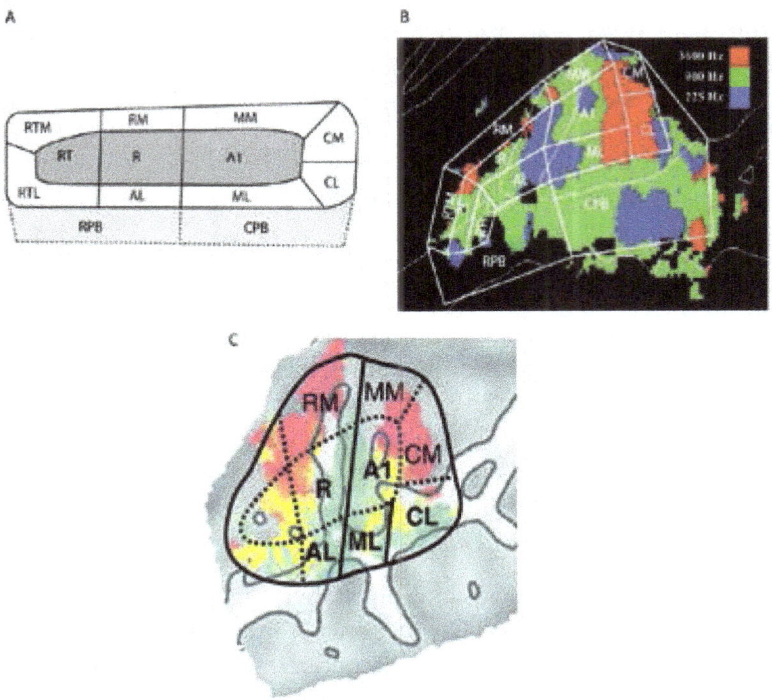

Figure 2. A. Overview of auditory fields in the primate brain showing core areas (A1, R, RT), belt areas (CL, CM, ML, MM, RM, AL, RTL, RTM) and proposed parabelt areas (RPB, CPB); adapted from Kaas et al. (2000). B. The same representation of auditory cortical fields superimposed on tonotopic data in human auditory cortex; adapted from Woods et al., (2009). C. Auditory cortical fields superimposed on tonotopic data; adapted from Humphries et al. (2010). Abbreviations for auditory fields: A1 = primary auditory cortex; R = rostral, T = temporal, M= middle; A = anterior; L = lateral, C=caudal, PB = parabelt.

4.2. Animal studies of tinnitus

Evidence for changes in the firing patterns of neurons in the central auditory system (Figure 3) as a possible substrate of tinnitus is mainly based on animal models. Noise trauma and ototoxic drugs, which are known to cause peripheral hearing loss and tinnitus in humans, result in behavioral responses in animals that seem consistent with the presence of tinnitus. One of these substrates is a change in the spontaneous firing rates of auditory neurons (Eggermont & Roberts, 2004). Since an increased (stimulus-driven) firing rate in auditory neurons typically corresponds to the presence of sound source, an increased spontaneous firing rate could also lead to an auditory percept, i.e., tinnitus. Alternatively, the temporal pattern of spontaneous neural activity could change by increased synchrony of activity across auditory neurons (Noreña & Eggermont 2003; Seki & Eggermont, 2003). The third candidate is a reorganization of the tonotopic map in auditory neurons in the central auditory system (Eggermont 2006; Mühlnickel et al., 1998; Seki & Eggermont, 2003). Although such changes themselves may not directly correspond to tinnitus, they may contribute to abnormal neural activity. For example, cortical reorganization may lead to the over-representation of frequencies corresponding to the frequency at the edge of a high-frequency sloping hearing loss (Eggermont, 2006; Rajan & Irvine, 1998). In other words, auditory-nerve or lower-brainstem neurons that are tuned to an edge frequency could be excessively projected to a region of the auditory cortex. fMRI can be used to identify mechanisms that underlie the generation of tinnitus in humans. Section 4.3 describes the application of fMRI and discusses the outcomes of selected studies.

4.3. Functional magnetic resonance imaging of tinnitus in humans

Although there is much evidence for neural changes based on animal models, there is little corresponding evidence for tinnitus in humans. fMRI is expected to be sensitive to changes in the overall neuronal activity and may reveal changes in neural activity patterns. Yet, given the temporal resolution of typical fMRI studies, changes in synchronous neural activity or spontaneous firing rates may not be apparent from fMRI data. The BOLD signal is a relative measure of tissue properties and so 'activity' cannot be measured directly nor quantified. Instead, fMRI paradigms rely on modulating the hemodynamic response, reflected by neural activity in two (or more) conditions, which allows them to detect differences between states (Ogawa et al., 1990).

Given that tinnitus tends to be a continuous phantom percept, several paradigms have been applied to modulate it in some way. One approach examines sound-evoked responses in tinnitus and control participants, while the second method relies on the ability of a subgroup of people with tinnitus to manipulate their experience by somatic modulation. Examples of include forceful head and neck contractions (Levine, 1999), oral facial movements like jaw clenching or jaw protrusion (Pinchoff et al., 1998), electrical stimulation of the median nerve (Møller et al., 1992) and cutaneous stimulation (Cacace et al., 1999a; 1999b). Other paradigms that could be considered are i) the rapid change of gaze or tonic lateral gaze causing or modulating tinnitus, ii) pharmaceutical interventions that causes a temporal change of the tinnitus (e.g., lidocaine), and, iii) residual inhibition, which refers to the reduc-

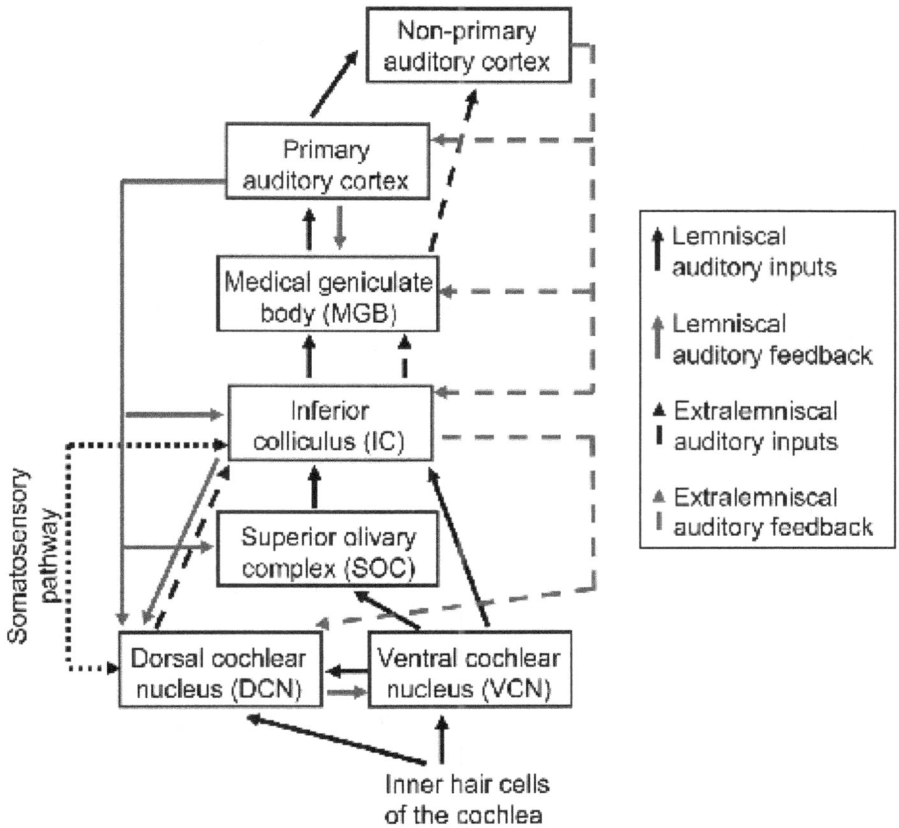

Figure 3. Schematic outline of the auditory system redrawn from Eggermont & Roberts (2004). Inner hairs cells of the cochlea decompose multi-frequency signals into an output that is spatially organised according to frequency (tonotopy). Auditory nerve fibers send inputs to dorsal and ventral cochlear nuclei which both show tonotopic maps. The lemniscal pathway (solid black line) propagates this frequency-specific information throughout all structures. The central auditory system is characterized by strong reciprocal connections (grey lines). The interconnected feedback loops allow the cortex to modulate activity. Changes in dorsal cochlear nucleus, in turn, will directly affect the processing of lemniscal activity at the level of the ventral cochlear nucleus and inferior colliculus. This enables a strong synergy between changes occurring in cortex and brainstem.

tion of the loudness of tinnitus following the offset of an external acoustical stimulus (Roberts, 2007). A review of these paradigms is given by Lanting et al. (2009). Here, we highlight the contribution of fMRI to the current understanding of central mechanisms of tinnitus and explain how interpretations of neuroimaging data may help developing a better understanding of its diverse pathophysiology and of the functional interplay between sensory, cognitive and affective systems.

4.4. Effects of tinnitus on patterns of sound-evoked activity

Compared to non-tinnitus controls, people with unilateral tinnitus initially appeared to show an abnormally small signal change in the inferior colliculus contralateral to the tinnitus percept, but not ipsilateral (Melcher et al., 2000). These findings were interpreted as evidence that tinnitus corresponds with abnormally elevated baseline neural activity on the contralateral side. When an external stimulus is presented, the hemodynamic response reaches saturation, resulting in a reduced difference between the 'sound' and 'silence' conditions. A potential confound to these observed patterns of sound-related activity was the influence of ambient background noise. Hence, in a new experiment, this variable was examined by repeating the study with the noisy helium pump either switched on or off (Melcher et al., 2009). All participants had normal hearing. With the pump off, the tinnitus group showed greater stimulus-evoked activation of the inferior colliculus than the non-tinnitus group. With the pump on, the tinnitus group showed reduced activation compared to controls. This result indicates some degree of auditory response saturation in the brains of people with tinnitus. A possible explanation is that a compensatory mechanism of central auditory gain has increased the response amplitudes close to their maximum limit. Lanting et al. (2008) used a sparse temporal sampling paradigm, minimizing the interaction between the scanner noise, the noise of the pump and auditory brain activity. Stimuli consisted of monaural dynamic rippled broadband noise stimuli at two intensity levels (40 dB and 70 dB SPL). Responses were measured at the level of auditory cortex and inferior colliculus of subjects with unilateral tinnitus and near-normal hearing. These were compared with those of people without tinnitus. This study demonstrated abnormally elevated responses in the inferior colliculus in people with tinnitus subjects compared to controls. Figure 4 shows increased sound-evoked responses, a reduced response lateralization (i.e., stimuli presented to the contralateral and ipsilateral ear gave roughly the same signal change) and a disturbed intensity level dependency in subjects with tinnitus compared to subjects without tinnitus at the level of the inferior colliculus (Lanting et al., 2008).

In summary, the first study by Melcher (Melcher et al., 2000) found *decreased* responses in inferior colliculus on the opposite side to the unilateral tinnitus percept, while the other two studies found overall *increased* responses (Lanting et al., 2008; Melcher et al., 2009). At first sight, these three results appear to be contradictory, but a key methodological difference may account for the discrepancy. While Lanting applied sparse temporal sampling, Melcher scanned continuously. Therefore, Melcher's experiments were performed in high levels of ambient scanner noise which may have caused inferior colliculus to respond excessively to this source of background noise and hence reduce the BOLD response to the experimental sound stimuli. The three papers are thus consistent with the interpretation that the inferior colliculus of people with tinnitus displays a disproportionate response to sound, whether it is ambient sound or experimentally controlled sound.

Although sound-evoked responses appear elevated in people with tinnitus, hyperacusis could be an important alternative explanation. This condition is defined as an abnormal sensitivity to sound and is manifest as a diminished level of sound tolerance possibly elevating sound-evoked responses in the auditory brain. Hyperacusis is often co-morbid with tinnitus (Baguley, 2003). A recent study assessed the neural correlates of hyperacusis, recruiting 13 people with tinnitus and 14 people with no tinnitus (Gu et al., 2010). Hyperacusis was assessed using minimum loudness discomfort levels and a validated questionnaire. Severity of sound level tolerance (i.e. hyperacusis) was correlated with

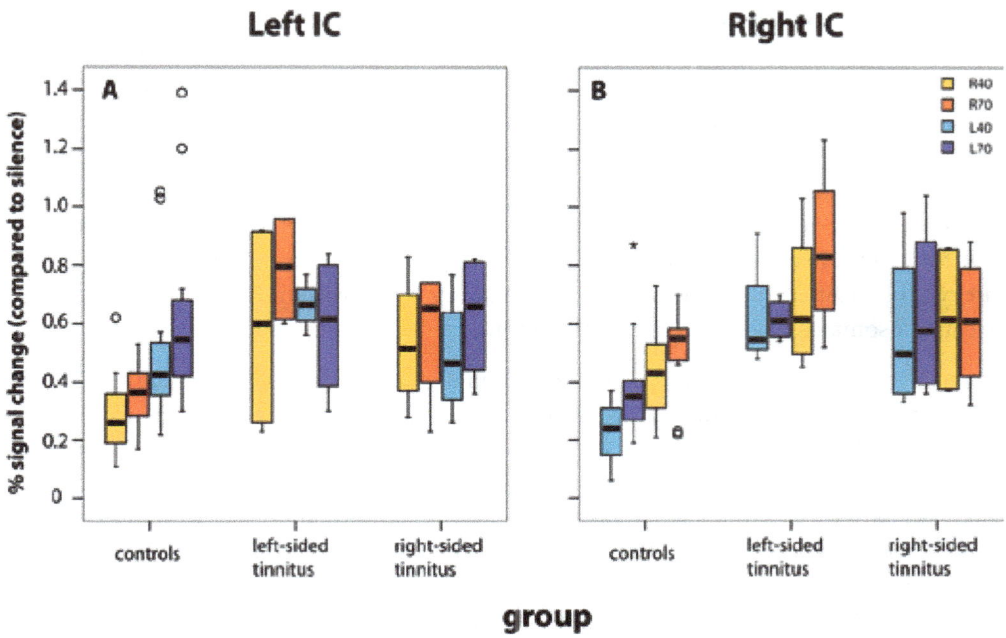

Figure 4. Sound-evoked responses measured in left (**A**) and right (**B**) inferior colliculus (IC). The pattern of evoked responses for the side of presentation (left or right ear) and the sound intensity (40 dB and 70 dB SPL) is different for subjects with unilateral tinnitus as compared to controls. Adapted from Lanting et al. (2008)

elevated activity in the auditory midbrain, thalamus, and primary auditory cortex, despite a fixed sound stimulation level. Sound-evoked activity in the inferior colliculus and medial geniculate body was more associated with hyperacusis than tinnitus, while in primary auditory cortex it was more associated with tinnitus than hyperacusis. Previous findings of increased sound-evoked responses in the inferior colliculus of people with tinnitus (Lanting et al., 2008; Melcher et al., 2009) are most likely to be due to the hypersensitivity to an external sound stimulus than tinnitus per se.

In conclusion, although fMRI has shown general increases in sound-evoked activity in tinnitus, it is more likely to be associated with hyperacusis. Any hypothesized reorganization of tonotopic maps in the auditory cortex has not yet been demonstrated, mostly due to the fact that tonotopic mapping is a relative new field. With the increasing availability of ultra high-field fMRI, this is a promising area for further research.

5. Cross-modal integration in tinnitus

In addition to auditory nerve input, dorsal cochlear nucleus is also innervated by fibers from various parts of the somatosensory system, so this structure is a multi-modal processing station that is considered part of the extralemniscal auditory pathway (Figure 3). Parts of inferior colliculus, medial geniculate body and non-primary auditory cortex are all characterized by sensitivity to somatosensory stimuli (Eggermont & Roberts, 2004). As mentioned in Section 4.3, somatosensory manoeuvers can elicit or modulate tinnitus. Somatic modulation of tinnitus may therefore be considered a special case of multisensory integration—a phenomenon, in which one (sensory) modality influences another. The observation that some people with tinnitus can modulate the loudness or pitch of their tinnitus might be explained by changes in normal multisensory integration. Noise-induced hearing-loss, for example, has been reported to alter the normal somatosensory input (Shore et al., 2008). Somatosensory input to the cochlear nucleus increased after hearing loss, changing the balance of somatosensory and auditory input at the level of the brainstem, which in turn might be the neural correlate of somatosensory modulation of tinnitus.

To investigate this proposed model of cross-modal integration, Lanting et al. (2010) studied two groups: people with tinnitus and matched controls. Tinnitus participants were selected according to their ability to change the psychoacoustical characteristics of their tinnitus by jaw protrusion. Unimodal fMRI responses to sound stimuli and jaw protrusion alone were measured, as well as the response obtained in multimodal condition. To minimize motion artifacts, a sparse sampling method (inter-scan interval = 10 s) was used in which the protrusion started 4 s after the beginning of the acquisition and ended 1.5 s before the next acquisition. Since the jaw was always fully relaxed during scan acquisitions, the task did not degrade data quality. Results showed responses to jaw protrusion throughout the central auditory pathway, in both groups. Auditory responses to jaw protrusion presumably account for the modulation of tinnitus by these manoeuvers. Interestingly, responses in cochlear nucleus and inferior colliculus were greater in people with tinnitus than in controls, suggesting an abnormal auditory-somatic interaction in the patient group. This increased sensitivity to somatosensory inputs may correspond to neuroplastic changes, triggered by pathological change of either the somatosensory or auditory input pathways to dorsal cochlear nucleus (see Figure 3 and also Shore, 2011) that, in turn, lead to compensatory shifts in the balance of excitation and inhibition often attributed to tinnitus.

6. Functional and structural assessments of candidature for cochlear implantation

Hearing loss is the most common sensory deficit. Approximately 1.5% of children and 60% of over-70s have hearing loss and, as the average age of the population increases, the social, economic and psychological impact of hearing loss is likely to become more of a burden. Hearing after mild to moderate deafness can be regained through acoustic amplification with a hearing aid, whilst more severe to profound hearing loss can be partially restored by replacing the non-functioning inner ear with a CI.

A CI is a surgically-implanted auditory prosthesis that provides a sense of hearing to deaf individuals. As part of a preoperative clinical evaluation, computerized-tomography (CT) and MRI are both routinely used to assess CI candidates and to aid pre-operative planning and patient counselling. CT provides excellent structural information about bony detail and is useful for assessing congenital malformations that would affect the course of the facial nerve. MRI on the other hand can visualize soft-tissue with high resolution and is used to evaluate the integrity of the auditory nerve and the patency of the cochlea. Traditional CI candidates were adults with such profound hearing loss they could not benefit from any acoustic hearing. Over the past 25 years CI candidature has been relaxed, to include children and infants in whom auditory deprivation has the most severe developmental consequences. More recently, CIs have been used to treat individuals with some residual acoustic hearing in one or both ears. To date, nearly 200,000 individuals worldwide have been implanted with a CI, approximately half of those being children.

6.1. Prognostic indicators of cochlear implant performance

Although many CI users are able to develop age-appropriate communication and language skills without the need for visual cues, outcomes vary considerably between individuals. A number of factors have been found to correlate with speech outcomes following cochlear implantation (Blamey et al., 1996; Miyamoto et al., 1994). Pre-linguistically deaf adults generally perform more poorly than post-linguistically deaf adults (Busby et al., 1993a; 1993b; Eddington et al., 1978), whilst a long duration of deafness prior to implantation is generally detrimental to performance (O'Donoghue et al., 2000; Sarant et al., 2001). Also, it has been shown that auditory experience can improve clinical performance of cochlear implant users (Blamey et al., 1996; Gantz et al., 1993; Rubinstein et al., 1999). However, individuals with remarkably similar hearing experiences can often have markedly different speech comprehension skills. For example, older pre-linguistically deaf children can occasionally succeed very well in understanding speech, whilst the majority do not (Schramm et al., 2002). Therefore, whilst a number of factors that influence the clinical performance of cochlear implants have been identified, the field currently lacks accurate predictors of cochlear implant performance that can be applied to an individual. Such a prognostic tool, could help direct limited health-care resources towards effective clinical care.

Current national guidelines within the UK suggest that unilateral cochlear implantation is recommended for people with severe to profound hearing loss who do not receive adequate benefit from an acoustic hearing aid. Within this group, simultaneous bilateral cochlear implantation is recommended for i) pre-linguistically deaf children, ii) individuals who are blind, and iii) those who are at risk of cochlear ossification. Therefore, sensitive prognostic tools could be used to mould this crude patient pathway to meet the needs of individual patients, whilst providing realistic indicators of potential outcomes and requirements for rehabilitation.

Behavioural assessments of hearing with a CI are difficult to assess in very young children, as well as individuals with significant physical and/or developmental delay. Therefore, some investigators have focused on developing objective, non-invasive measures of CI function. Electrically-evoked compound action potentials (ECAPs) and electrically-evoked auditory brainstem responses (EABRs) are both routinely used to measure CI function at the level of the auditory nerve and brainstem, respectively. Whilst ECAPs and EABRs are useful clinical tools to ensure that the stimulus levels provided by the CI processor are within the range of perception, there is little evidence to suggest that they correlate well with speech and language outcomes (Miller et al., 2008).

Ultimately, CI users are likely to develop good speech and language skills provided accurate auditory information reaches the auditory cortex. For this reason, attempts have been made to assess functional activation of the auditory cortex with a CI. A number of methods can be used to assess cortical responsiveness to auditory stimulation. However, most of these methods have significant limitations when they are applied to a paediatric CI population.

Earlier in this chapter we discussed the advantages of fMRI in auditory research: a technique that permits the mapping of auditory responses with fine topographic detail, as well multiple observations over time, within both adult and paediatric populations. However, the surgically-implanted magnetic component of a CI device is incompatible with the high magnetic field generated by most MRI scanners. Traditionally, prior to considering MRI, it was necessary to surgically-remove the magnet after cochlear implantation. Recently it has been shown that CI patients can undergo MRI using a low (1.5) Tesla scanner, provided the implanted device is tightly bound before scanning (Crane et al., 2010). Patients in this study received an implant on one side. Although Crane and colleagues observed no magnet displacement whilst visualizing the contralateral- and part of the ipsilateral-internal auditory canal, the artefact surrounding the implanted device (~7x5 cm) precluded functional imaging of the cortex on that side. Similarly, magnetoencephalography (MEG) is limited by the magnetic field associated with current CI devices.

Electroencephalography (EEG) is also used to investigate auditory-evoked cortical potentials. However, the electrical artefact generated by the CI confounds these recordings. Although algorithms have been developed to minimize the effect of CI-generated electrical signals in EEG recordings (Debener et al., 2008), stimulus parameters are generally limited to short-duration sounds such as clicks (Gilley et al., 2006). Responses to longer sounds, including speech and language stimuli, are difficult to extract from the electrical artefact. Functional activation of the auditory cortex can also be assessed using PET that involves the use of ionizing radiation. Due to the cumulative effects of radiation exposure, this technique is not ideal for longitudinal studies, particularly in children.

Sevy et al. (2010) recently demonstrated a relatively novel imaging technique called 'near-infrared spectroscopy' (NIRS) could be used to assess cortical responses to auditory stimulation in children with cochlear implants. NIRS measures relative changes in the tissue contraction, oxy-haemoglobin, deoxy-haemoglobin and total haemoglobin in the cerebral cortex through beaming infra-red light. One of the greatest advantages of this approach is that the optical signals from the auditory cortex are not influenced by the magnetic fields that plague fMRI and MEG recordings. Unlike EEG, NIRS is not affected by CI-generated electrical artifacts. Subjects experience no discomfort with NIRS, as it is a non-invasive test that only requires contacting small optical fibre tips onto the scalp. There are no known risks associated with NIRS. Therefore, unlike PET, it is suitable for multiple measurements in paediatric populations. Although, NIRS provides sufficient resolution to measure evoked responses that are confined to auditory regions of the brain, this spatial resolution (within 1-2 cm of the activated area) is less than that of fMRI. Regardless, compared with alternative techniques, NIRS seems highly suited to assess the responsiveness of the auditory cortex before and after cochlear implantation in paediatric populations.

7. Cross-modal reorganization in the deaf brain

Animal neurophysiology has demonstrated that when sensory neurons lose their input (e.g. vision, touch or hearing) they do not become 'silent'. Instead, they change their responsiveness. In the case of (noise-induced) sensorineural high-frequency hearing loss, neurons previously responding to high frequencies respond to low frequencies (Rajan et al., 1993; Robertson & Irvin, 1989). In the case of complete deafness, neurons become rewired to previously unconnected neurons from another sensory modality (Lomber et al., 2010; Rauschecker et al., 1995).

Cross-modal reorganization refers to the takeover of the processing of sensory information using new cortical pathways. It may be of clinical relevance for hearing-impaired individuals and individuals with a cochlear implant: some people with congenital hearing loss show 'supra-normal' visual abilities (Bavelier et al., 2006; Neville & Lawson, 1987). Furthermore, congenital deafness is known to induce rewiring of inputs within the auditory cortex (Allman et al., 2009; Auer et al., 2007; Finney et al., 2001; 2003; Levänen et al., 1998; Lomber et al., 2010; Nishimura et al., 1999) that plays a vital role in allowing us to process speech and naturally occurring sounds. Recently, Lomber et al. (2010) used cortical cooling techniques in deaf cats to suggest that enhanced visual performance is caused by cross-modal reorganization of the posterior auditory cortex.

Currently, it is not clear whether this rewiring is beneficial to hearing with a cochlear implant (potentially acting as an instructive map to 'train' the reinstated hearing pathways) or detrimental to hearing (by taking away resources from the auditory brain). Regardless, it remains possible that cross-modal reorganization following deafness may prove to be a clinically-useful predictor of performance following cochlear implantation. Lee et al. (2001) used F-18 fluorodeoxyglucose PET to examine resting-state brain activity in pre-lingually deaf individuals. Results indicated an association between hypometabolism in the auditory cortex and the amount of improvement in hearing after cochlear implantation. They speculated that the hypometabolism may be related to cross-modal plasticity and that the individual status of auditory rewiring might be used as an effective predictor of an individual's speech performance following cochlear implantation. More recently, Rouger et al. (2011) demonstrated cross-modal responses in post-lingually deaf adults with cochlear implants engaged in a visual speech reading task using PET brain imaging. Furthermore, they suggested that cross-modal reorganization diminishes in post-lingually deaf adults with CIs with increasing time after implantation (up to at least one year later), towards the levels seen in normal-hearing individuals (Rouger et al., 2011). Doucet et al. (2006) compared cortical evoked potentials between adults with good and poor speech outcomes following cochlear implantation. They found that poor performers exhibited broader, anteriorly-distributed evoked potentials whereas the good performers showed significantly higher amplitudes of the P2 component over the primary visual cortex. Furthermore, Buckley et al. (2006) suggested that cortical responsiveness to visual and auditory evoked potentials accounts for a significant amount of the variability observed in speech perception performance in adults with cochlear implants with pre-lingual, but not post-lingual, hearing loss. Although, approximately half of cochlear implant recipients are children worldwide, currently, little is known about cross-modal brain reorganization during development.

8. Conclusion and future directions

While the results from a number of functional imaging studies in humans provide preliminary insights into plasticity within the central auditory pathway, more information is needed to understand the patterns of neural reorganization and the mechanisms underpinning those changes. This is an exciting time as novel imaging techniques, such as ultra-high field fMRI and NIRS, open new possibilities for investigating the effects of hearing loss, cochlear implantation and tinnitus on the developing and the mature brain. From our review, three key questions capture avenues of future research that are likely to impact on clinical practice: i) What are the separate effects of deafness, hyperacusis, tinnitus and cochlear implantation on central auditory plasticity, including cross-modal reorganization? ii) What are the perceptual consequences of that reorganization, and iii) How does brain reorganization affect and/or predict treatment outcome?

An ultimate goal for functional imaging is to provide the information necessary for evidence-based healthcare, such as targeting tinnitus treatments to specific neural sites of its generation and predicting outcomes following cochlear implantation. Currently, imaging of the central auditory pathway is not used for routine clinical purposes in Ear, Nose and Throat or Audiology clinics. It is our hope that research using imaging techniques may provide valuable insights into mechanisms underlying tinnitus and the variable speech outcomes following cochlear implantation in humans that may tailor our treatment towards the requirements of the individual.

Author details

Deborah A. Hall[1], Cornelis P. Lanting[2] and Douglas E.H. Hartley[3]

1 NIHR National Biomedical Research Unit in Hearing, Nottingham, UK

2 MRC Institute of Hearing Research, Nottingham, UK

3 Department of Otorhinolaryngology, Nottingham University, UK

References

[1] Allman, B.L., Keniston, L.P., & Meredith, M.A. (2009). Adult deafness induces somatosensory conversion of ferret auditory cortex. *Proceedings of the National Academy of Sciences in the United States of America*, 106, 14, pp. 5925-5930.

[2] Auer, E.T., Bernstein, L.E., Sungkarat, W., & Singh, M. (2007). Vibrotactile activation of the auditory cortices in deaf versus hearing adults. *Neuroreport*, 18, 7, pp. 645-648.

[3] Axelsson, A., & Ringdahl, A. (1989). Tinnitus--a study of its prevalence and characteristics. *British Journal of Audiology*, 23, 1, pp. 53-62.

[4] Baguley. D.M. (2003). Hyperacusis. *J R Soc Med*, 96, pp. 582-585.

[5] Baumann, S., Griffiths, T.D., Sun, L., Petkov, C.I., Thiele, A., & Rees, A. (2011). Orthogonal representation of sound dimensions in the primate midbrain. *Nature Neuroscience*, 14, 4, pp. 31-33.

[6] Bavelier, D., Dye, M.W.G., & Hauser, P.C. (2006). Do deaf individuals see better? *Trends in Cognitive Sciences*, 10, 11, pp. 512-518

[7] Berliner, K.I., Shelton, C., Hitselberger, W.E., & Luxford, W.M. (1992). Acoustic tumours: effect of surgical removal on tinnitus. *The American Journal of Otology*, 13, 1, pp. 13- 17.

[8] Bilecen, D., Scheffler, K., Schmid, N., Tschopp, K., & Seelig, J. (1998). Tonotopic organization of the human auditory cortex as detected by BOLD-FMRI. *Hearing Research*, 126, 1- 2, pp. 19-27.

[9] Bilecen, D., Seifritz, E., Scheffler, K., Henning, J., & Schulte, A.C. (2002). Amplitopicity of the human auditory cortex: an fMRI study. *NeuroImage*, 17, 2, pp. 710-718.

[10] Blackman, G., & Hall, D.A. (2011). Reducing the effects of background noise during auditory functional magnetic resonance imaging of speech processing: Qualitative and quantitative comparisons between two image acquisition schemes and noise cancellation. *Journal of Speech, Language and Hearing Research*. 54, pp. 693–704.

[11] Blamey, P., Arndt, P., Bergeron, F., Bredberg, G., Brimacombe, J., Facer, G., Larky, J., Lindstrom, B., Nedzelski, J., Paterson, A., Shipp, D., Staller, S., & Whitford, L., (1996). Factors affecting auditory performance of postlinguistically deaf adults using cochlear implants. *Audiology & Neuro-otology*, 1, 5, pp. 293-306.

[12] Buckley, K.A., & Tobey, E.A. (2011). Cross-modal plasticity and perception in pre- and postlingually deaf cochlear implant users. *Ear and Hearing*, 32, 1, pp. 2-15.

[13] Busby, P.A., Tong Y.C., & Clark G.M. (1993a). Electrode position, repetition rate, and speech-perception by early-deafened and late-deafened cochlear implant patients. *The Journal of the Acoustical Society of America*, 93, 2, pp. 1058-1067.

[14] Busby, P.A., Tong Y.C., & Clark G.M. (1993b). The perception of temporal modulations by cochlear implant patients. *The Journal of the Acoustical Society of America*, 94, 1, pp. 124-131.

[15] Cacace, A.T., Cousins, J.P., Parnes, S.M., Semenoff, D., Holmes, T., McFarland D.J., Davenport, C., Stegbauer, K., & Lovely, T.J. (1999a). Cutaneous-evoked tinnitus. I. Phenomenology, psychophysics and functional imaging. *Audiology & Neuro-otology*, 4, 5, pp. 247-257.

[16] Cacace, A.T., Cousins, J.P., Parnes, S.M., McFarland, D.J., Semenoff, D., Holmes, T., Davenport, C., Stegbauer, K., & Lovely, T.J. (1999b). Cutaneous-evoked tinnitus. II. Review of neuroanatomical, physiological and functional imaging studies. *Audiology & Neuro-otology*, 4, 5, pp. 258-268.

[17] Crane, B. T., Gottschalk, B., Kraut, M., Aygun, N., & Niparko, J. K. (2010). Magnetic resonance imaging at 1.5 T after cochlear implantation. *Otology Neurotology, 31*, 8, 1215-1220.

[18] Debener, S., Hine, J., Bleeck, S., & Eyles, J. (2008). Source localization of auditory evoked potentials after cochlear implantation. *Psychophysiology, 45*, 1, 20-24.

[19] Detre, J.A., & Wang, J. (2002). Technical aspects and utility of fMRI using BOLD and ASL. *Clinical Neurophysiology*, 113, 5, pp. 621-634.

[20] Doucet, M.E., Bergeron, F., Lassonde, M., Ferron, P., & Lepore, F. (2006). Cross-modal reorganization and speech perception in cochlear implant users. *Brain*, 129, pp. 3376-3383.

[21] Duong, T.Q., Yacoub, E., Adriany, G., Hu, X.P., Ugurbil, K., & Kim, S.G. (2003). Microvascular BOLD contribution at 4 and 7 T in the human brain: Gradient-echo and spin-echo fMRI with suppression of blood effects. *Magnetic Resonance in Medicine*, 49, 6, pp. 1019-1027.

[22] Eddington, D.K., Dobelle, W.H., Brackmann, D.E., Mladejovsky, M.G., & Parkin, J.L., (1978). Auditory prostheses research with multiple channel intracochlear stimulation in man. *The Annals of Otology, Rhinology, and Laryngology*, 87, 6.2, pp. 1-39.

[23] Edmister, W.B., Talavage, T.M., Ledden, P.J., & Weisskoff R.M. (1999). Improved auditory cortex imaging using clustered volume acquisitions. *Human Brain Mapping*, 7, pp. 89-97.

[24] Eggermont, J.J. (2006). Cortical tonotopic map reorganisation and its implications for treatment of tinnitus. *Acta Oto-laryngologica. Supplementum*, 556, pp. 9-12.

[25] Eggermont, J.J., & Roberts, L.E. (2004). The neuroscience of tinnitus. *Trends in Neurosciences*, 27, 11, pp. 676-682.

[26] Ehret, G., (1978). Stiffness gradient along the basilar membrane as a basis for spatial frequency analysis within the cochlea. *The Journal of the Acoustical Society of America,* 64, 6, pp. 1723-1726.

[27] Engel, S., Glover, G.H., & Wandell, B. (1997). Retinotopic organization in human visual cortex and the spatial precision of functional MRI. *Cerebral Cortex,* 7, 2, pp. 181-192.

[28] Finney, E.M., Fine, I., & Dobkins, K.R. (2001). Visual stimuli activate cortex in the deaf. *Nature Neuroscience,* 4, 12, pp. 1171-1173.

[29] Finney, E.M., Clementz, B.A., Hickok, G., & Dobkins, K.R. (2003). Visual Stimuli activate auditory cortex in deaf subjects: evidence from MEG. *Neuroreport,* 14, 11, pp. 1425- 1427.

[30] Formisano, E., Kim, D.S., Di Salle, F., Van de Moortele, P, F., Ugurbil, K., & Goebel, R. (2003). Mirror-symmetric tonotopic maps in human primary auditory cortex. *Neuron,* 40, 4, pp. 859-869.

[31] Foster, J.R., Hall, D.A., Summerfield, A.Q., Palmer, A.R., & Bowtell, R.W. (2000). Sound-level measurements and calculations of safe noise dosage during fMRI at 3T. *Journal of Magnetic Resonance Imaging,* 12, pp. 157-163.

[32] Gaab, N., Gabrieli, J.D.E., & Glover, G.H. (2007). Assessing the influence of scanner background noise on auditory processing. I. An fMRI study comparing three experimental designs with varying degrees of scanner noise. *Human Brain Mapping,* 28, 8, pp. 703-720.

[33] Gantz, B.J., Woodworth, G.G., Knutson, J.F., Abbas, P.J., & Tyler, R.S. (1993) Multivariate predictors of success with cochlear implants. *Advances in Oto-Rhino-Laryngology,* 48, pp. 153-167.

[34] Gilley, P. M., Sharma, A., Dorman, M., Finley, C. C., Panch, A. S., & Martin, K. (2006). Minimization of cochlear implant stimulus artifact in cortical auditory evoked potentials. *Clinical Neurophysiology, 117,* 8, 1772-1782.

[35] Giraud A.L., Truy, E., & Frackowiak, R. (2001). Imaging plasticity in cochlear implant patients. *Audiology & Neuro-otology,* 6, 6, pp. 381-393.

[36] Goense, J.B.M., Ku, S.-P., Merkle, H., Tolias, A.S., & Logothetis, N.K. (2008). fMRI of the temporal lobe of the awake monkey at 7 T. *NeuroImage,* 39, 3, pp. 1081-1093.

[37] Gu, J.W., Halpin, C.F., Nam, E.-C., Levine, R., & Melcher, J.R. (2010). Tinnitus, diminished sound-level tolerance, and elevated auditory activity in humans with clinically normal hearing sensitivity. *Journal of Neurophysiology,* 104, 6, pp. 3361-3370.

[38] Hackett, T.A., Preuss, T.M., & Kaas, J.H. (2001). Architectonic identification of the core region in auditory cortex of macaques, chimpanzees, and humans. *Journal of Comparative Neurology,* 222, pp. 197-222.

[39] Hall, D.A., Haggard, M.P., Akeroyd, M.A., Palmer, A.R., Summerfield, A.Q., Elliott, M.R., Gurney, E., & Bowtell, R.W. (1999). Sparse temporal sampling in auditory fMRI. *Human Brain Mapping,* 7, 3, pp. 213-223.

[40] Hall, D.A., Chambers, J., Foster, J., Akeroyd, M.A., Coxon, R., & Palmer, A.R. (2009). Acoustic, psychophysical, and neuroimaging measurements of the effectiveness of active cancellation during auditory functional magnetic resonance imaging. *The Journal of the Acoustical Society of America* 125, 1, pp. 347–359.

[41] Hart, H.C., Hall, D.A., & Palmer, A.R. (2003). The sound-level-dependent growth in the extent of fMRI activation in Heschl's gyrus is different for low- and high-frequency tones. *Hearing Research,* 179, 1-2, pp. 104-112.

[42] Howard, M.A., Volkov, I.O., Abbas, P.J., Damasio, H., Ollendieck, M.C., & Granner, M.A. (1996). A chronic microelectrode investigation of the tonotopic organization of human auditory cortex. *Brain Research,* 724, 2, pp. 260-264.

[43] Humphries, C., Liebenthal, E., & Binder, J.R. (2010). Tonotopic organization of human auditory cortex. *NeuroImage,* 50, 3, pp. 1202-1211.

[44] Jäncke, L., Wüstenberg, T., Schulze, K., & Heinze, H.J. (2002). Asymmetric hemodynamic responses of the human auditory cortex to monaural and binaural stimulation. *Hearing Research,* 170, 1-2, pp. 166-178.

[45] Kaas, J.H., & Hackett, T. (2000). Subdivisions of auditory cortex and processing streams in primates. *Proceedings of the National Academy of Sciences of the United States of America,* 97, 22, pp. 11793-11799.

[46] Kaltenbach, J.A., Zhang, J., & Finlayson, P. (2005). Tinnitus as a plastic phenomenon and its possible neural underpinnings in the dorsal cochlear nucleus. *Hearing Research,* 206, 1-2, pp. 200-226.

[47] Komiya, H., & Eggermont, J.J. (2000). Spontaneous firing activity of cortical neurons in adult cats with reorganized tonotopic map following pure-tone trauma. *Acta Oto-laryngologica,* 120, 6, pp. 750-756.

[48] Langers, D.R.M., Backes, W.H., & Van Dijk, P. (2007). Representation of lateralization and tonotopy in primary versus secondary human auditory cortex. *NeuroImage,* 34, 1, pp. 264-273.

[49] Lanting, C.P., De Kleine, E., Bartels, H., & Van Dijk, P. (2008). Functional imaging of unilateral tinnitus using fMRI. *Acta Oto-laryngologica,* 128, 4, pp. 415-21.

[50] Lanting, C.P., De Kleine, E., & Van Dijk, P. (2009). Neural activity underlying tinnitus generation: results from PET and fMRI. *Hearing Research,* 255, 1-2, pp. 1-13.

[51] Lanting, C.P., De Kleine, E., Eppinga, R.N., & Van Dijk, P (2010). Neural correlates of human somatosensory integration in tinnitus. *Hearing Research,* 267, 1-2, pp. 78-88.

[52] Lauter, J.L., Herscovitch, P., Formby, C., & Raichle, M.E. (1985). Tonotopic organization in human auditory cortex revealed by positron emission tomography. *Hearing Research,* 20, 3, pp. 199-205.

[53] Lee, D. S., Lee, J. S., Oh, S. H., Kim, S. K., Kim, J. W., Chung, J. K., et al. (2001). Cross-modal plasticity and cochlear implants. *Nature, 409,* 6817, 149-150.

[54] Levänen, S., Jousmäki, V., & Hari, R. (1998). Vibration-induced auditory-cortex activation in a congenitally deaf adult. *Current Biology,* 8, 15, pp. 869-872.

[55] Levine, R.A. (1999). Somatic (craniocervical) tinnitus and the dorsal cochlear nucleus hypothesis. *American Journal of Otolaryngology,* 20, 6, pp. 351-362.

[56] Lockwood, A.H. Salvi, R.J., Coad, M.L., Arnold, S.A., Wack, D.S., Murphy, B.W., & Burkard, R.F. (1999). The functional anatomy of the normal human auditory system: responses to 0.5 and 4.0 kHz tones at varied intensities. *Cerebral Cortex,* 9, 1, pp. 65-76.

[57] Logothetis, N.K., Pauls, J., Augath, M., Trinath, T., & Oeltermann, A. (2001). Neurophysiological investigation of the basis of the fMRI signal. *Nature,* 412, 6843, pp. 150-157.

[58] Lomber, S.G., Meredith, M.A., & Kral, A. (2010). Cross-modal plasticity in specific auditory cortices underlies visual compensations in the deaf. *Nature Neuroscience,* 13, 11, pp. 1421-U163.

[59] Lu, H., Golay, X., Pekar, J.J., & Van Zijl, P.C.M. (2003). Functional magnetic resonance imaging based on changes in vascular space occupancy. *Magnetic Resonance in Medicine,* 50, 2, pp. 263-274.

[60] Mechefske, C.M., Geris, R., Gati, J.S., & Rutt, B.K. (2002). Acoustic noise reduction in a 4 T MRI scanner. *Magnetic Resonance Materials in Physics, Biology and Medicine,* 13, 3, pp. 172-176.

[61] Melcher, J.R., Sigalovsky, I.S., Guinan, J.J., & Levine, R.A. (2000). Lateralized tinnitus studied with functional magnetic resonance imaging: abnormal inferior colliculus activation. *Journal of Neurophysiology,* 83, 2, pp. 1058-1072.

[62] Melcher, J.R., Levine, R.A., Bergevin, C., & Norris, B. (2009). The auditory midbrain of people with tinnitus: abnormal sound-evoked activity revisited. *Hearing Research,* 257, 1-2, pp.63-74.

[63] Merzenich, M.M., Knight, P.L., & Roth, G.L. (1975). Representation of cochlea within primary auditory cortex in the cat. *Journal of Neurophysiology,* 38, 2, pp. 231-249.

[64] Miller, J. D., Watson, C. S., Kistler, D. J., Wightman, F. L., & Preminger, J. E. (2008). Preliminary evaluation of the speech perception assessment and training system (SPATS) with hearing-aid and cochlear-implant users. *Proc Meet Acoust, 2,* 1, 1-9.

[65] Miyamoto, R. T., Osberger, M. J., Cunningham, L., Kirk, K. I., Myres, W. A., Robbins, A. M., et al. (1994). Single-channel to multichannel conversions in pediatric cochlear implant recipients. *American Journal of Otology, 15,* 1, 40-45; discussion 45-46.

[66] Morel, A., Garraghty, P.E., & Kaas, J.H., (1993). Tonotopic organization, architectonic fields, and connections of auditory cortex in macaque monkeys. *The Journal of Comparative Neurology*, 335, 3, pp. 437-459.

[67] Møller, A.R., Møller, M.B., & Yokota, M. (1992). Some forms of tinnitus may involve the extralemniscal auditory pathway. *The Laryngoscope*, 102, 10, pp. 1165-1171.

[68] Mühlnickel, W., Elbert, T., Taub, E., & Flor, H. (1998). Reorganisation of auditory cortex in tinnitus. *Proceedings of the National Academy of Sciences of the United States of America*, 95, 17, pp. 10340-10343.

[69] Neville, H. J., & Lawson, D. (1987). Attention to central and peripheral visual space in a movement detection task: an event-related potential and behavioral study. II. Congenitally deaf adults. *Brain Research, 405,* 2, 268-283.

[70] Nicolas-Puel, C., Akbaraly, T., Lloyd, R., Berr, C., Uziel, A., Rebillard, G., & Puel, J-L. (2006). Characteristics of tinnitus in a population of 555 patients: Specificities of tinnitus induced by noise trauma. *The International Tinnitus Journal*, 12, 1, pp. 64-70.

[71] Nishimura, H., Hashikawa, K., Doi, K., Iwaki, T., Watanabe, Y., Kusuoka, H., et al. (1999). Sign language 'heard' in the auditory cortex. *Nature, 397,* 6715, 116.

[72] Noreña, A.J., & Eggermont, J.J. (2003). Changes in spontaneous neural activity immediately after an acoustic trauma: implications for neural correlates of tinnitus. *Hearing Research*, 183, 1-2, pp. 137-153.

[73] O'Donoghue, G.M., Nikolopoulos, T.P., & Archbold, S.M. (2000). Determinants of speech perception in children after chochlear implantation. *Lancet*, 356, 9228, pp. 466-468.

[74] Ogawa, S., Lee, T.M., Kay, A.R., & Tank, D.W. (1990). Brain magnetic resonance imaging with contrast dependent on blood oxygenation. *Proceedings of the National Academy of Sciences of the United States of America*, 87, 24, pp. 9868-9872.

[75] Ojemann, J.G., Akbudak, E., Snyder, A.Z., McKinstry, R.C., Raichle, M.E., & Conturo, T.E. (1997). Anatomic localization and quantitative analysis of gradient refocused echoplanar fMRI susceptibility artifacts. *NeuroImage*, 6, 3, pp. 156-167.

[76] Paltoglou, A.E., Sumner, C.J., & Hall, D.A. (2011). Mapping feature-sensitivity and attentional modulation in human auditory cortex with functional magnetic resonance imaging. *The European Journal of Neuroscience*, 33, 9, pp. 1733-1741.

[77] Parkes, L.M., Schwarzbach, J.V., Bouts, A.A., Deckers, R.H.R., Pullens, P., Kerskens, C.M., & Norris, D.G. (2005). Quantifying the spatial resolution of the gradient echo

and spin echo BOLD response at 3 Tesla. *Magnetic Resonance in Medicine*, 54, 6, pp. 1465-1472.

[78] Petkov, C.I., Kayser, C., Augath, M., & Logothetis, N.K. (2006). Functional imaging reveals numerous fields in the monkey auditory cortex. *PLoS Biology*, 4, 7, pp. e215.

[79] Pinchoff, R.J., Burkard, R.F., Salvi, R.J., Coad, M.L., & Lockwood, A.H. (1998). Modulation of tinnitus by voluntary jaw movements. *The American Journal of Otology*, 19, 6, pp. 785-789.

[80] Polimeni, J.R., Fischl, B., Greve, D.N., & Wald, L.L. (2010). Laminar analysis of 7T BOLD using an imposed spatial activation pattern in human V1. *NeuroImage*, 52, 4, pp. 1334-1346.

[81] Price, D.L., de Wilde, J.P., Papadaki, A.M., Curran, J.S., & Kitney, R.I. (2001). Investigation of acoustic noise on 15 MRI scanners from 0.2 T to 3 T. *Journal of Magnetic Resonance Imaging*, 13, pp. 288-293.

[82] Rajan, R., Irvine, D.R.F., Wise, L.Z., & Heil, P. (1993). Effect of unilateral partial cochlear lesions in adult cats on the representation of lesioned and unlesioned cochleas in primary auditory-cortex. *Journal of Comparative Neurology*, 338, 1, pp. 17-49.

[83] Rajan, R., & Irvine, D.R. (1998) Neuronal responses across cortical field A1 in plasticity induced by peripheral auditory organ damage. *Audiology & Neuro-otology*, 3, 2-3, pp. 123-144.

[84] Rauschecker, J.P. (1995). Compensatory plasticity and sensory substitution in the cerebralcortex. *Trends in Neurosciences*, 18, 1, pp. 36-43

[85] Rauschecker, J.P., & Tian, B. (2000). Mechanisms and streams for processing of "what" and "where" in auditory cortex. *Proceedings of the National Academy of Sciences of the United States of America*, 97, 22, pp. 11800-11806.

[86] Roberts, L.E. (2007). Residual inhibition. *Progress in Brain Research*, 166, pp.487-495.

[87] Robertson, D., & Irvine, D.R.F. (1989). Plasticity of frequency organization in auditory-cortex of guinea-pigs with partial unilateral deafness. *Journal of Comparative Neurology*, 282, 3, pp. 456-471.

[88] Rouger, J., Lagleyre, S., Demonet, J. F., Fraysse, B., Deguine, O., & Barone, P. (2011). Evolution of crossmodal reorganization of the voice area in cochlear-implanted deaf patients. *Human Brain Mapping*, doi: 10.1002/hbm.21331.

[89] Rubinstein, J.T., Parkinson, W.S., Tyler, R.S., & Gantz, B.J. (1999). Residual Speech recognition and cochlear implant performance: Effects of implantation criteria. *American Journal of Otology*, 20, 4, pp. 445-452.

[90] Sarant, J.Z., Blamey, P.J., Dowell, R.C., Clark, G.M., & Gibson, W.P.R. (2001). Variation in speech perception scores among children with cochlear implants. *Ear and Hearing*, 22, 1, pp. 18-28.

[91] Schönwiesner, M., Von Cramon, D.Y., & Rübsamen, R. (2002). Is it tonotopy after all? *NeuroImage*, 17, 3, pp. 1144-11461.

[92] Schramm, D., Fitzpatrick, E., & Seguin, C. (2002). Cochlear implantation for adolescents and adults with prelinguistic deafness. *Otology & Neurotology*, 23, 5, pp. 698-703.

[93] Seki, S., & Eggermont, J. J. (2003). Changes in spontaneous firing rate and neural synchrony in cat primary auditory cortex after localized tone-induced hearing loss. *Hearing Research*, 180, 1-2, pp. 28-38.

[94] Sereda, M., Hall, Deborah., Bosnyak, D.J., Edmondson-Jones, M., Roberts, L.E., Adjamian, P., & Palmer, A.R. (2011). Re-examining the relationship between audiometric profile and tinnitus pitch. *International Journal of Audiology*, 50, 5, pp. 303-312.

[95] Sevy, A.B.G., Bortfeld, H., Huppert, T.J., Beauchamp, M.S., Tonini, R.E., & Oghalai, J.S. (2010). Neuroimaging with near-infrared spectroscopy demonstrates speechevoked activity in the auditory cortex in deaf children following cochlear implantation. *Hearing Research*, 270, 1-2, pp. 39-47.

[96] Shellock, F.G., Morisoli, S., & Kanal, E. (1993). MR procedures and biomedical implants, materials, and devices - 1993 update. *Radiology*, 189, 2, pp. 587-599.

[97] Shmuel, A., Yacoub, E., Chaimow, D., Logothetis, N.K, & Ugurbil, K. (2007). Spatiotemporal point-spread function of fMRI signal in human gray matter at 7 Tesla. *NeuroImage*, 35, 2, pp. 539-552.

[98] Shore, S.E. (2011). Plasticity of somatosensory inputs to the cochlear nucleus - Implications for tinnitus. *Hearing Research*, 18, 281, 1-2, pp. 38-46.

[99] Shore, S.E., Koehler, S., Oldakowski, M., Hughes, L.F., & Syed, S. (2008). Dorsal cochlear nucleus responses to somatosensory stimulation are enhanced after noise-induced hearing loss. *The European Journal of Neuroscience*, 27, 1, pp. 155-168.

[100] Striem-Amit, E., Hertz, U., & Amedi, A. (2011). Extensive cochleotopic mapping of human auditory cortical fields obtained with phase-encoding fMRI. *PloS One*, 6, 3, pp. e17832.

[101] Talavage, T.M., Edmister, W.B., Ledden, P.J., & Weisskoff, R.M. (1999). Quantitative assessment of auditory cortex responses induced by imager acoustic noise. *Human Brain Mapping*, 7, 2, pp. 79-88.

[102] Talavage, T.M, Ledden, P.J, Benson, R.R., Rosen, B.R., & Melcher, J.R. (2000). Frequencydependent responses exhibited by multiple regions in human auditory cortex. *Hearing Research*, 150, 1-2, pp. 225-244.

[103] Talavage, T.M., & Edmister, W.B. (2004). Nonlinearity of fMRI responses in human auditory cortex. *Human Brain Mapping*, 22, 3, pp. 216-228.

[104] Talavage, T.M., Sereno, M.I., Melcher, J.R., Ledden, P.J., Rosen, B.R., & Dale, A.M. (2004). Tonotopic organization in human auditory cortex revealed by progressions of frequency sensitivity. *Journal of Neurophysiology*, 91, 3, pp. 1282-96.

[105] Van der Zwaag, W., Francis, S., Head, K., Peters, A., Gowland, P., Morris, P., & Bowtell, R. (2009). fMRI at 1.5, 3 and 7 T: Characterising BOLD signal changes. *NeuroImage*, 47, 4, pp.1425-1434.

[106] Warnking, J. (2002). fMRI retinotopic mapping—step by step. *NeuroImage*, 17, 4, pp. 1665- 1683.

[107] Weisskoff, R.M., Zuo, C.S., Boxerman, J.L., & Rosen, B.R. (1994). Microscopic susceptibility variation and transverse relaxation: theory and experiment. *Magnetic Resonance in Medicine*, 31, 6, pp. 601-610.

[108] Wessinger, C.M., Buonocore, M.H., Kussmaul, C.L., & Mangun, G.R. (1997). Tonotopy in human auditory cortex examined with functional magnetic resonance imaging. *Human Brain Mapping, 5, 1,* pp.18-25.

[109] Woods, D.L, Stecker, G.C., Rinne, T., Herron, T.J., Cate, A.D., Yund, E.W., Liao, I., & Kang, X. (2009). Functional maps of human auditory cortex: effects of acoustic features and attention. *PloS ONE, 4, 4,* pp. e5183.

[110] Yacoub, E., Shmuelm A., Pfeuffer, J., Van de Moortele, P.F., Adriany, G., Andersen, P., Vaughan, J.T., Merkle, H., Ugurbil, K., & Hu, X.P. (2001). Imaging brain function in humans at 7 Tesla. Magnetic Resonance in Medicine, 45, 4, pp. 588-594.

4

Developmental Plasticity: fMRI Investigations into Human Visual Cortex

Alyssa A. Brewer and Brian Barton

1. Introduction

The ultimate goal of many fields of neuroscience research is to harness the ability for the human brain to reorganize, as an understanding of how to induce plasticity in cortex could foster the development of treatments of such devastating conditions as paralysis, neurodegenerative disease and stroke. The specifics of the timing and types of reorganization possible in cortical sensorimotor maps have generated tremendous interest, both in the adult and juvenile brain. While it is clear that cortical representations in human are able to undergo significant reorganization during development (an early critical period of life) (e.g., [1-4]), the extent of reorganization possible in the developing human brain is still not fully known. In addition, there are likely differences in the timing and degree of reorganization possible across the different sensory modalities [5-11]. This chapter will focus on examples of plasticity in the visual cortex of the developing human arising from congenital disorders, with specific attention to the use of functional magnetic resonance imaging (fMRI) in in vivo measurements of these cortical changes.

1.1. The definition of plasticity

The phenomenon we refer to as 'structural plasticity' will be defined as the long-term reorganization of human visual cortex due to a structural change such as the growth of new axons [5] (Table 1). This type of reorganization is generally expected to be permanent and to take weeks or months to accomplish [12]. 'Structural plasticity' is to be differentiated from 'adaptation', which we use here to refer to rapid changes in visual processing arising from the normal organization of the visual system and not a result of long-term reorganization (see [5] for a detailed discussion of terms).

Phenomena of adaptation are expected to be immediate and completely reversible. Furthermore, these two terms are to be separated from 'functional plasticity', which we will use to describe longer-term reorganization of human visual cortex, primarily due to re-weighting or unmasking of extant neural connections rather than to more extensive structural changes like the growth of new axons. Functional plasticity is expected to take days to weeks to accomplish, and it is still unclear how permanent it can be. At one point or another, each of these terms has been described using the term 'plasticity', and we would like to put an end to this non-specificity, as it leads to misunderstandings regarding each phenomenon.

1.2. Overview of developmental plasticity in the visual cortex of animal models

Many aspects of the development of the visual system have been extensively studied in animal models such as monkey and cat. The mammalian visual system develops in a balance between intrinsic, genetically-guided factors and activity-based experience [13-17]. The ability of the brain to wire and rewire itself based on visual input is known as experience-dependent plasticity (a form of structural plasticity) and plays a key role in determining the final organization of adult visual cortex [1, 12, 15, 18]. The following descriptions of visual cortex development in animal models can serve here as examples of what processes may underlie the visual cortex reorganization described in this chapter for the developing human.

In human and monkey, visual information travels from the retina through the lateral geniculate nucleus (LGN) of the thalamus to primary visual cortex (area V1) in the posterior occipital lobe [19]. In the adult primate, the inputs from each eye are organized into separate groups within V1 called ocular dominance (OD) columns [20]. Emerging from a literature which viewed the immature brain as a haphazardly wired structure that undergoes large-scale remodeling at birth to form OD columns, Hubel and Wiesel were surprised to find that the OD columns within primary visual cortex are actually organized at birth in an adult-like pattern [21-23]. Several subsequent studies investigated whether visual experience (e.g., light stimulation) is necessary for development of the mature pattern of OD columns seen in the infant brain [22-25]. Horton and Hocking [20] finally resolved the issue with heroic measurements of completely dark-reared infant macaque monkeys; the OD columns in these monkeys with no visual experience are organized like those measured in the adult macaque. Other features of cortical functional architecture, such as orientation tuning and orientation columns, are also present before any visual experience [15].

Further experiments investigating how this initial functional architecture is formed have unveiled activity-dependent processes that operate even before the retinal photoreceptors are functional and play a key role in determining the OD organization [16]. In utero, spontaneous coordinated waves of retinal ganglion cell action potentials are required for the development of normal OD and orientation columns [13, 15, 26, 27]. Thus, patterned retinal inputs to the cortex modify initially imprecise connections to produce an organized visual topography prior to the visual experience.

In turn, visual experience during an early critical period of life can profoundly alter the cortical visual topography formed by the in utero retinal activity [14, 18]. For example, if one eye is

Measurement	Structural Plasticity	Functional Plasticity	Adaptation
Temporal scale of cause	Longer than inciting factor	Longer than inciting factor	Short (~tracking input statistics)
Temporal scale of effect	Weeks to months	Days to weeks	Short (~tracking input statistics)
Anatomical connectivity	New connections	Likely re-weighted existing connections	Unlikely to change
Receptive field: Location	May change	May change	May change
Receptive field: Size	May change	May change	May change
Receptive field: Gain	May change	May change	May change
Reversibility	Not typical	Yes, in days to weeks	Yes, within a short time

Table 1. Characteristics of Plasticity and Adaptation. This table delineates core characteristics of three types of 'plasticity': structural plasticity, functional plasticity, and adaptation. Differentiating between each of the three can be difficult, because many measurements do not distinguish one type from another. In addition, there are not always sharp distinctions between the three phenomena. Confusion and controversy have often arisen from the non-specific use of the term 'plasticity' to describe these different cortical changes. This table is adapted and expanded from Box 1 in [5], a prominent review of plasticity and stability of the visual system.

deprived of vision for several weeks in infancy, then most of the mature visual cortical neurons are responsive only to stimuli presented to the eye that remained open; the cortical territory normally devoted to the closed eye is greatly diminished [18, 21]. This reorganization causes a loss of perception in the eye that was closed, as seen in cases of congenital cataracts leading to amblyopia and life-long blindness [28-31].

1.3. Using the topography of visual cortex to track changes in human development

These examples of visual cortical development were studied in animal models using such invasive techniques as electrophysiology and histology. How can we study cortical changes in the living, developing human? One technique that is proving very effective is to measure visual field maps (VFMs) in human visual cortex with functional magnetic resonance imaging (fMRI) to study cortical reorganization in response to abnormal visual input [5].

Human visual cortex is organized into distinct VFMs whose locations and properties provide important information about visual computations [32-35]. In each retinotopically-organized VFM, neurons whose visual receptive fields lie next to one another in visual space are located next to one another in cortex, forming one complete representation of contralateral visual space. By taking advantage of the knowledge of the retinotopic organization of visual input, multiple cortical VFMs can be measured using fMRI with respect to the two orthogonal dimensions needed to identify a unique location in visual space: eccentricity and polar angle (Figs. 3A, 4A, 5A). Each VFM subserves a specific computation or set of computations; locating these VFMs allows for the systematic exploration of these computations across visual cortex [33, 36].

Understanding the organization of these maps provides a baseline for studying reorganization following abnormal development or cortical damage. This chapter will review a series of studies of human developmental visual plasticity that capitalize on our ability to measure these VFMs with a high level of detail in individual subjects. We examine genetic, retinal, and cortical alterations that lead to reorganization of the cortical VFM organization. These examples of cortical developmental plasticity give us insight into the flexibility and constraints present in the human visual system.

2. Methods

2.1. General fMRI methods

Measurements of VFMs in human require very precise fMRI measurements and highly detailed, individual subject analysis [32, 34]. Before delving into the details of the two main types of fMRI experimental techniques used to measure VFMs, it is vital to remember that all fMRI techniques are empowered and limited by four common factors: the properties of fMRI in general, subject biology, experimental stimuli, and statistical analysis. Regardless of the cleverness of the experimental design, basic errors in any of these categories run the risk of rendering an entire study irrelevant due to inaccurate or misinterpreted results [37]. We will briefly review these factors with respect to their importance to visual field mapping.

2.1.1. Properties of fMRI

Let's begin with the basics of fMRI. When neurons are active consequent to task-induced or spontaneous neural metabolic modulations, the ratio of diamagnetic, oxygenated hemoglobin to paramagnetic, deoxygenated hemoglobin in nearby blood increases after a few seconds with a characteristic profile, called the hemodynamic response function (HRF; for reviews and more details, see [38-41]). fMRI is a technique that takes advantage of such blood oxygen-level dependent (BOLD) activity in the brain by applying a strong magnetic field and encoding positions in space through slight differences in magnetic field strength and phase [40, 42]. This allows for a very specific spatial readout of brain activity (on the order of 1mm^3, often in the 1-4 mm^3 range), but the hemodynamic response is on the order of seconds, which limits the ability of fMRI to distinguish fine temporal differences [43].

Scanners suitable for human research commonly have a magnetic field strength of 1, 1.5, 3, or 4 Tesla (T), though access to 7T scanners is becoming more common. The field strength affects many aspects of the scanning parameters that can be chosen, but there is a basic trade-off between spatial resolution and signal-to-noise ratio (SNR), although different field strengths may also suffer from differing distortions or artifacts [44-46]. Lower field strength gives researchers a lower SNR, which forces researchers to use larger voxels. A larger voxel size increases SNR, because signal can be averaged across a greater number of active neurons within a voxel. However, large voxels also reduce spatial detail, which is important for advanced fMRI techniques such as those used for visual field mapping [34, 38, 47]. A key element for making careful, accurate measurements of plasticity in human cortex is to be able to acquire both high spatial resolution images and high SNR. Naturally, there are many other details to consider in the scanning parameters, but these are outside the scope of the chapter.

2.1.2. Subject cortical biology

The basic properties of fMRI scanners quickly become more complicated when biological factors are taken into account [39, 48, 49]. Air cavities, like the frontal sinuses or the ear canals, can create 'blow-out' artifacts in the images of the nearby portions of brain by locally distorting the magnetic fields [50]. Although less relevant for most measurements of visual cortex, it is a factor that should not be ignored. For example, if one were to compare visual activity in primary visual cortex to visual activity near these distorted regions, one may make incorrect inferences about activity level differences that have little to do with the experiment but instead are driven by these distortions [34, 38, 39, 48, 49, 51].

Another consideration is the arterial and venial physiology of individual subjects. Large draining veins may create distortions in the fMRI signal arising from neighboring cortex [52]. These distortions are unpredictable due both to the sensitivity of these distortions to the relative magnetic gradients and to the high variability of the venous system across individuals. For example, Winawer et al. [53] demonstrated the role for a 'venous eclipse' in the difficulties in measuring of the contiguous hV4 hemifield representation on the human ventral occipital cortex. These difficulties led to several years of confusion and controversy regarding the VFM organization in this region [33, 54-59].

It is also important to take the cortical anatomy of the individual subject into account. Although it is becoming more common practice in some fields to segment out white from gray matter and consider only activity occurring in gray matter, this is still not the standard approach [39]. As far as is currently known, the primary neural computations take place in gray matter; therefore, one should only consider activity in biologically relevant tissue, particularly when comparing regions of interest that could, without considering only gray matter, include different amounts of white matter as frequently occurs in typical slice-based analysis [60]. It should also be noted that not all white-gray matter segmentation is created equal—there are several algorithms used to parcel them out, but all require hand-editing for appropriate accuracy, which can be time intensive [32, 61-63].

2.1.3. Experimental stimuli

For any field of visual neuroimaging research, one must be incredibly careful in the choice of experimental stimuli, especially when contrasting activity between two or more types of stimuli. First, one must take into account the retinotopic nature of large portions of visual cortex [32-34, 64] and present stimuli in retinotopically consistent locations (unless activity is being measured for different locations of the visual field). Next, stimuli must be chosen that are equivalent on every aspect except those of interest. Unaccounted-for features can explain the results of interest when low-level features of stimuli are ignored in favor of interpreting data in terms of perceptual categories (e.g., [65, 66]).

2.1.4. Statistical analysis

In the unending search for statistical significance, researchers often use some variety of spatial averaging across subjects in order to increase their statistical power. There are two primary approaches to spatial brain averaging: morph individual subject brains onto a template brain or average locally based on local anatomical landmarks. From a behavioral experimental perspective, this may seem as reasonable as averaging together d-prime scores for individual subjects, but that is far from the case. One must take into account the inter-subject biological variability, not just in the location of veins, but of every aspect of the brain. Individual, neurologically normal subjects may have extra, missing, differently sized or differently folded gyri and sulci [67, 68]. The cortical surface of primary visual cortex, V1, can vary by a factor of ~2.5 among normal subjects, which not only affects the measurement of V1, but of all neighboring regions as a result of the displacement with respect to the underlying anatomy [69]. Although likely less problematic for vision, handedness has also been implicated in differences between hemispheric organization [70, 71]. Also, overall brain size can vary not only by gender, but by skull and body size. Additionally, skull shape can vary, shifting locations of individual brain regions due to the brain displacement relative to other subjects [72]. Obviously this is not an exhaustive list of normal variation, and it doesn't even take into account the wide variety of possibilities for damage in people who self-report being neurologically normal—or the differences between patients with similar neurological conditions within a particular study of visual plasticity.

Despite these issues, the vast majority of researchers use spatial averaging. The only truly viable solution is functional averaging, which is where regions of interest (ROIs) are defined based on functional data, then data from corresponding ROIs across subjects are averaged together. For example, if one wanted to study color activity in hV4, one would first use a visual field mapping technique to map hV4 in each subject (see Travelling Wave Retinotopy and Population Receptive Field Modeling sections below), then average together color activity for each subject from their individually defined hV4 maps [32, 54]. In this way, each subject's unique brain is taken into account rather than being distorted to approximate a template, and the relevant information is still averaged across subjects.

Finally, let us consider another common practice: spatial smoothing. This is when researchers average together activity in nearby voxels, often using a several-millimeter Gaussian kernel. What this allows researchers to do is to smooth the data for each voxel, reducing overall signal variability. However, such smoothing eliminates detailed information in the process. While this may be acceptable when one's technique cannot utilize detailed spatial information, it is disastrous when applied to detailed information such as that contained in visual field maps [33, 58].

2.2. Travelling wave retinotopy

Travelling Wave Retinotopy (TWR) was developed to measure retinotopically organized visual cortex (also known as visual field maps, VFMs). To do so, TWR takes advantage of knowledge gleaned from electrophysiological measurements of visual cortex in animal models about the structure and stimulus preferences of VFMs. In short, a VFM is a visual area with a complete representation of visual space, where neurons that represent adjacent locations on the retina (and thus visual space) are also adjacent in cortex. Because many computations are required to create our visual experience, our brains have many specialized VFMs which perform one or more of those computations across the entire visual scene (e.g., motion perception happens throughout our visual field, not just in the upper left quadrant).

Taking advantage of this knowledge, TWR uses two types of stimuli to measure the two orthogonal dimensions of visual space: eccentricity (i.e., center to periphery) and polar angle (i.e., around the clock) [32, 34, 73-76] (Figs. 3A, 4A). These stimuli tile across as much of the visual field as possible given field of view limitations with the MR scanner. The first stimulus is designed to elicit each voxel's preferred eccentricity by presenting a high-contrast flickering stimulus shaped like a ring, expanding in discrete even steps from the center of vision (fixation) to the periphery. The second is designed to elicit each voxel's preferred polar angle by presenting a high-contrast flickering stimulus shaped like a wedge that extends from the fovea to periphery, which rotates in discrete even steps around the fixation point. A checkerboard pattern commonly comprises the high contrast stimulus, as this pattern maximally stimulates V1; however, any pattern of interest can theoretically be used [77]. In each scan, only one type of stimulus is presented (rings or wedges), and all of visual space is cycled through several times with each stimulus (Fig. 1). Typically, several scans are then averaged together for each stimulus type. The type of activity driven by these stimuli physically appears to be a wave that travels from one end of the VFM to the other along iso-angle or iso–eccentricity lines, giving TWR its name.

The design of TWR presents all eccentricities or polar angles at a given frequency per scan (typically 6-8), which allows the use of Fourier analysis. First, TWR only considers activity that is at the signal frequency (typically 6-8 cycles/scan), excluding low-frequency physiological noise, among other things. A coherence analysis is then performed, where the strength at the signal frequency is divided by the strength at the other frequencies, and only voxels with coherence above a threshold are further evaluated (typically 0.15 to 0.30 coherence) [32, 34]. Finally, a phase is assigned to each voxel, which corresponds to a particular eccentricity or polar angle preference (Fig. 1).

Between these measurements of eccentricity and polar angle, TWR provides an estimate of the preferred RF center of the population of neurons with visual RFs in each voxel (Fig. 2). This technique is excellent at driving activity in early retinotopic areas (e.g., V1, V2, V3, hV4), in which neural RFs are relatively small [73, 74, 78, 79]. However, VFMs with larger neural RFs (e.g., regions in lateral-occipital cortex) are more difficult to measure, because the voxels respond to large swaths of the visual field [33, 78-80]. Even with large receptive fields, regions can still be retinotopically organized with retinotopically dispersed, preferred receptive field centers [32]. This large response field means that several TWR stimulus positions can similarly activate such a region. Because TWR analysis relies on measuring cortical responses in sync with the stimulus movement, regions that activate to a specific set of multiple stimulus positions may appear to have lower or no retinotopic responses, even with retinotopically dispersed RF centers.

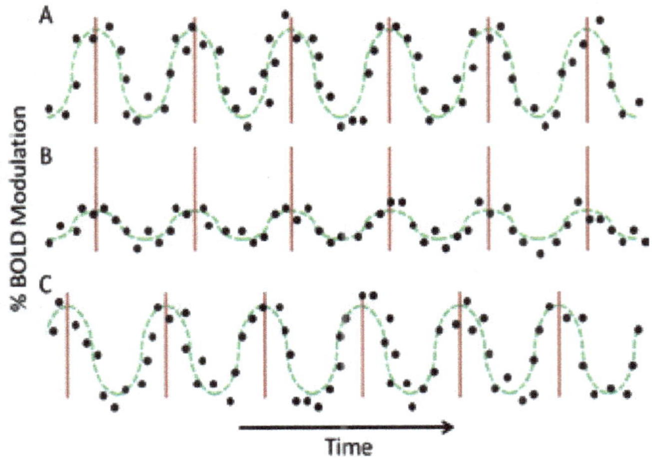

Figure 1. Visual Field Mapping Time Series Analysis. Each row represents the activity and analysis of a time series of a single 6-cycle scan of one type of experimental stimuli (expanding rings or rotating wedges) for a single voxel. Black dots indicate simulated raw data points of % BOLD modulation. The red lines indicate the peak activations per cycle for an imaginary set of voxels, which are the measurements used by the TWR analysis. The green dotted line represents a sinusoidal fit of the simulated data points, which are the measurements used by pRF modeling. Rows (A) and (B) represent time series of voxels with identical peak responses, indicating identical stimulus selectivity. However, (B) has much lower %BOLD modulation than (A), which could be due to two common factors: differences in local vasculature or broader receptive field tuning for (B) than (A). Rows (A) and (C) represent time series of voxels with identical %BOLD modulation, but different peak responses, which indicate different stimulus selectivity (i.e., different 'phases' of response). For example, (A) might represent a voxel with a preferred eccentricity tuning of 5° eccentric to fixation, whereas (C) might have a preferred tuning of only 2° eccentric to fixation.

Additionally, VFMs that have a larger degree of RF scatter within each voxel are more difficult to measure for the same reasons as large neural RFs. As a result of the power of TWR, it has become the standard workhorse for localizing and measuring the spatial details of VFMs. Relative to other neuroimaging methods like general condition contrast (GCC) approaches, TWR provides an unprecedented amount of detail [32, 33, 77]. For example, while the GCC may reveal the location of a large cluster of voxels that has been termed the human motion complex, hMT+, TWR reveals several distinct, highly organized VFMs within that large voxel cluster [64, 81].

2.3. Population receptive field modeling

The most recently developed technique of those covered in this chapter is population receptive field (pRF) modeling [78]. Once it had become clear that there were serious limits to the ability of TWR to deal with VFMs with large RFs, researchers at Stanford University decided that the best solution was to use a model of the pRFs of each voxel in VFMs [78]. This approach arose in part from previous work in several studies [30, 57, 79, 82, 83], which measured receptive fields in human and macaque visual cortex. The logic of pRF modeling is that, because VFMs are retinotopically organized, the population of RFs in each voxel of a VFM is expected to have similar preferred centers and sizes, allowing their combined pRFs to be estimated as a single, two-dimensional Gaussian RF (Fig. 2). Despite the fact that there is some variability in the neural RFs of each voxel in terms of their preferred center and size, termed RF scatter, the pRF provides a good, if somewhat slightly larger, estimate of the individual neural RFs in the voxel [78, 81, 84].

The advantages of the method are generally stated in comparison to the field standard for measuring VFMs, TWR. Not only does pRF modeling allow for the measurement of the preferred centers of the pRF of a voxel like TWR, but it also measures the spatial spread of the pRF, allows for the use of any stimulus that systematically tiles visual space, and takes less scan time to do, as it can use a single stimulus like a moving bar to measure both dimensions of visual space.

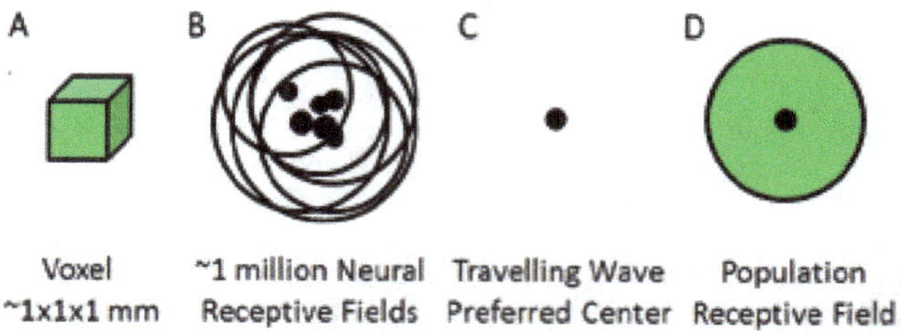

Figure 2. Measurements of an Individual Voxel. (A) A typical voxel recorded from a 3T MRI scanner is on the order of 1 mm3, though often slightly larger (2-3 mm3). (B) Within each typical voxel, there are on the order of ~1 million neurons, depending on the size of the voxel. For voxels in retinotopic visual cortex, the neurons each have similarly located spatial receptive fields (black outlines) with preferred centers (black dots). (C) TWR takes advantage of the fact that nearby neurons in retinotopic cortex have similar preferred centers in order to estimate a population preferred center for the population of neurons in a given voxel. (D) pRF modeling takes advantage of the fact that nearby neurons in retinotopic cortex have similar receptive fields in order to estimate not only a preferred center, but also a pRF for the population of neurons in a given voxel.

To accomplish this, the pRF model first creates a database of all possible pRF sizes and centers given the field of view of the stimulus used. Then, the model creates an expected HRF profile for each of the pRF possibilities based on an assumed or individually measured HRF. Finally, the model uses a least-squares fitting method to iteratively test each of the pRF possibilities for each voxel independently against the actual data collected [78]. Whichever pRF best fits the data is then assigned as the pRF for that voxel. Voxels are discarded if they do not have above a threshold of variance explained by the model. Although it is technically possible to use any stimulus that traverses the entire field of view, typically the stimuli take one of two forms. First is a slightly modified version of the TWR stimuli, in which neutral gray blank periods are inserted at an off-frequency from the stimulus frequency (e.g., 4 instead of 6-8 cycles/scan, so they are separable in the Fourier analysis). The second and increasingly common stimulus is a high-contrast flickering checkerboard moving bar stimulus that steps across the field of view in the 8 cardinal directions, again with several interspersed neutral gray blank periods. In theory, one could also tile visual space using any stimulus of interest, if the aforementioned stimuli do not drive the cortical region well. Since they were designed to drive activity in early visual cortex, it is possible other stimuli may perform better in higher-order VFMs [85, 86].

Because pRF modeling has proven so successful, we expect that it will eventually replace TWR as the standard method for measuring VFMs. Moreover, pRF modeling has an excellent future in the measurement of the details of pRFs, which is particularly important for the measurement of visual plasticity in humans. So far, the technique has primarily used a two-dimensional Gaussian profile for the pRF estimates, but researchers are working on the use of center-surround Gaussian pRFs, multiple location pRFs, and non-classical pRF shapes, which may allow for better pRF estimation as time continues [87]. For its purpose, the limitations of the pRF modeling method are essentially the measurement limitations of the scanner and stimuli used. In the future, it is likely that pRF modeling will be very successful when used in isolation, but also excellent to use in conjunction with other techniques.

3. Developmental plasticity following congenital lesions

Cortical reorganization is generally accepted by neuroscientists as a fact of life during development. Along the way to adulthood, neural structures grow, sprout, connect, and are pruned in a series of complex cascades and critical periods. In short, cortical reorganization not only happens during development, it's rampant. Perhaps that is why there is less controversy surrounding claims of cortical plasticity as a result of congenital abnormalities. As a rule, the developing brain is more plastic than the adult brain, but in both cases, the brain is striking a balance between plasticity and stability [5].

For the visual system, the balance is decidedly skewed towards stability, except in the earlier stages of development [88]. Stability is very useful for the visual system in the adult, because there are very few circumstances under which changes in properties of neurons in visual cortex such as their spatial representations is beneficial after development [6]. In fact, in most circumstances, it would be costly and destructive to change visual circuitry in the brain. In effect, each portion of visual space has its own processing pipeline through the visual hierarchy, which is possible only if independent processing channels for each portion of space are maintained. If the visual system were highly plastic, portions of the visual field would necessarily be cross-wiring these processing pipelines, disrupting the processing hierarchy in chaotic fashion wherever a crossing occurred. Contrast this with the memory systems of the brain, which could not possibly function without a high degree of plasticity to encode memories and associate them with one another (e.g., [89]). Of course, memory systems are not entirely plastic, as memories must also be maintained, but the balance point between plasticity and stability is quite different from that of the visual system.

In the congenital disorders described, developmental alterations of the organization of visual input to cortex are expected to drive the reorganization of visual representations in visual cortex. This reorganization of cortical visual representations might occur in one or more of the following ways (e.g., [5, 90]). First, major changes in the visual input to cortex may lead to a total disruption of retinotopic organization in visual cortex. Second, major retinal changes may lead to a reorganization of a section of cortical visual representation in response to a loss of retinal activity for a portion of visual space. Third, altered visual pathways could lead to a restriction of the field of view as cortical maps reach a limit on how much of the contra- and ipsilateral hemifields could be represented in each hemisphere. Fourth, changes in the crossing of the visual pathways could lead to larger-than-normal, contiguous representations of visual space representing more than the normal contralateral hemifield. Finally, such changes in visual pathways could produce overlapped visual field representations, in which an abnormal representation of the ipsilateral visual field is superimposed on the representation of the normal contralateral visual field. In a single congenital disorder affecting the visual system, one or even several such changes in cortical visual representations could theoretically be present. Measurements of what types of reorganization actually appear in these disorders highlight the capabilities for adaptation to altered visual inputs in human visual cortex.

The abnormal drivers of developmental plasticity in the visual system can be grouped into three major categories. The first are retinal lesions, in which visual information about a location is never present in the visual system because of a functional failure in retinal circuitry. The second are altered visual pathways, in which visual information is misrouted from the retina to its intended thalamic or cortical targets. Finally, we have cortical lesions, in which visual information enters the visual system, but undergoes abnormal processing due to a disruption in the cortical processing hierarchy. The following sections will describe examples from each category that were studied in human subjects using fMRI.

3.1. Congenital retinal lesions can produce changes in cortical visuospatial representations.

3.1.1. Rod monochromatism

Two primary classes of photoreceptors tile the human retina: cones, which are maximally responsive under normal lighting (photopic) conditions, and rods, which are maximally responsive under very low lighting (scotopic) conditions [91]. The cones are highly concentrated in the fovea of each retina, whereas the concentration of rods drops dramatically and becomes zero within a radius of ~0.6-0.8° of visual angle about the eyes' fixation point [91-93]. While the rod-free fovea occupies <1% of the retina, the cortical representation of this retinal region occupies roughly 20% of primary visual cortex [94].

Under scotopic conditions, normal subjects perceive a scotoma ~2-4° of visual angle in diameter at the center of their vision [93, 95-97]. This rod scotoma, like the blind spot, is functionally equivalent to a retinal lesion—light falls on a location in the retina but is not processed due to a lack of active photoreceptors (Fig. 3AB). Recent research indicates that the rod scotoma in normal adults does not fill-in lines or patterns or color, as rods alone do not give rise to color [97], but does fill-in diffusely lit surfaces [98]. The differences in filling-in properties of the rod scotoma from those of the blind spot likely are due to the differences in their cortical receptive field sizes (small vs. large), their ocularity (binocular vs. monocular), their retinal locations (central vs. peripheral), and their physical exposures (infrequent vs. constant). Regardless, the cortical representation of the rod scotoma provides a natural testing ground for hypotheses regarding visual plasticity in response to retinal lesions.

Because we have invented many clever ways of maintaining photopic conditions outside of natural sunlight, modern humans are exposed to scotopic vision, and the rod scotoma, rather infrequently. Under normal conditions, occasional exposure to the rod scotoma, with cones inactive and rods active, throughout development and adulthood is not enough to induce cortical plasticity. For example, in adulthood, cortical representations of the fovea do not shift after prolonged exposure of one week to purely scotopic conditions. This was tested by Baseler et al. [95], who used TWR under photopic and scotopic conditions in normal subjects to map out the portions of V1 that represent the rod scotoma. They found no evidence for reorganization in these normal subjects either in the short term or after one week of adaptation. In fact, the region representing the rod-free fovea under photopic conditions was simply inactive under scotopic conditions, as expected from a lack of signal from the retina (Fig. 3AB).

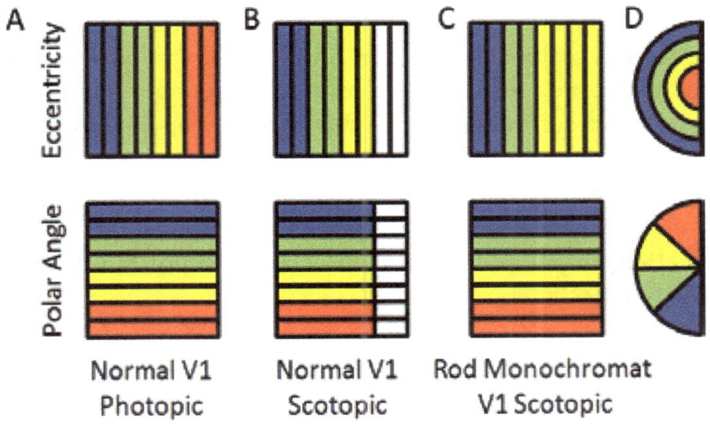

Figure 3. Visual Field Maps in Normal and Rod Monochromat Subjects. (A) Top: Eccentricity gradient for a VFM in a subject with normal vision viewing the stimulus under photopic (daylight) light conditions. Note the gradient running from the center to more peripheral eccentricities runs from right to left. This gradient would be orthogonal to the polar angle gradient in the bottom panel, such that each iso-eccentricity line has a representation of the full range of polar angles. The combination of the orthogonal gradients in top and bottom panels forms one complete representation of a hemifield of visual space. This forms one half of a complete VFM, with the corresponding half being located in the opposite hemisphere of the brain. Because the hemifield represented in this cartoon is the left (see legend in (D)), this map would be located in the right hemisphere. The colors denote positions in visual space represented in each cortical location. Note that the red colors depicting the center of space are represented in this cartoon VFM for a normal subject under photopic conditions. (B) Top: Eccentricity gradient for a VFM in a subject with normal vision viewing the stimulus under scotopic (starlight) light conditions. Bottom: Polar angle gradient of the same VFM, in the same subject under scotopic conditions. Note that the red colors depicting the center of space are not represented in the eccentricity gradient, nor are the corresponding locations of the polar angle gradient. The reason is that, under scotopic conditions, a normal subject has a "rod scotoma" at the center of their gaze where there are few-to-no rod photoreceptors; thus the portions of the VFM representing the center of gaze are not activated. (C) Top: Eccentricity gradient for a VFM in a rod monochromat under scotopic conditions. Bottom: Polar angle gradient for a VFM in a rod monochromat under scotopic conditions. Note that the red colors in the top panel of (A) have been replaced with yellow colors of (C), and that the corresponding locations in the lower panel of (C) are active, unlike the same location in the bottom panel of (B). The reason for this is that the rod monochromat's VFM has reorganized, such that regions of the VFM that would have represented the rod-free fovea now represents regions just outside. (D) Top: Visual space legend for eccentricity. Each color represents an iso-eccentricity line in the left visual hemifield. Bottom: Visual space legend for polar angle. Each color represents an iso-polar angle line in the left visual hemifield.

What if, instead, you were exposed to the rod scotoma for every moment your eyes were open since birth? Would the cortical region that would normally represent the rod-free fovea remain inactive, or would this region of cortex reorganize to represent a still-active, rod-driven region of the retina? These questions can be investigated in a particular group of subjects called rod monochromats, who lack retinal cone function. This loss of cone function is due to a specific genetic mutation in the cone cells that disrupts the phototransduction cascade in all three types of cone photoreceptors [99, 100]; the cones are present in the retina in normal locations and density, but do not respond to stimulation by light [101]. As a result, rod monochromats depend upon only their rod photoreceptors to see and, as such, have been constantly exposed to the rod scotoma throughout development and into adulthood.

Baseler et al. [95] also used TWR under photopic and scotopic conditions to map out the region of V1 devoted to processing the rod scotoma in rod monochromats. In contrast to the results in normal subjects, their measurements showed that the rod monochromats had significant activity under both photopic and scotopic conditions in the region of V1 that would be expected to represent the rod-free scotoma (Fig. 3C). In addition, this cortical activity now represented parafoveal input; this cortical region had reorganized in rod monochromats to receive input from the region of retina surrounding the rod-free fovea. This result indicates that constant exposure to the rod scotoma throughout development leads to cortical reorganization, while infrequent exposure does not.

3.2. Genetic mutations that alter the optic nerves lead to significant alterations in cortical visual field map organization.

3.2.1. Albinism

The most obvious abnormality associated with albinism is the lack of normal pigmentation of the skin, hair, and eyes due to a defect in melanin production [102]. A lesser-known abnormality is albinism's disruptive effect on the development of the visual pathways, in which abnormal projections from each temporal retina carry additional ipsilateral information to each V1 [103-105]. Typically, each cortical hemisphere primarily represents the one contralateral hemifield of visual space (Fig. 4A), but with the abnormal projections in albinism each hemisphere represents a greater span of the visual field from the ipsilateral eye [106] (Fig. 4B). The question, then, is what happens with that information? Is the abnormal ipsilateral information simply suppressed, such that a normal contralateral hemifield representation is maintained in visual cortex, but with, perhaps, abnormal visual perception from the missing ipsilateral coverage? Or, do the projections lead to integrated representations of the ipsilateral information from the temporal retina? If the latter, how are these ipsilateral visual representations integrated into the normal contralateral ones?

Previous electrophysiological research in non-primate albino mammals has suggested that the genetic mutations that underlie albinism can drive different degrees of topographical reorganization in cortex (for review, see [105]). In one organizational pattern measured primarily in Siamese cats and albino ferrets that is called the 'Boston' pattern, the abnormal pathways are reorganized within the projections from the thalamus to cortex, which leads to a contiguous

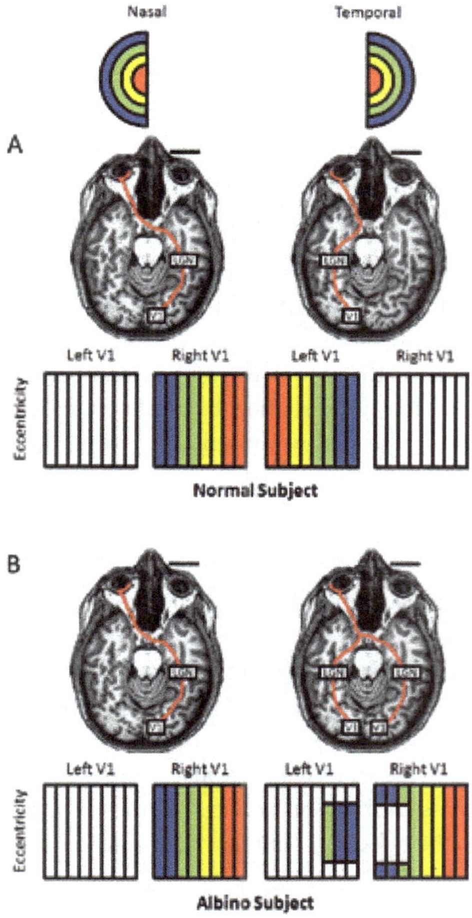

Figure 4. Visual Field Projections in Normal and Albino Subjects. In all panels, the right eye is covered with an eye patch, and only information from the left eye reaches visual cortex. The left column concerns cases where the left side of visual space, which corresponds to the nasal retina of the left eye, is stimulated. The right column concerns cases where the right side of visual space, which corresponds to the temporal retina of the left eye, is stimulated. Top row: Eccentricity visual space legend. Each color represents an iso-eccentricity line in the visual hemifield. (A) Normal subject. Top row: Information flow from the retina to visual cortex. Note that the left side of visual space (nasal retina, left column) is passed to the right hemisphere, whereas the right side of visual space (temporal retina, right column) is passed to the left hemisphere. Bottom row: Eccentricity gradient response for left and right V1. Colors represent locations in visual space denoted by the legend at the top of the figure. Note that the left side of visual space (nasal retina, left column) is represented in right V1, whereas the right side of visual space (temporal retina, right column) is represented in left V1. (B) Albino subject. Top row: Information flow from the retina to visual cortex. Note that the left side of visual space (nasal retina, left column) is passed to the right hemisphere, as in the normal subject in (A). However, unlike the normal subject in (A), the majority of the right side of visual space (temporal retina, right column) is passed to the right hemisphere. Also note that a weakened, residual normal pathway still projects a portion of the left side of visual space (temporal retina, right column) to the left hemisphere. Bottom row: Eccentricity gradient response for left and right V1. Colors represent locations in visual space denoted by the legend at the top of the figure. Note that the left side of visual space (nasal retina, left column) is represented in right V1, as in the normal subject in (A). However, unlike the normal subject in (A), the majority of the right side of visual space (temporal retina, right column) is represented in right V1. Some of the right visual field is still represented in left V1, but not at all at the scale as the normal subject in (A).

representation of the abnormal and normal representations of visual space within visual cortex [105, 107-109]. In a second pattern called 'Midwestern' that is also seen in these mammals, the abnormal visual projections continue from the thalamus into visual cortex without reordering into a contiguous map with concurrent cortical suppression of the abnormally projecting pathways [105, 110]. The visual perceptual dysfunction in these patterns appears in some measurements to include a lack of behavioral sensitivity to the temporal retina [107, 111]. Both patterns have actually been measured within the primary visual cortex of the same animal [112].

The third and rarest pattern, called the 'true albino' pattern, has been measured in one non-human primate as well as a few albino mammals. These electrophysiological measurements suggested that this pattern lacks the reordering of inputs into cortex, forming a superimposed set of inputs from nasal and temporal retinae, but unlike the cortical suppression suggested in the 'Midwestern' pattern, these superimposed inputs are functional [113].

The use of electrophysiology in these studies makes the analysis of the broad organization of visual space across a cortical region difficult. The differing organizational patterns within discrete sections of primary visual cortex in individual albino animals highlights the importance of being able to examine larger regions of the cortical topography than provided by electrophysiological measurements. Functional MRI, however, provides excellent spatial resolution for visual field measurements across a broad field of view, the type of measurement necessary to fully examine the cortical pattern of the representations of visual space across larger swaths of cortex than possible with electrophysiology. In addition, fMRI more easily allows for analysis across a greater number of subjects, important to fully understand the extent of variations possible across individual subjects. Finally, the non-invasive nature of fMRI permits investigation into the effects of albinism on human cortical development.

A recent fMRI study by Hoffman et al. [114] used TWR to map out the cortical representations of visual space in VFMs V1, V2, and V3 in human subjects with ocular or oculocutaneous albinism. They found that the ipsilateral information from the temporal retina is abnormally represented in cortex and forms a mirror-image map in V1 that is superimposed on top of the normal contralateral representation from the nasal retinal projections, following the 'true albino pattern' [113] (Fig. 4; also see [104, 106]). This causes each voxel in V1 to represent two visual field locations that are mirrored around the vertical meridian. A similar pattern of integration was measured in VFMs V2 and V3. Together with the previous study in non-human primate, these results suggest that the developmental mechanisms that subserve the reorganization of thalamocortical projections in non-primate albino mammals are not active in albino primate, leading to a more exclusive 'true albino' pattern of topographical integration in primates.

A few further studies have explored how this abnormal integration of the retinal projections into early visual cortex representations relates to the deficits in visual perception described in albinism. In contrast to the results seen in several animal studies [107, 111], Hoffman et al. [115, 116] and Klemen et al. [117] found no visual field deficits related to the abnormal visual projections and cortical representations. Thus, human albinism presents an excellent example of how intra-cortical self-organization during development allows abnormal representations to still subserve normal visual perception.

3.2.2. *Achiasma*

Albinism provided an example of how partial misrouting of the temporal retinal fibers can be successfully integrated into cortical topography as a mirror-symmetric map superimposed on the normal contralateral map. But what happens with a complete misrouting of the temporal retinal fibers? Is there a limit to the extent of such integration? Another relatively recently discovered congenital disorder called achiasma allows us to investigate these questions [118, 119].

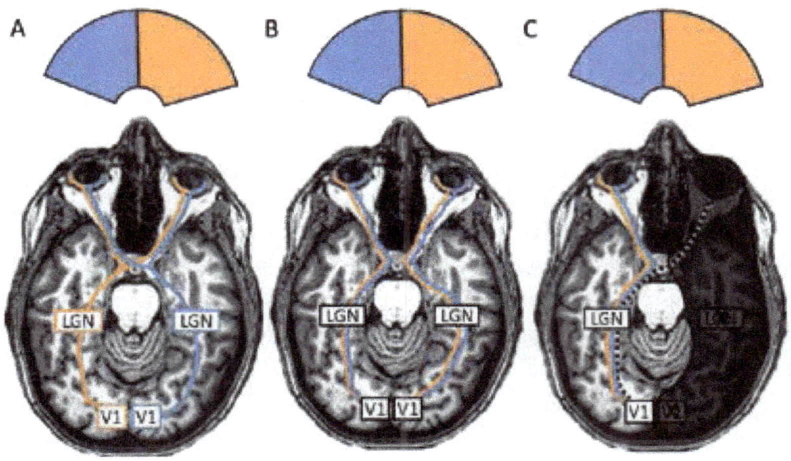

Figure 5. Visual Field Projections in Normal, Achiasmatic, and Missing Hemisphere Subjects. In all panels, blue represents the left half of visual space and tan represents the right side (top panel). (A) Normal subject. An image falling on the retinae is separated into nasal and temporal components in each eye. The part of the image within the left hemifield (blue) falls on the nasal retina in the left eye and the temporal retina in the right eye. The information from these two sections of each retina representing the left hemifield is transmitted through the optic nerve to the optic chiasm. To keep the correct hemifield information together for collective cortical processing, the axons from the nasal retina of the left eye cross over to the right optic tract at the optic chiasm, while the axons from the temporal retina of the right eye remain on the right side. Together, these sets of fibers carrying left hemifield image information then project first to the right lateral geniculate nucleus (LGN) of the thalamus and then through the optic radiations to V1 at the occipital pole of the right cortical hemisphere. Retinotopic organization is preserved along these pathways and then integrated into specific maps within visual cortex under the guidance of molecular cues and patterns of coordinated activity. The same pathways operate in reverse for the right hemifield (tan). Note that this results in one complete representation of visual space distributed across both hemispheres. (B) Achiasmatic subject. Because the fibers from the temporal retinae failed to properly cross at the expected region of the optic chiasm, information from each eye is passed only to the ipsilateral hemisphere. Thus, information from the left eye remains in the left hemisphere and information from the right eye remains in the right hemisphere. Note that this forms two complete representations of the full field of visual space, one for each eye, in each hemisphere. (C) Missing hemisphere subject. The development of the right hemisphere terminated in utero; therefore information from the left eye cannot possibly be passed to the right hemisphere. Instead, like achiasmatic subjects, the information remains in the ipsilateral hemisphere. Note that this means the entire visual field must be represented in the left hemisphere, resulting in one complete representation of visual space. The dotted black and white line represents possible remnants of connections to an undeveloped right eye.

Normally, molecular cues guide the axons of the retinal ganglion cells to either cross (temporal retinal fibers) to form the optic chiasm or to remain ipsilateral (nasal retinal fibers) (Figs. 4A, 5A). In individuals with achiasma, this crossing fails, with axons across each entire retina projecting through the ipsilateral thalamus to the ipsilateral cortical hemisphere (Fig. 5B) [118, 119]. The behavioral effects of this disorder can include deficits related to ocular instability (e.g., nystagmus, problems with stereopsis) [120 122].

Functional MRI was first used to investigate the topographical changes in achiasma by Victor et al. [120]. This study used a full field visual stimulus to show that stimulation of each eye produced functional activity within only the ipsilateral hemisphere. In addition, they found that the stimulation of each hemisphere produced overlapping activity within primary visual cortex. Their subjects had few visual deficits, other than problems related to ocular instability. These findings suggest successful integration of the misrouted visual pathways into the cortical topography. However, the pattern of cortical integration could not be determined from these methods.

With the development of higher resolution fMRI methods like TWR [34, 74] and pRF modeling [78], researchers have since been able to investigate more details about the topographical integration as well as changes in receptive field properties of regions within V1. A very recent study by Hoffman et al. [122] used both TWR and pRF to reveal that the congenital changes in achiasma drive developmental reorganization much like that seen in albinism. The complete misrouting of temporal retinal fibers was able to be successfully integrated as an overlapping, functional map of the ipsilateral visual field on top of that of the contralateral field (Fig. 5B). Further, the pRF measurements gave the first glimpse into human receptive field changes in these congenital disorders of visual pathway misrouting. Their results demonstrate pRFs that represent bilateral regions of the visual field in both striate and extrastriate VFMs along the medial occipital lobe.

Hoffman et al. [122] further used diffusion tensor imaging (DTI) to measure the general topography of the geniculostriate and occipital callosal connections in their achiasmatic subjects. Previous studies in achiasmatic dogs showed that the misrouted fibers formed retinotopic maps of opposing hemifields in adjacent layers of the LGN of the thalamus, suggesting no regorganization of geniculostriate pathways. The DTI measurements in human confirmed both that there were no significant changes in the input tracts to visual cortex as well as grossly normal topography in the inter-hemispheric callosal connections between the VFMs along the calcarine sulci. Together with the fMRI topographical and receptive field measurements, these findings by Hoffman et al. [122] suggest that the majority of the developmental reorganization in achiasma occurs in the intra-cortical local wiring within visual cortex.

3.3. How does the visual cortex reorganize following a massive cortical lesion in utero?

3.3.1. Missing hemisphere

In our last section, a dramatic recent example of a cortical lesion in utero allows us to examine the effects of a massive structural change to cortex on the development of cortical visual field representations. Muckli et al. [123] used TWR to study VFMs in a girl whose right cerebral hemisphere was completely absent at birth (Fig. 5C). She has only a rudimentary right eye and right optic nerve, but no right optic tract. Despite this extensive cortical loss and absent right eye, this subject has mostly normal visual function in both hemifields, with a mild left hemiplegia. Her spared bilateral visual functions suggest an enormous degree of developmental cortical reorganization [124].

In this very unusual case, the right hemisphere failed to develop around the seventh week of gestation due to an in utero lesion. Therefore, no crossing of temporal retinal fibers to the contralateral LGN and cerebral hemisphere was possible. Instead, the axons from the left retina carrying information from the entire visual scene (both hemifields) could only project to the occipital lobe of the left hemisphere (Fig. 5C).

In this situation, what happens with the integration of the retinal fibers from the single eye? As with the development of the visual pathways in congenital disorders with grossly intact cortical structures, four primary possibilities exist. The first could be termed 'normal' development, in which the contralateral visual field develops as usual and no ipsilateral representation is created, leading to a full left hemianopsia. The second is the opposite of the first, such that only the ipsilateral field is represented, leading to total right hemianopsia following suppression of the normal contralateral representation. The third is that contiguous VFMs, representing both hemifields, develop either as complete maps or in patches in place of contralateral hemifields. Finally, superimposed or interdigitated representations of the contralateral and ipsilateral hemifields may develop, as seen in albinism and achiasma. In addition, it is possible that more than one of these organizational structures could exist concurrently among VFMs, as seen in some non-primate albino mammals.

Interestingly, the TWR measurements by Muckli et al. [123] demonstrate such a concurrent existence of more than one organizational pattern in her intact left hemisphere. In V1, contiguous representations of both the contra- and ipsilateral visual fields were superimposed within the calcarine sulcus. However, discrete islands of ipsilateral quarterfield representations were also measured along the vertical meridian of V2 and V3, with a distortion of the contralateral visual field representations.

Why in this case do we see full field maps in addition to the superposition found in albinism and achiasma? Perhaps reorganization at an earlier stage of the visual pathways has occurred here. Muckli et al. [123] examined the organization of the visual field representations in the remaining left LGN. Unlike the reorganization seen in albinism [114] and achiasma [122] in which the contra- and ipsilateral representations remained segregated in the LGN, the measurements in this subject appeared to be fully overlapping, suggesting a greater degree of reorganization at this stage of visual processing. Similar LGN reorganization was measured in some albino cats and ferrets, which also had at least sections of contiguous full field visual field representations in their primary visual cortex [107-110].

The organization of the visual field representations is reflected in the extent of her preserved visual function. First, the fact that she has intact vision in the ipsilateral, right visual field demonstrates that the novel ipsilateral visual field representations are functionally relevant.

Second, visual perimetry mapping showed that both the right and left visual fields were centrally intact, but that both were somewhat restricted. Interestingly, the insertion of the ipsilateral islands into the contralateral representations resulted in both distortions of the cortical contralateral representations as well as concurrent distortions of her functional contralateral visual field. This restriction was more prominent in the upper visual field of both fields, in accord with the greater distortion of the contralateral visual field representation on the ventral cortical surface. The different patterns of self-organization in these VFMs in this unique case demonstrate a surprisingly flexible developmental restructuring in response to massive cortical loss.

4. Conclusion

This chapter has examined fMRI measurements of naturally-occurring cortical reorganization due to congenital abnormalities in the developing human visual system. These examples of retinal and genetic changes and cortical loss highlight the roles of plasticity and stability in the developing visual system. In these congenital conditions, the abnormally represented visual information has become available for grossly normal visual perception, despite limited compensatory alterations in the relatively stable geniculostriate projections. Together, these studies suggest that instead of large-scale reorganizations of the afferent visual pathways, relatively less drastic intra-cortical mechanisms underlie such developmental plasticity.

The next essential expansion of these findings is to apply our understanding of developmental plasticity to the controversial field of plasticity in adult sensory systems. Several aspects of cortical organization are thought to remain plastic into adulthood, allowing cortical sensori-motor maps to be modified continuously by experience. This dynamic nature of cortical circuitry is important for learning, as well as for repair following nervous system injury. Studies of the extent of cortical reorganization in adult primate visual cortex in response to changes in sensory input have produced quite disparate results, however (e.g., [1, 2, 125-138]). The ability to control cortical reorganization in the adult either by harnessing existing adult mechanisms for plasticity or by reactivating mechanisms of developmental plasticity would be a tremendous advancement in the treatment of cortical damage and neurodegenerative disease. The understanding of the balance of plasticity and stability in the human visual system arising from the examination of such congenital visual disorders as described here will be a key element of our progress towards this goal.

Acknowledgements

This work was supported by University of California, Irvine, startup funds to A.A.B.

Author details

Alyssa A. Brewer* and Brian Barton

*Address all correspondence to: aabrewer@uci.edu

Center for Cognitive Neuroscience and Department of Cognitive Sciences, University of California, Irvine, CA, USA

References

[1] J. C. Horton and D. R. Hocking, "Timing of the critical period for plasticity of ocular dominance columns in macaque striate cortex," J Neurosci, vol. 17, pp. 3684-709, May 15 1997.

[2] J. C. Horton and D. R. Hocking, "Effect of early monocular enucleation upon ocular dominance columns and cytochrome oxidase activity in monkey and human visual cortex," Vis Neurosci, vol. 15, pp. 289-303, Mar-Apr 1998.

[3] D. D. O'Leary, N. L. Ruff, and R. H. Dyck, "Development, critical period plasticity, and adult reorganizations of mammalian somatosensory systems," Curr Opin Neurobiol, vol. 4, pp. 535-44, Aug 1994.

[4] T. K. Hensch, "Critical period plasticity in local cortical circuits," Nat Rev Neurosci, vol. 6, pp. 877-88, Nov 2005.

[5] B. A. Wandell and S. M. Smirnakis, "Plasticity and stability of visual field maps in adult primary visual cortex," Nat Rev Neurosci, vol. 10, pp. 873-84, Dec 2009.

[6] S. M. Smirnakis, A. A. Brewer, M. C. Schmid, A. S. Tolias, A. Schuz, M. Augath, W. Inhoffen, B. A. Wandell, and N. K. Logothetis, "Lack of long-term cortical reorganization after macaque retinal lesions," Nature, vol. 435, pp. 300-7, May 19 2005.

[7] D. V. Buonomano and M. M. Merzenich, "Cortical plasticity: from synapses to maps," Annu Rev Neurosci, vol. 21, pp. 149-86, 1998.

[8] M. M. Merzenich, R. J. Nelson, M. P. Stryker, M. S. Cynader, A. Schoppmann, and J. M. Zook, "Somatosensory cortical map changes following digit amputation in adult monkeys," J Comp Neurol, vol. 224, pp. 591-605, Apr 20 1984.

[9] J. H. Kaas, M. M. Merzenich, and H. P. Killackey, "The reorganization of somatosensory cortex following peripheral nerve damage in adult and developing mammals," Annu Rev Neurosci, vol. 6, pp. 325-56, 1983.

[10] L. G. Cohen, P. Celnik, A. Pascual-Leone, B. Corwell, L. Falz, J. Dambrosia, M. Honda, N. Sadato, C. Gerloff, M. D. Catala, and M. Hallett, "Functional relevance of cross-modal plasticity in blind humans," Nature, vol. 389, pp. 180-3, Sep 11 1997.

[11] K. Fox and R. O. Wong, "A comparison of experience-dependent plasticity in the visual and somatosensory systems," Neuron, vol. 48, pp. 465-77, Nov 3 2005.

[12] C. D. Gilbert, W. Li, and V. Piech, "Perceptual learning and adult cortical plasticity," J Physiol, vol. 587, pp. 2743-51, Jun 15 2009.

[13] C. J. Shatz, "Emergence of order in visual system development," Proc Natl Acad Sci U S A, vol. 93, pp. 602-8, Jan 23 1996.

[14] D. H. Hubel, T. N. Wiesel, and S. LeVay, "Plasticity of ocular dominance columns in monkey striate cortex," Philos Trans R Soc Lond B Biol Sci, vol. 278, pp. 377-409, Apr 26 1977.

[15] B. Chapman, I. Godecke, and T. Bonhoeffer, "Development of orientation preference in the mammalian visual cortex," J Neurobiol, vol. 41, pp. 18-24, Oct 1999.

[16] M. Weliky and L. C. Katz, "Correlational structure of spontaneous neuronal activity in the developing lateral geniculate nucleus in vivo [see comments]," Science, vol. 285, pp. 599-604, 1999.

[17] L. C. Katz and C. J. Shatz, "Synaptic activity and the construction of cortical circuits," Science, vol. 274, pp. 1133-8, Nov 15 1996.

[18] C. J. Shatz and M. P. Stryker, "Ocular dominance in layer IV of the cat's visual cortex and the effects of monocular deprivation," J Physiol, vol. 281, pp. 267-83, Aug 1978.

[19] D. C. Van Essen, "Behind the optic nerve: an inside view of the primate visual system," Trans Am Ophthalmol Soc, vol. 93, pp. 123-33, 1995.

[20] J. C. Horton and D. R. Hocking, "An adult-like pattern of ocular dominance columns in striate cortex of newborn monkeys prior to visual experience.," Journal of Neuroscience, vol. 16, pp. 1791-1807, 1996.

[21] D. H. Hubel and T. N. Wiesel, "Receptive Fields of Cells in Striate Cortex of Very Young, Visually Inexperienced Kittens," J Neurophysiol, vol. 26, pp. 994-1002, Nov 1963.

[22] D. H. Hubel, T. N. Wiesel, and S. LeVay, "Functional architecture of area 17 in normal and monocularly deprived macaque monkeys," Cold Spring Harb Symp Quant Biol, vol. 40, pp. 581-9, 1976.

[23] T. N. Wiesel and D. H. Hubel, "Ordered arrangement of orientation columns in monkeys lacking visual experience," J Comp Neurol, vol. 158, pp. 307-18, Dec 1 1974.

[24] S. LeVay, M. P. Stryker, and C. J. Shatz, "Ocular dominance columns and their development in layer IV of the cat's visual cortex: a quantitative study.," Journal of Comparative Neurology, vol. 179, pp. 223-244, 1978.

[25] P. Rakic and M. S. Lidow, "Distribution and density of mnoamine receptor s in the primate visual cortex devoid of retinal input from early embryonic stagesemut f," J. Neuroscience, vol. 15, pp. 256-2574, 1995.

[26] D. Stellwagen, C. J. Shatz, and M. B. Feller, "Dynamics of retinal waves are controlled by cyclic AMP," Neuron, vol. 24, pp. 673-85, Nov 1999.

[27] M. P. Stryker and W. A. Harris, "Binocular impulse blockade prevents the formation of ocular dominance columns in cat visual cortex," J Neurosci, vol. 6, pp. 2117-33, Aug 1986.

[28] C. Zetterstrom, A. Lundvall, and M. Kugelberg, "Cataracts in children," J Cataract Refract Surg, vol. 31, pp. 824-40, Apr 2005.

[29] S. Awaya and S. Miyake, "Form vision deprivation amblyopia: further observations," Graefes Arch Clin Exp Ophthalmol, vol. 226, pp. 132-6, 1988.

[30] X. Li, S. O. Dumoulin, B. Mansouri, and R. F. Hess, "The fidelity of the cortical retinotopic map in human amblyopia," Eur J Neurosci, vol. 25, pp. 1265-77, Mar 2007.

[31] X. Li, S. O. Dumoulin, B. Mansouri, and R. F. Hess, "Cortical deficits in human amblyopia: their regional distribution and their relationship to the contrast detection deficit," Invest Ophthalmol Vis Sci, vol. 48, pp. 1575-91, Apr 2007.

[32] A. A. Brewer and B. Barton, "Visual field map organization in human visual cortex," in Visual Cortex - Current Status and Perspectives, S. Molotchnikoff and J. Rouat, Eds., ed: InTech, 2012, pp. 30-60.

[33] B. A. Wandell, A. A. Brewer, and R. F. Dougherty, "Visual field map clusters in human cortex," Philos Trans R Soc Lond B Biol Sci, vol. 360, pp. 693-707, Apr 29 2005.

[34] B. A. Wandell, S. O. Dumoulin, and A. A. Brewer, "Visual field maps in human cortex," Neuron, vol. 56, pp. 366-83, Oct 25 2007.

[35] D. C. Van Essen, "Organization of Visual Areas in Macaque and Human Cerebral Cortex," in The Visual Neurosciences, L. M. Chalupa and J. S. Werner, Eds., ed Boston: Bradford Books, 2003.

[36] J. H. Kaas, "Topographic Maps are Fundamental to Sensory Processing," Brain Research Bulletin, vol. 44, pp. 107–112, 1997.

[37] S. Zeki, "Improbable areas in the visual brain," Trends Neurosci, vol. 26, pp. 23-6, Jan 2003.

[38] B. A. Wandell and J. Winawer, "Imaging retinotopic maps in the human brain," Vision Res, Aug 6 2010.

[39] N. K. Logothetis and B. A. Wandell, "Interpreting the BOLD signal," Annu Rev Physiol, vol. 66, pp. 735-69, 2004.

[40] S. Ogawa, T. M. Lee, A. R. Kay, and D. W. Tank, "Brain magnetic resonance imaging with contrast dependent on blood oxygenation," Proc Natl Acad Sci U S A, vol. 87, pp. 9868-72, Dec 1990.

[41] D. J. Heeger and D. Ress, "What does fMRI tell us about neuronal activity?," Nat Rev Neurosci, vol. 3, pp. 142-51, Feb 2002.

[42] P. A. Bandettini, E. C. Wong, R. S. Hinks, R. S. Tikofsky, and J. S. Hyde, "Time course EPI of human brain function during task activation," Magn Reson Med, vol. 25, pp. 390-7, Jun 1992.

[43] A. K. Liu, J. W. Belliveau, and A. M. Dale, "Spatiotemporal imaging of human brain activity using functional MRI constrained magnetoencephalography data: Monte Carlo simulations," Proc Natl Acad Sci U S A, vol. 95, pp. 8945-50, Jul 21 1998.

[44] M. B. Hoffmann, J. Stadler, M. Kanowski, and O. Speck, "Retinotopic mapping of the human visual cortex at a magnetic field strength of 7T," Clin Neurophysiol, vol. 120, pp. 108-16, Jan 2009.

[45] J. D. Swisher, J. C. Gatenby, J. C. Gore, B. A. Wolfe, C. H. Moon, S. G. Kim, and F. Tong, "Multiscale pattern analysis of orientation-selective activity in the primary visual cortex," J Neurosci, vol. 30, pp. 325-30, Jan 6 2010.

[46] C. Triantafyllou, R. D. Hoge, G. Krueger, C. J. Wiggins, A. Potthast, G. C. Wiggins, and L. L. Wald, "Comparison of physiological noise at 1.5 T, 3 T and 7 T and optimization of fMRI acquisition parameters," Neuroimage, vol. 26, pp. 243-50, May 15 2005.

[47] E. Disbrow, T. P. Roberts, D. Slutsky, and L. Krubitzer, "The use of fMRI for determining the topographic organization of cortical fields in human and nonhuman primates," Brain Res, vol. 829, pp. 167-73, May 22 1999.

[48] N. K. Logothetis, "What we can do and what we cannot do with fMRI," Nature, vol. 453, pp. 869-78, Jun 12 2008.

[49] Y. Ejima, S. Takahashi, H. Yamamoto, M. Fukunaga, C. Tanaka, T. Ebisu, and M. Umeda, "Interindividual and interspecies variations of the extrastriate visual cortex," Neuroreport, vol. 14, pp. 1579-83, Aug 26 2003.

[50] N. K. Chen and A. M. Wyrwicz, "Correction for EPI distortions using multi-echo gradient-echo imaging," Magn Reson Med, vol. 41, pp. 1206-13, Jun 1999.

[51] M. Lauritzen, "Relationship of spikes, synaptic activity, and local changes of cerebral blood flow," J Cereb Blood Flow Metab, vol. 21, pp. 1367-83, Dec 2001.

[52] A. Seiyama, J. Seki, H. C. Tanabe, I. Sase, A. Takatsuki, S. Miyauchi, H. Eda, S. Hayashi, T. Imaruoka, T. Iwakura, and T. Yanagida, "Circulatory basis of fMRI signals: re-

lationship between changes in the hemodynamic parameters and BOLD signal intensity," Neuroimage, vol. 21, pp. 1204-14, Apr 2004.

[53] J. Winawer, H. Horiguchi, R. A. Sayres, K. Amano, and B. A. Wandell, "Mapping hV4 and ventral occipital cortex: the venous eclipse," J Vis, vol. 10, p. 1, 2010.

[54] A. A. Brewer, J. Liu, A. R. Wade, and B. A. Wandell, "Visual field maps and stimulus selectivity in human ventral occipital cortex," Nat Neurosci, vol. 8, pp. 1102-9, Aug 2005.

[55] K. A. Hansen, K. N. Kay, and J. L. Gallant, "Topographic organization in and near human visual area V4," J Neurosci, vol. 27, pp. 11896-911, Oct 31 2007.

[56] A. R. Wade, A. A. Brewer, J. W. Rieger, and B. A. Wandell, "Functional measurements of human ventral occipital cortex: retinotopy and colour," Philos Trans R Soc Lond B Biol Sci, vol. 357, pp. 963-73, Aug 29 2002.

[57] J. Larsson and D. J. Heeger, "Two retinotopic visual areas in human lateral occipital cortex," J Neurosci, vol. 26, pp. 13128-42, Dec 20 2006.

[58] R. B. Tootell and N. Hadjikhani, "Where is 'dorsal V4' in human visual cortex? Retinotopic, topographic and functional evidence," Cereb Cortex, vol. 11, pp. 298-311, Apr 2001.

[59] N. Hadjikhani, A. K. Liu, A. M. Dale, P. Cavanagh, and R. B. Tootell, "Retinotopy and color sensitivity in human visual cortical area V8," Nat Neurosci, vol. 1, pp. 235-41, Jul 1998.

[60] B. A. Wandell, S. Chial, and B. Backus, "Visualization and Measurement of the Cortical Surface," J. of Cognitive Neuroscience, vol. 12, pp. 739-52, 2000.

[61] P. C. Teo, G. Sapiro, and B. A. Wandell, "Creating connected representations of cortical gray matter for functional MRI visualization," IEEE Trans Med Imaging, vol. 16, pp. 852-63, Dec 1997.

[62] D. C. Van Essen, J. W. Lewis, H. A. Drury, N. Hadjikhani, R. B. Tootell, M. Bakircioglu, and M. I. Miller, "Mapping visual cortex in monkeys and humans using surface-based atlases," Vision Res, vol. 41, pp. 1359-78, 2001.

[63] A. M. Dale, B. Fischl, and M. I. Sereno, "Cortical surface-based analysis. I. Segmentation and surface reconstruction," Neuroimage, vol. 9, pp. 179-94, Feb 1999.

[64] H. Kolster, R. Peeters, and G. A. Orban, "The retinotopic organization of the human middle temporal area MT/V5 and its cortical neighbors," J Neurosci, vol. 30, pp. 9801-20, Jul 21 2010.

[65] X. Yue, B. S. Cassidy, K. J. Devaney, D. J. Holt, and R. B. Tootell, "Lower-level stimulus features strongly influence responses in the fusiform face area," Cereb Cortex, vol. 21, pp. 35-47, Jan 2011.

[66] T. Liu, F. Pestilli, and M. Carrasco, "Transient attention enhances perceptual performance and FMRI response in human visual cortex," Neuron, vol. 45, pp. 469-77, Feb 3 2005.

[67] J. S. Peper, R. M. Brouwer, D. I. Boomsma, R. S. Kahn, and H. E. Hulshoff Pol, "Genetic influences on human brain structure: a review of brain imaging studies in twins," Hum Brain Mapp, vol. 28, pp. 464-73, Jun 2007.

[68] W. F. Baare, H. E. Hulshoff Pol, D. I. Boomsma, D. Posthuma, E. J. de Geus, H. G. Schnack, N. E. van Haren, C. J. van Oel, and R. S. Kahn, "Quantitative genetic modeling of variation in human brain morphology," Cereb Cortex, vol. 11, pp. 816-24, Sep 2001.

[69] R. F. Dougherty, V. M. Koch, A. A. Brewer, B. Fischer, J. Modersitzki, and B. A. Wandell, "Visual field representations and locations of visual areas V1/2/3 in human visual cortex," J Vis, vol. 3, pp. 586-98, 2003.

[70] M. P. Bryden, H. Hecaen, and M. DeAgostini, "Patterns of cerebral organization," Brain Lang, vol. 20, pp. 249-62, Nov 1983.

[71] R. A. Harshman, E. Hampson, and S. A. Berenbaum, "Individual differences in cognitive abilities and brain organization, Part I: Sex and handedness differences in ability," Can J Psychol, vol. 37, pp. 144-92, Mar 1983.

[72] J. H. Kaas, "The evolution of the complex sensory and motor systems of the human brain," Brain Res Bull, vol. 75, pp. 384-90, Mar 18 2008.

[73] S. A. Engel, G. H. Glover, and B. A. Wandell, "Retinotopic organization in human visual cortex and the spatial precision of functional MRI," Cereb Cortex, vol. 7, pp. 181-92, Mar 1997.

[74] S. A. Engel, D. E. Rumelhart, B. A. Wandell, A. T. Lee, G. H. Glover, E. J. Chichilnisky, and M. N. Shadlen, "fMRI of human visual cortex," Nature, vol. 369, p. 525, Jun 16 1994.

[75] M. I. Sereno, A. M. Dale, J. B. Reppas, K. K. Kwong, J. W. Belliveau, T. J. Brady, B. R. Rosen, and R. B. Tootell, "Borders of multiple visual areas in humans revealed by functional magnetic resonance imaging," Science, vol. 268, pp. 889-93, May 12 1995.

[76] E. A. DeYoe, G. J. Carman, P. Bandettini, S. Glickman, J. Wieser, R. Cox, D. Miller, and J. Neitz, "Mapping striate and extrastriate visual areas in human cerebral cortex," Proc. Natl. Acad. Sci. (USA), vol. 93, pp. 2382-2386, 1996.

[77] S. A. Engel, "The development and use of phase-encoded functional MRI designs," Neuroimage, vol. 62, pp. 1195 - 200, Aug 15 2012.

[78] S. O. Dumoulin and B. A. Wandell, "Population receptive field estimates in human visual cortex," Neuroimage, vol. 39, pp. 647-60, Jan 15 2008.

[79] A. T. Smith, K. D. Singh, A. L. Williams, and M. W. Greenlee, "Estimating receptive field size from fMRI data in human striate and extrastriate visual cortex," Cereb Cortex, vol. 11, pp. 1182-90, Dec 2001.

[80] B. A. Wandell and J. Winawer, "Imaging retinotopic maps in the human brain," Vision Res, vol. 51, pp. 718-37, Apr 13 2011.

[81] K. Amano, B. A. Wandell, and S. O. Dumoulin, "Visual field maps, population receptive field sizes, and visual field coverage in the human MT+ complex," Journal of Neurophysiology, vol. 102, pp. 2704-18, Nov 2009.

[82] J. D. Victor, K. Purpura, E. Katz, and B. Mao, "Population encoding of spatial frequency, orientation, and color in macaque V1," J Neurophysiol, vol. 72, pp. 2151-66, Nov 1994.

[83] R. B. Tootell, J. D. Mendola, N. K. Hadjikhani, P. J. Ledden, A. K. Liu, J. B. Reppas, M. I. Sereno, and A. M. Dale, "Functional analysis of V3A and related areas in human visual cortex," J Neurosci, vol. 17, pp. 7060-78, Sep 15 1997.

[84] B. M. Harvey and S. O. Dumoulin, "The relationship between cortical magnification factor and population receptive field size in human visual cortex: constancies in cortical architecture," J Neurosci, vol. 31, pp. 13604-12, Sep 21 2011.

[85] M. I. Sereno, H. H. Yu, and E. K. Vogel, "Mapping Retinotopy in Higher Level Extrastriate Visual Areas in Humans," in Society for Neuroscience, San Diego, 2001.

[86] M. I. Sereno, S. Pitzalis, and A. Martinez, "Mapping of contralateral space in retinotopic coordinates by a parietal cortical area in humans," Science, vol. 294, pp. 1350-4, Nov 9 2001.

[87] W. Zuiderbaan, B. M. Harvey, and S. O. Dumoulin, "Modeling center-surround configurations in population receptive fields using fMRI," J Vis, vol. 12, p. 10, 2012.

[88] H. J. Neville and D. Bavelier, "Variability of developmental plasticity," in Mechanisms of Cognitive Develoment: Behavioral and Neural Perspectives, J. L. McClelland and R. S. Siegler, Eds., ed New Jersey: Lawrence Erlbaum Associates, Inc., 2001.

[89] M. M. Merzenich and K. Sameshima, "Cortical plasticity and memory," Curr Opin Neurobiol, vol. 3, pp. 187-96, Apr 1993.

[90] P. Sinha and M. Meng, "Superimposed hemifields in primary visual cortex of achiasmic individuals," Neuron, vol. 75, pp. 353-5, Aug 9 2012.

[91] C. A. Curcio, K. R. Sloan, R. E. Kalina, and A. E. Hendrickson, "Human photoreceptor topography," J Comp Neurol, vol. 292, pp. 497-523, Feb 22 1990.

[92] C. A. Curcio, K. R. S. Jr., O. Pakcer, A. E. Hendrickson, and R. E. Kalina, "Distribution of cones in human and monkey retina: individual variaibility and radial asymmetry," in Science, 1987, pp. 579-581.

[93] K. R. Duffy and D. H. Hubel, "Receptive field properties of neurons in the primary visual cortex under photopic and scotopic lighting conditions," Vision Res, vol. 47, pp. 2569-74, Sep 2007.

[94] J. C. Horton and W. F. Hoyt, "The representation of the visual field in human striate cortex. A revision of the classic Holmes map," Arch Ophthalmol, vol. 109, pp. 816-24, Jun 1991.

[95] H. A. Baseler, A. A. Brewer, L. T. Sharpe, A. B. Morland, H. Jagle, and B. A. Wandell, "Reorganization of human cortical maps caused by inherited photoreceptor abnormalities," Nat Neurosci, vol. 5, pp. 364-70, Apr 2002.

[96] N. Hadjikhani and R. B. Tootell, "Projection of rods and cones within human visual cortex," Hum Brain Mapp, vol. 9, pp. 55-63, 2000.

[97] D. H. Hubel, "Vision in dim light," Nature, vol. 388, pp. 32-3, Jul 3 1997.

[98] D. H. Hubel, P. D. Howe, A. M. Duffy, and A. Hernandez, "Scotopic foveal afterimages," Perception, vol. 38, pp. 313-6, 2009.

[99] S. Kohl, B. Baumann, M. Broghammer, H. Jagle, P. Sieving, U. Kellner, R. Spegal, M. Anastasi, E. Zrenner, L. T. Sharpe, and B. Wissinger, "Mutations in the CNGB3 gene encoding the beta-subunit of the cone photoreceptor cGMP-gated channel are responsible for achromatopsia (ACHM3) linked to chromosome 8q21," Hum Mol Genet, vol. 9, pp. 2107-16, Sep 1 2000.

[100] S. Kohl, T. Marx, I. Giddings, H. Jagle, S. G. Jacobson, E. Apfelstedt-Sylla, E. Zrenner, L. T. Sharpe, and B. Wissinger, "Total colourblindness is caused by mutations in the gene encoding the alpha-subunit of the cone photoreceptor cGMP-gated cation channel," Nat Genet, vol. 19, pp. 257-9, Jul 1998.

[101] M. Glickstein and G. G. Heath, "Receptors in the monochromat eye," Vision Res, vol. 15, pp. 633-6, Jun 1975.

[102] J. L. Rees, "Genetics of hair and skin color," Annu Rev Genet, vol. 37, pp. 67-90, 2003.

[103] P. Hedera, S. Lai, E. M. Haacke, A. J. Lerner, A. L. Hopkins, J. S. Lewin, and R. P. Friedland, "Abnormal connectivity of the visual pathways in human albinos demonstrated by susceptibility-sensitized MRI," Neurology, vol. 44, pp. 1921-6, Oct 1994.

[104] A. B. Morland, M. B. Hoffmann, M. Neveu, and G. E. Holder, "Abnormal visual projection in a human albino studied with functional magnetic resonance imaging and visual evoked potentials," J Neurol Neurosurg Psychiatry, vol. 72, pp. 523-6, Apr 2002.

[105] R. W. Guillery, "Neural abnormalities of albinos," Trends in Neurosciences, vol. 9, pp. 364-367, 1986.

[106] A. B. Morland, H. A. Baseler, M. B. Hoffmann, L. T. Sharpe, and B. A. Wandell, "Abnormal retinotopic representations in human visual cortex revealed by fMRI," Acta Psychol (Amst), vol. 107, pp. 229-47, Apr 2001.

[107] R. W. Guillery, V. A. Casagrande, and M. D. Oberdorfer, "Congenitally abnormal vision in Siamese cats," Nature, vol. 252, pp. 195-9, Nov 15 1974.

[108] D. H. Hubel and T. N. Wiesel, "Aberrant visual projections in the Siamese cat," J Physiol, vol. 218, pp. 33-62, Oct 1971.

[109] K. Huang and R. W. Guillery, "A demonstration of two distinct geniculocortical projection patterns in albino ferrets," Brain Res, vol. 352, pp. 213-20, Jun 1985.

[110] J. H. Kaas and R. W. Guillery, "The transfer of abnormal visual field representations from the dorsal lateral geniculate nucleus to the visual cortex in Siamese cats," Brain Res, vol. 59, pp. 61-95, Sep 14 1973.

[111] E. I. Elekessy, J. E. Campion, and G. H. Henry, "Differences between the visual fields of Siamese and common cats," Vision Res, vol. 13, pp. 2533-43, Dec 1973.

[112] M. L. Cooper and G. G. Blasdel, "Regional variation in the representation of the visual field in the visual cortex of the Siamese cat," J Comp Neurol, vol. 193, pp. 237-53, Sep 1 1980.

[113] R. W. Guillery, T. L. Hickey, J. H. Kaas, D. J. Felleman, E. J. Debruyn, and D. L. Sparks, "Abnormal central visual pathways in the brain of an albino green monkey (Cercopithecus aethiops)," J Comp Neurol, vol. 226, pp. 165-83, Jun 20 1984.

[114] M. B. Hoffmann, D. J. Tolhurst, A. T. Moore, and A. B. Morland, "Organization of the visual cortex in human albinism," J Neurosci, vol. 23, pp. 8921-30, Oct 1 2003.

[115] M. B. Hoffmann, P. S. Seufert, and L. C. Schmidtborn, "Perceptual relevance of abnormal visual field representations: static visual field perimetry in human albinism," Br J Ophthalmol, vol. 91, pp. 509-13, Apr 2007.

[116] M. B. Hoffmann, B. Lorenz, A. B. Morland, and L. C. Schmidtborn, "Misrouting of the optic nerves in albinism: estimation of the extent with visual evoked potentials," Invest Ophthalmol Vis Sci, vol. 46, pp. 3892-8, Oct 2005.

[117] J. Klemen, M. B. Hoffmann, and C. D. Chambers, "Cortical plasticity in the face of congenitally altered input into V1," Cortex, Mar 23 2012.

[118] P. Apkarian, L. Bour, and P. G. Barth, "A unique achiasmatic anomaly detected in non-albinos with misrouted retinal fugal projections," Eur J Neurosci, vol. 6, pp. 501-7, Mar 1 1994.

[119] P. Apkarian, L. J. Bour, P. G. Barth, L. Wenniger-Prick, and B. Verbeeten, Jr., "Non-decussating retinal-fugal fibre syndrome. An inborn achiasmatic malformation associated with visuotopic misrouting, visual evoked potential ipsilateral asymmetry and nystagmus," Brain, vol. 118 (Pt 5), pp. 1195-216, Oct 1995.

[120] J. D. Victor, P. Apkarian, J. Hirsch, M. M. Conte, M. Packard, N. R. Relkin, K. H. Kim, and R. M. Shapley, "Visual function and brain organization in non-decussating retinal-fugal fibre syndrome," Cereb Cortex, vol. 10, pp. 2-22, Jan 2000.

[121] S. Prakash, S. O. Dumoulin, N. Fischbein, B. A. Wandell, and Y. J. Liao, "Congenital achiasma and see-saw nystagmus in VACTERL syndrome," J Neuroophthalmol, vol. 30, pp. 45-8, Mar 2010.

[122] M. B. Hoffmann, F. R. Kaule, N. Levin, Y. Masuda, A. Kumar, I. Gottlob, H. Horiguchi, R. F. Dougherty, J. Stadler, B. Wolynski, O. Speck, M. Kanowski, Y. J. Liao, B. A. Wandell, and S. O. Dumoulin, "Plasticity and stability of the visual system in human achiasma," Neuron, vol. 75, pp. 393-401, Aug 9 2012.

[123] L. Muckli, M. J. Naumer, and W. Singer, "Bilateral visual field maps in a patient with only one hemisphere," Proc Natl Acad Sci U S A, vol. 106, pp. 13034-9, Aug 4 2009.

[124] A. A. Brewer, "Visual maps: To merge or not to merge," Curr Biol, vol. 19, pp. R945-7, Nov 3 2009.

[125] C. Darian-Smith and C. D. Gilbert, "Axonal sprouting accompanies functional reorganization in adult cat striate cortex.," Nature, vol. 368, pp. 737-740, 1994.

[126] G. C. DeAngelis, A. Anzai, I. Ohzawa, and R. D. Freeman, "Receptive field structure in the visual cortex: does selective stimulation induce plasticity?," Proc Natl Acad Sci U S A, vol. 92, pp. 9682-6, Oct 10 1995.

[127] J. C. Horton and D. R. Hocking, "Monocular core zones and binocular border strips in primate striate cortex revealed by the contrasting effects of enucleation, eyelid suture, and retinal laser lesions on cytochrome oxidase activity," J Neurosci, vol. 18, pp. 5433-55, Jul 15 1998.

[128] J. H. Kaas, "Plasticity of sensory and motor maps in adult mammals.," Annual Review of Neuroscience, vol. 14, pp. 137-167, 1991.

[129] C. I. Baker, E. Peli, N. Knouf, and N. G. Kanwisher, "Reorganization of visual processing in macular degeneration," J Neurosci, vol. 25, pp. 614-8, Jan 19 2005.

[130] C. D. Gilbert and T. N. Wiesel, "Receptive field dynamics in adult primary visual cortex," Nature, vol. 356, pp. 150-2, Mar 12 1992.

[131] Y. M. Chino, J. H. Kaas, E. L. Smith, 3rd, A. L. Langston, and H. Cheng, "Rapid reorganization of cortical maps in adult cats following restricted deafferentation in retina," Vision Res, vol. 32, pp. 789-96, May 1992.

[132] C. Darian-Smith and C. D. Gilbert, "Topographic reorganization in the striate cortex of the adult cat and monkey is cortically mediated," J Neurosci, vol. 15, pp. 1631-47, Mar 1995.

[133] A. Das and C. D. Gilbert, "Topography of contextual modulations mediated by short-range interactions in primary visual cortex," Nature, vol. 399, pp. 655-61, Jun 17 1999.

[134] A. Das and C. D. Gilbert, "Long-range horizontal connections and their role in cortical reorganization revealed by optical recording of cat primary visual cortex," Nature, vol. 375, pp. 780-4, Jun 29 1995.

[135] J. S. Sunness, T. Liu, and S. Yantis, "Retinotopic mapping of the visual cortex using functional magnetic resonance imaging in a patient with central scotomas from atrophic macular degeneration," Ophthalmology, vol. 111, pp. 1595-8, Aug 2004.

[136] J. H. Kaas, L. A. Krubitzer, Y. M. Chino, A. L. Langston, E. H. Polley, and N. Blair, "Reorganization of retinotopic cortical maps in adult mammals after lesions of the retina," Science, vol. 248, pp. 229-31, Apr 13 1990.

[137] H. A. Baseler, A. B. Morland, and B. A. Wandell, "Topographic organization of human visual areas in the absence of input from primary cortex," J Neurosci, vol. 19, pp. 2619-27, Apr 1 1999.

[138] C. D. Gilbert, "Adult cortical dynamics," Physiol Rev, vol. 78, pp. 467-85, Apr 1998.

5

Feedback Regulation of Limb Position Characterized Using fMRI

Aaron J. Suminski and Robert A. Scheidt

1. Introduction

Functional magnetic resonance imaging (FMRI) is a powerful tool for exploring the neural basis of sensory control of movement and it has profitably been used to study simple actions like finger-tapping (Rao et al., 1996), compensation for visual feedback distortions during movement (Imamizu et al., 2000) and regulation of isometric force (Peck et al., 2001; Kawato et al., 2003; Vaillancourt et al., 2003). However, use of FMRI to image neural mechanisms contributing to more complex motor tasks like stabilization of limb position in the face of environmental perturbation has been limited because such tasks require mechanically-active, MRI-compatible devices capable to perturb the limb in a controlled manner. Here, we present a case study on the development and validation of a MRI-compatible device specifically for use in studying sensorimotor control in the presence of environmental perturbations. We then demonstrate the device in a functional imaging study of limb posture regulation wherein healthy human subjects stabilized their wrists against predictable and unpredictable loads. In particular, we sought to understand how the brain uses somatosensory information to adjust behavioral strategies for load compensation.

We anticipated that multiple strategies might be used to stabilize the limb against perturbation, and that distinct neural mechanisms would implement these strategies. We therefore hypothesized that at least two distinct neural mechanisms contribute to the stabilization of wrist position in the presence of persistent environmental perturbations. A first mechanism likely mediates the online control of endpoint position (not joint torque) via feedback control. Feedback control attempts to adjust motor commands to cancel deviations of the limb from its desired state. Thus we expect regions contributing to feedback control of wrist position to show increased FMRI BOLD response in the presence of positioning errors, independent of joint torque magnitude. Moreover, temporal variations in the BOLD response in these regions should correlate with variations in wrist position on a moment-by-moment basis. A second mechanism likely monitors performance over a longer timeframe than an online feedback controller. This mechanism would initiate discrete, conditional, corrective actions when feedback control fails to eliminate persistent errors. Regions contributing to this higher-order evaluation of performance should demonstrate BOLD responses that reflect changes in positioning errors with a longer temporal integration period than that used for moment-by-moment feedback control.

Portions of this chapter have appeared previously in separate publications (Suminski et al., 2007b; Suminski et al., 2007a).

2. Development of a MRI-compatible manipulandum

Devices intended for use in MRI environments must: 1) satisfy noise tolerance and size limitations imposed by MR scanner technologies, and 2) be constructed of MR compatible materials (Schenck, 1996; Chinzei et al.). The large static magnetic field generated by the scanner precludes use of ferromagnetic materials that would otherwise be attracted into the scanner bore, compromising safety of both the research subject and the scanner. It is also essential that all actuators and sensors in the device be impervious to rapidly switching imaging gradients and that device operation does not disturb the homogeneity of the magnetic field, which would lead to image distortion. Finally, the device must have a small form factor, capable to fit inside the scanner bore without causing subject discomfort. To date, a small number of such robotic devices have been developed for use in neuroscience research or rehabilitation applications (Suminski et al., 2002; Ganesh et al.,2004; Diedrichsen et al., 2005; Flueckiger et al., 2005; Khanicheh et al., 2005; Gassert et al., 2006; Khanicheh et al., 2008; Yu et al., 2008). In this section we describe the design, performance characteristics and validation of a novel, MR compatible, 1 degree-of-freedom (DOF), pneumatically actuated robot for motor control research (Fig. 1). Our aim was to create a device able to both monitor and perturb wrist motion during FMRI, and to demonstrate device safety and efficacy as a tool for the study of complex motor behavior in human subjects.

2.1. Device design and performance characteristics

We used a pneumatic actuator to exert computer-controlled torques about the wrist because this type of actuator can be MR compatible, small, light-weight and back-driveable. A single bellows-type actuator was enclosed within a curved volume. This actuator transmits force from compressed air to a wall rigidly attached to the device's handle. Pressurizing the actuator generates an extensor torque about the subject's right wrist whereas pulling a vacuum within the actuator imparts a flexor torque. Air pressure within the actuator is sensed by a pressure transducer (26PC Series, Honeywell International, Inc., Morristown, NJ), amplified (x25) and low-pass filtered (20Hz cutoff frequency) in hardware. Joint angle is sensed with an optical encoder (HEDM-6540, Agilent Technologies, Inc., Palo Alto, CA) located on the underside of the device. The device monitors wrist position to within 0.05° and wrist torque to within 0.001

Nm. Only the manipulandum, pressure transducer, optical encoder and necessary instrumentation are located within the MR environment; all other control components are located in the scanner control room. The manipulandum can accommodate both right- and left-handed individuals, providing 80° range of motion at the wrist (40° flexion to 40° extension). Pressure within the actuator is regulated by a Proportion Air QB3 electro-pneumatic pressure valve (Proportion-Air Inc., McCordsville, IN). Wrist angle and actuator pressure data are acquired at a rate of 1000 samples per second. Commands to the pressure valve are generated at the same rate.

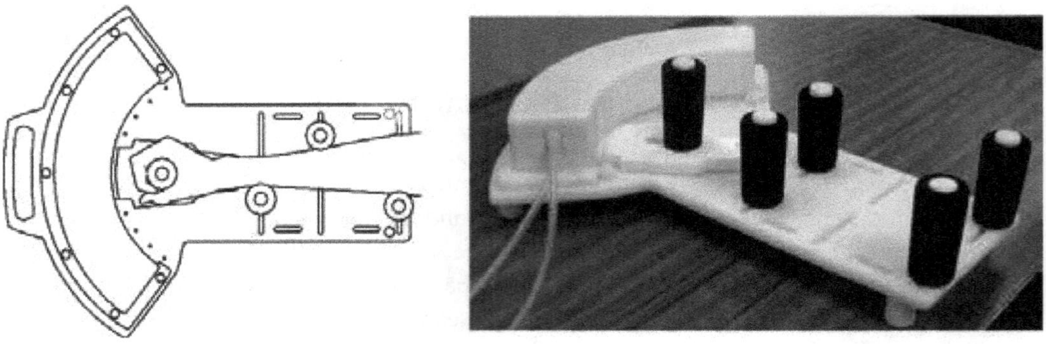

Figure 1. Schematic representation and a photograph of the 1 DOF pneumatic manipulandum.

We implemented a proportional-integral-derivative (PID) controller to improve the ability of the device to quickly and accurately regulate pressure within the pneumatic actuator.

$$P_C(t) = K_P e(t) + K_I \int e(t)dt + K_D \dot{e}(t) \tag{1}$$

where $P_C(t)$ is the commanded actuator pressure in units of psi, e(t) is the difference between the measured and desired actuator pressure in units of psi, K_P is the proportional gain, K_I is the integral gain, and K_D is the derivative gain. Ziegler-Nichols tuning rules were used to tune the controller (Ziegler and Nichols, 1942), yielding the following gain values: $K_P = 3.3$, $K_I = 14$, and $K_D = 0.055$. Under PID control, step response rise times (10% to 90% steady state) were 77ms and 90ms for 1 and 2 PSI step changes, respectively, with modest overshoot (19%; Fig. 2A). Due to time required to transmit air from the MRI control room to the actuator, we observed an average time delay (command onset to 10% steady state) of 62ms for both step responses.

We identified the bandwidth of the closed-loop system by assessing the system's ability to track changes in commanded actuator pressure having a 1 PSI peak-to-peak 'chirp' profile sweeping from 0 to 5Hz. The device is able to track commanded pressure changes within ±15% of the peak pressure up to 1.6 Hz (Fig. 2B). These frequency response characteristics allow the robot to apply torsional spring-like loads about the wrist. By way of demonstration, we commanded the robot to apply two separate position-dependent loads (0.075 and 0.15 Nm/°)

and estimated the realized spring constants obtained during 25° flexion/extension movements performed by a representative human subject. The estimated stiffness of the two spring-like loads, obtained by fitting a linear model to the joint torque vs. joint angle data, were 0.059 and 0.134 Nm/° respectively, yielding an average error of 16%. In both cases, the torque-angle relationships were linear, with regression r^2 values exceeding 96% and 99% for the 0.075 and 0.15 Nm/° loads, respectively (Fig. 2C).

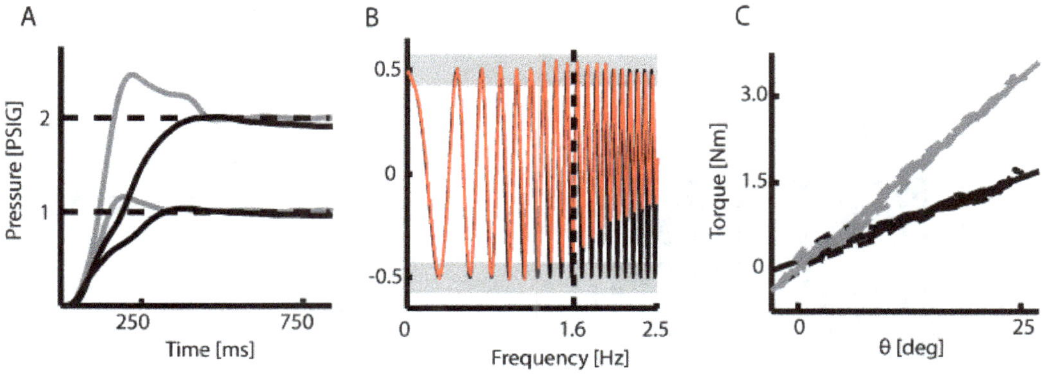

Figure 2. (A) Responses of the robot to 1 and 2 PSI step changes in pressure under open loop control (i.e. no pressure feedback to controller; black lines) and closed loop PID control (i.e. real-time feedback of actual actuator pressure to the controller; gray lines). (B) The frequency response of the system under closed loop control (red line) was identified by assessing the system's ability to track a desired actuator pressure signal sweeping from 0 to 5Hz (black line). The upper bound on the system's bandwidth was defined to be the frequency at which the controller was unable to regulate the actuator pressure within 15% of the peak commanded pressure (horizontal gray bars). (C) Spring constants for two simulated loads (0.075 and 0.15 Nm/°; dashed black and gray lines, respectively) estimated by fitting a line to the joint torque and wrist angle data (solid lines). Figure adapted from Suminski et al., 2007a.

2.2. MR-compatibility testing

We validated the simultaneous acquisition of manipulandum data and FMRI images by scanning a spherical head phantom both with and without the robotic device in a 3.0T GE Excite HD MR scanner (General Electric Healthcare, Milwaukee, WI). The phantom (Fig. 3A, P; GE Model #: 2359877) was supported within a split transmit/receive quadrature head coil (Fig. 3A, HC; GE Model #: 2376114). A gradient echo, echo planar imaging (EPI) pulse sequence (29 contiguous sagittal slices; echo time (TE) = 25ms, inter-scan period (TR) = 2s, flip angle = 77°, field of view (FOV) = 24cm, 64 x 64 matrix; 3.75x3.75x6 mm spatial resolution) was used to verify: 1) that operation of the robot during scanning does not induce significant artifacts in functional images, and 2) that the robot can measure pressure and joint angle without contamination from gradient switching noise during EPI.

Validation testing used a blocked experimental design (Duration = 270s). During "Motion" states, the computer cycled the device's handle through a sinusoidal trajectory (0.25 cycles per second) whereas the device remained motionless during "No Motion" states (50% duty cycle; period = 60s). Raw, complex k-space data (I and Q channels) were collected to allow analysis

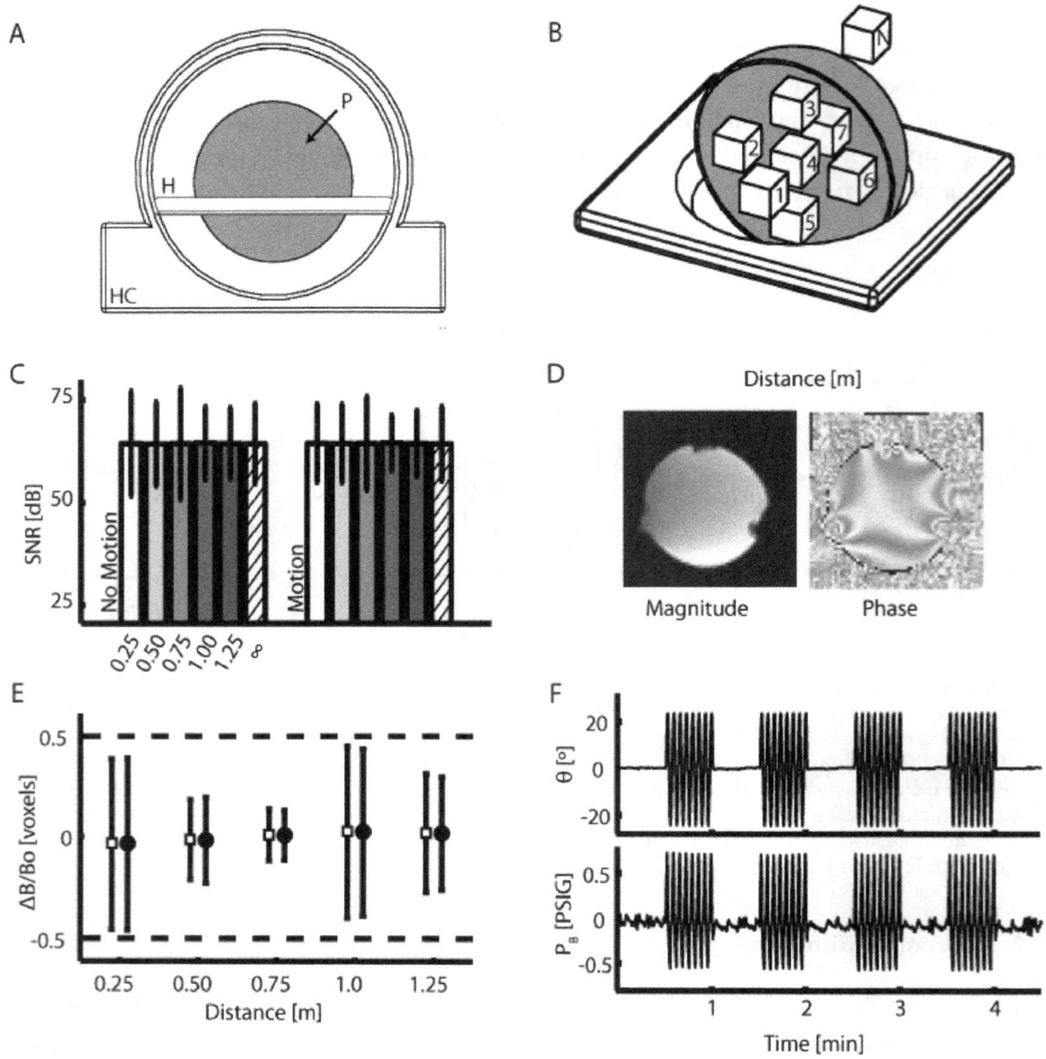

Figure 3. (A) Set-up of the head coil (HC), phantom holder (H), and phantom (P). (B) Holder and phantom cut-away showing details of ROIs used to calculate signal-to-noise ratio (SNR) and field homogeneity. (C) SNR for ROI 3 vs. device operating distance measured from the center of the imaging volume. Error bars represent 95% confidence intervals about the mean SNR at each distance. (D) Sagittal slice of magnitude and phase images of the phantom. Susceptibility artifact in the lower portion of the images was caused by the phantom holder, and was seen in images both with and without the manipulandum in the scanner. (E) Estimate of field homogeneity in ROI 3 from phase data collected in the "No Motion" (open squares) and "Motion" (filled circles) states. We were interested in the distribution of homogeneity values, so error bars in this panel represent ± 2 SD about the mean and thus 95% of the data lie within these bounds. (F) Representative wrist angle and bellows pressure time series collected when the device was 0.50 m from the imaging volume. Angle and pressure measurements are not adversely effected by scanner operation. Figure adapted from Suminski et al., 2007a.

of both magnitude and phase MR images. We quantified the effects of simultaneous operation of the robot and scanner during "Motion" and "No Motion" states by imaging the phantom with the robot at 6 distances from the center of the imaging volume (0.25m, 0.50m, 0.75m, 1.0m, and 1.25m) as well as in a control condition with the robot operating in the scanner control room (∞). The phantom was sampled using 7 equal-volume regions of interest (ROI) distributed within its spherical boundary to test whether the robot induced amplitude and phase anisotropies during scanning.

We computed three measures to assess compatibility of the robot and MR scanner; two evaluated MR signal quality during robot operation in the "Motion" and "No Motion" states and the third evaluated the effects of echo planar imaging on measurements of handle position and actuator pressure. First, we calculated the signal to noise ratio (SNR) within each ROI for each robot-distance condition using the magnitude images:

$$SNR_{ROI} = \frac{\mu_{ROI}}{0.665 * \sigma_{noise}} \tag{2}$$

μ_{ROI} is the time series average within a given ROI, and σ_{noise} is an estimate of noise obtained by calculating the standard deviation of the time series in the magnitude images in an identically sized ROI located outside the phantom (Fig. 3B; ROI "N"). The factor 0.665 corrected for changes in the statistical distribution of σ_{noise} caused by calculating the magnitude image from the original complex MR data (Haacke et al., 1999). Values of SNR varied across the seven ROIs but were insensitive to the robot's distance within each ROI (eg. Fig 3C). Three-way ANOVA found main effects of both ROI location ($p < 0.0005$) and robot distance ($p < 0.0005$) but no effect of robot motion state ($p = 0.929$). Comparison of SNR at each of the five distances relative to the control condition (∞) revealed a small but significant 0.64 dB and 0.90 dB *increase* in SNR at 1.0 m and 1.25 m as compared to control ($p < 0.05$), but no change in SNR for the other distances ($p > 0.7$). Thus, we found no systematic degradation of functional MR SNR as a function of robot distance from the imaging volume.

Second, we used the phase images to quantify changes in magnetic field homogeneity induced by robot operation within the scanner suite. We computed the average change in the static magnetic field for each ROI (ΔB_{ROI}):

$$\Delta B_{ROI} = \frac{\phi_{ROI}}{-\gamma T_E} \tag{3}$$

where, ϕ_{ROI} is the average change in each ROI's phase time series with respect to baseline (i.e. ∞), γ is the gyromagnetic ratio, and T_E is the echo time of the EPI sequence (Haacke et al., 1999). We then normalized ΔB_{ROI} to the magnitude of the static magnetic field (B_0 = 3.0T) yielding a unit-less quantity corresponding to the homogeneity of the magnetic field ($\Delta B/B_0$) in parts per million. This normalization process allows comparison of the field homogeneity and the bandwidth/voxel (39Hz or 0.32 ppm) of the EPI sequence. If introduction of the robot into the scanning environment disturbs the field homogeneity by > 0.16 ppm (i.e. ½ voxel), the actual and measured voxel locations would be inconsistent causing inaccuracy in the resultant images. As shown for a representative ROI (Fig. 3B), field inhomogeneity induced by the robot was well below ½ voxel at each distance in the "No Motion" and "Motion" conditions. One-sided t-tests rejected the hypothesis that the field distortion exceeded ½ voxel in either condition ($p < 0.0005$ in each case). Thus, image quality was not compromised by operating the robotic device within the MR scanner.

Finally, we quantified the effects of echo planar imaging on robot operation by calculating SNR for the actuator pressure (SNR_P) and wrist angle (SNR_A) signals while the computer drove the robot's handle through a sinusoidal trajectory:

$$SNR = 20^{*}\log_{10}\left(\frac{RMS_{Signal} - RMS_{Noise}}{RMS_{Noise}}\right) \tag{4}$$

Root mean squared (RMS) values of actuator pressure and joint angle were calculated during "Motion" and "No Motion" states to approximate signal and noise respectively. Neither joint angle nor pressure SNR varied systematically as a function of robot distance from the center of the scanner bore. Individual two-sample t-tests found no difference in SNR_A or SNR_P ($p > 0.705$) when compared to baseline measures obtained when the robot was operated outside the scanning environment (∞).

In conclusion, we have implemented a pneumatically actuated manipulandum that applies controlled joint torques and measures joint angle at the wrist. This device neither degrades fMRI signal quality nor is itself compromised by rapidly switching imaging gradients.

2.3. Comparison of the device with other MR-compatible devices

In the last decade, several robotic devices have been developed for use during MR scanning (see Gassert et al., 2008 for review). The 1 DOF manipulandum we developed compares favorably to other MR-compatible devices used in neuroscience research or rehabilitation applications. For example, the device developed by Hidler et al. (Hidler et al., 2006) only monitors the torque/force generated by a subject whereas our device can simulate dynamic environments by generating controlled torques about the wrist. Other MR-compatible devices can apply dynamic loads using Lorentz coils (Riener et al., 2005), ultrasonic motors (Flueckiger et al., 2005), electrorheological fluids (Khanicheh et al., 2008) or hydrostatic pistons (Gassert et al., 2006). However, in contrast to the device presented by Riener and colleagues, our device does not degrade image quality when operated less than 1m from the scanner's isocenter. Because the devices presented by Flueckinger (Flueckiger et al., 2005) and Gassert (Gassert et al., 2006) are not backdriveable, they can not simulate realistic dynamic loads during movements requiring rapid changes in direction whereas our device clearly can do so. Recently, Yu, et al. compared 1 DOF MR-compatible devices containing hydraulic and pneumatic actuators (Yu et al., 2008) and concluded that pneumatic actuation was favorable for fast, force controlled applications, whereas hydraulic actuation was best for applications requiring accurate position control (Yu et al., 2008). And while the 2 DOF device presented by Diedrichsen (Diedrichsen et al., 2005) offers the ability to perturb planar reaching movements of the arm, perturbation of proximal limb segments can lead to considerable head motion that must be accounted for during analysis of fMRI data (Diedrichsen and Shadmehr, 2005). In contrast, our current design limits motion to the wrist, which may lead to fewer head motion artifacts in the fMRI dataset.

3. Limb position regulation with proprioceptive feedback

For a first demonstration of the robot's utility, we examined how the brain uses proprioceptive feedback of limb position for the moment-by-moment (i.e. on-line) feedback stabilization of wrist position during a compensatory tracking task. Limb stabilization is important because meaningful interaction with the world frequently requires stabilization of hand-held items (eg. holding a young child's hand) and/or movement of such objects between stabilized positions or "postures" (eg. turning the steering wheel of a car). At any moment, task performance may be compromised due to environmental perturbations (eg. the car hitting a pothole) requiring corrective action to maintain desired performance.

The central nervous system can employ three strategies acting on different timescales to compensate for errors arising during stabilization. First, it may utilize feedback regulation of joint position via segmental (Sinkjaer and Hayashi, 1989) and transcortical ("long loop") reflex pathways (Evarts and Tanji, 1976; Strick, 1978; Evarts and Fromm, 1981) to minimize errors. Alternatively, subjects may increase the impedance of the limb via voluntary co-activation (Milner and Cloutier, 1993) of muscles whose actions oppose one another (i.e. antagonist muscles). Finally, subjects may generate discrete, feedforward, corrective movements when feedback mechanisms and impedance regulation fail to adequately reduce perceived errors (Haaland and Harrington, 1989; Fagg et al., 1998). These strategies are not mutually exclusive, but are complementary in two ways. First, they reduce performance errors over different timescales ranging from the short-latency mechanical responses of antagonist coactivation and reflex action to the reduction of persistent errors by discrete adjustment of behavioral goals. Second, they provide the flexibility in motor output needed to respond to task-dependent tradeoffs between accuracy and muscular effort, thus providing the behavioral basis for optimality in human motor control (Todorov and Jordan, 2002; Scott, 2004). Much is yet unknown about the neuromuscular control of limb position (i.e. posture stabilization), including which aspects of environmental perturbation are compensated on a moment-by-moment basis, and what performance criteria might cause a subject to generate a discrete corrective movement during stabilization.

Ten healthy right-handed volunteers (5 female) participated in two experimental sessions performed on separate days. They performed identical wrist stabilization tasks both days. In one session, subjects stabilized the wrist against robotic perturbation while inside a mock MR scanner. This allowed recording of electromyographic (EMG) data from task-relevant muscles. In the other session, subjects performed the experiment while undergoing FMRI scanning in a 1.5T General Electric Signa scanner equipped with a 3-axis local gradient head coil and an elliptical endcapped quadrature radiofrequency head coil. In both sessions, subjects rested supine in the scanner with their head constrained by foam padding to reduce head motion. With arms at their sides, subjects grasped the robot handle with their right hand. The handle and wrist axes of rotation were aligned and the frame of the device was secured to both the subject's forearm and the inner wall of the scanner bore for support.

3.1. Experimental procedure

Both sessions consisted of a blocked experimental design that alternated between periods of rest and active wrist stabilization. Each stabilization trial was conducted in 5 phases (Fig. 4). During the 30 s prior to stabilization (phase 1), the subject was instructed to relax while the robot held the hand in a comfortable resting posture of 40° flexion (θ_r). 3 s prior to the start of stabilization (phase 2), the robot moved the relaxed hand to the target posture (20° flexion) and held it there until the onset of the stabilization period. The purpose of this phase was to provide a salient haptic cue of the desired wrist angle about which subjects were to stabilize. During the 30 s stabilization period (phase 3), subjects were instructed to hold their wrist steady at the target angle during two experimental conditions in which the device was programmed to apply either a predictable, constant extensor torque about the wrist (*CT*, mean = 1.2 Nm) or unpredictable, pseudo-random extensor torques comprised of band-limited Gaussian "white" noise with a high-frequency cutoff of 1.6 Hz (*RT*; 1.2±1.1 Nm; mean ± SD). At the end of the stabilization period, subjects were instructed to relax while the robot moved the passive hand to its resting position at 40° flexion (phase 4), after which resting EMG continued to be monitored for 3 s (phase 5). Direct view of the wrist was precluded and subjects received no visual feedback of hand motion during stabilization phase 3. Instead, subjects viewed a stationary fixation target that was back-projected onto a screen located at their feet and was visible using prism glasses. The fixation target moved in concert with the hand during passive movement phases 2 and 4 and thus provided an implicit visual representation of the desired wrist angle during stabilization phase 3.

During each 3-minute imaging run, *CT* and *RT* stabilization trials were each presented one time in pseudo-random order, along with 30 s periods of inactivity (rest) preceding and following stabilization. Each subject performed 10 of these runs in each session. Whole-brain images were acquired using a single-shot, blipped gradient-echo echo-planar pulse sequence (19 contiguous sagittal 7-mm slices, TE = 40 ms, TR = 2.5 s, 90° flip angle, FOV = 24 cm, 64x64 matrix, 3.75-mm in-plane resolution). 72 whole-brain images were acquired in each run. BOLD contrast was used to image the hemodynamic related changes in the brain occurring during the two stabilization tasks. Before functional imaging, high-resolution 3D spoiled gradient recalled at steady-state T1-weighted anatomic images were collected for anatomic localization and co-registration (TE=5 ms, TR=24 ms, 40° flip angle, slice thickness=1.2 mm, FOV=24 cm, 256x192 matrix).

3.2. Behavioural correlates of stabilization

We found that that wrist torque perturbations elicited changes in wrist angle (θ) and wrist angular velocity ($d\theta/dt$) despite instruction to hold the hand steady. We quantified kinematic performance using the root mean square (RMS) stabilization error. Not unexpectedly, subjects

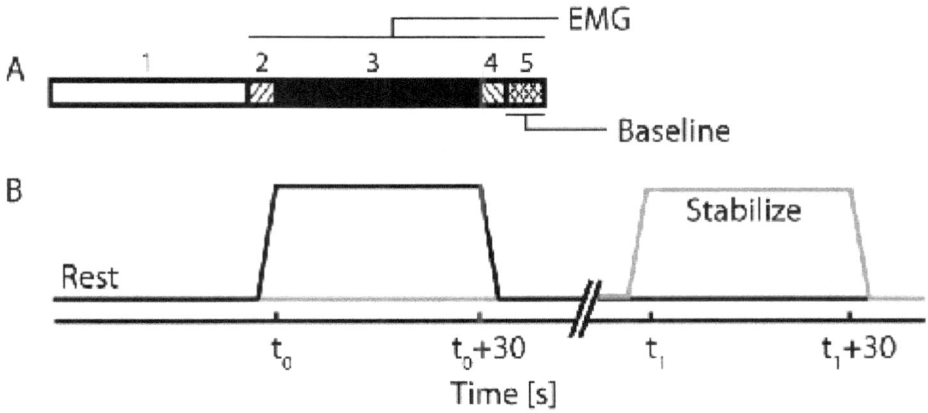

Figure 4. (A) Single stabilization trials were conducted in 5 phases. See text for details. (B) During each imaging run, subjects stabilized their wrist against constant (gray line) or pseudo-random (black line) extensor torque perturbations. Figure adapted from Suminski et al., 2007b.

were less able to maintain steady hand posture while perturbed by band-limited pseudo-random torques than by constant torques. Paired t-tests found greater errors in *RT* vs. *CT* trials ($p <= 0.0005$, both sessions). We also observed positional drift over time (a significant slope in the joint angle time series over the final 20 seconds a trial) in 91% of *RT* trials (88 of 96) and 75% of *CT* trials (72 of 95). The absolute magnitude of this drift was 0.155 ± 0.104 °/s and 0.017 ± 0.028 °/s in the *RT* and *CT* cases respectively.

Elevated Coactivity: We quantified coordination between muscles in the arm by estimating the amount of antagonist muscle co-activity at the wrist, elbow and shoulder joints using a coactivity measure also known as 'wasted contraction' (Thoroughman and Shadmehr, 1999) [***C(t)***]. We considered the anterior and postierior deltoid as shoulder antagonists, the biceps and triceps as elbow antagonists, and flexor carpi radialis and extensor carpi radialis as wrist antagonists. ANOVA and post-hoc Dunnet's t-tests found significant elevations in muscle co-activity values (Fig. 5A) during phase 3 ***RT*** stabilization at each joint ($p < 0.0005$) and during phase 3 ***CT*** stabilization at the wrist ($p = 0.03$). No significant EMG activity was observed at any joint during passive movement (phases 2 and 4) when compared to rest.

Feedback Regulation: We evaluated the contributions of reflex-mediated responses to wrist stabilization by analyzing the cross-correlation between wrist angular velocity and measured EMG responses in the ***RT*** condition. For wrist flexor FCR, we consistently observed increased EMG activity lagging wrist extension by 59.0 ± 44.2 ms (Fig. 5B-d). The timing of this load-dependent activity was within the range of delays expected for transcortical reflex compensation for muscle stretch (Evarts and Vaughn, 1978; Strick, 1978; Matthews, 1981). For wrist extensor ECR, we observed decreased EMG activity lagging wrist extension by 40.3 ± 23.7 ms (Fig. 5B-c). The sign and latency of these EMG changes are consistent with an unloading response mediated by spinal circuits (Sinkjaer et al., 2000). We also observed an increase in ECR activity with lag of 484.8 ± 118.3 ms (Fig. 5B-e) in 5 out of 10 subjects. This later response is consistent with a strategy of voluntary co-activation about the wrist since no contemporaneous decrease in flexor activity was observed.

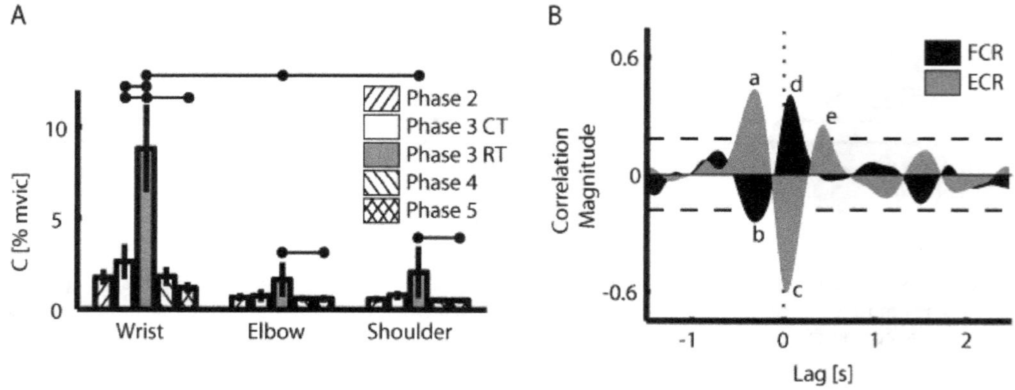

Figure 5. (A) Population average of antagonist muscle coactivity. Horizontal bars indicate significant differences between stabilization conditions ($p < 0.05$). Hatched bars: co-activity during phases 2, 4, and 5. White and gray bars: co-activity during periods of active stabilization against *CT* and *RT* respectively. Error bars indicate ± 2 SEM. (B) Cross-correlation of wrist angular velocity ($d\theta/dt$) and EMG from flexor carpi radialis (*FCR;* black) and extensor carpi radiallis (*ECR;* gray) for a representative subject. Significant correlations were observed with EMG both lagging/leading changes in $d\theta/dt$. Horizontal dashed lines: 95% confidence interval about zero correlation. Figure adapted from Suminski et al., 2007b.

Discrete Corrections: Consistent with expectation, we observed many rapid movements that did not appear to be a direct mechanical consequence of moment-by-moment fluctuations in the robot's commanded wrist torque. To identify the onset of discrete corrective movements, we first computed the average wrist angle trajectory for each subject in each condition. We then removed the trial-averaged trajectory from every individual trial to obtain a 'corrected' wrist angle time series. We considered as discrete corrections only those motions wherein the angular velocity of corrected wrist angle trajectories exceeded 5°/s if they occurred >1 second after the start of stabilization. Discrete corrective movements occurred in 95% of ***RT*** trials (91 of 96) and 19% of ***CT*** trials (18 of 95). The majority of corrective movements were directed appropriately to reduce positioning errors (56.1% and 80% of movements in the ***RT*** and ***CT*** cases, respectively).

In summary, the behavioral and electromyographic data revealed that subjects compensated for environmental perturbations using a combination of three readily identifiable strategies. Subjects modulated limb impedance via co-activation of agonist/antagonist muscle pairs spanning the wrist, elbow and shoulder. Correlation analysis found that subjects also invoke both spinal and supraspinal reflexes to compensate for the perturbations. Finally, subjects generated discrete corrective movements to reduce performance errors that likely accumulated due to the lack of visual feedback during stabilization (cf. Wann and Ibrahim, 1992). We next sought to characterize the neural mechanisms contributing to each of these strategies during experiments conducted within the MR scanner.

3.3. Neural correlates of stabilization

Functional images were generated and analyzed within the Analysis of Functional NeuroImages (AFNI) software package (Cox, 1996). The first three images in each run were discarded to allow for equilibration of the magnetic field. Individual run time series were then concatenated and aligned in three-dimensional space using an interactive, linear, least squares method. Voxel-wise multiple linear regression was used to determine the amount of FMRI signal contrast between the two task conditions (***CT*** and ***RT*** stabilization) and the resting baseline. The resulting functional images for ***RT*** and ***CT*** were interpolated to obtain a volumetric grid having 1mm^3 voxel volumes, coregistered, and then converted into the Talairach stereotaxic coordinate space (Talairach and Tournoux, 1988). To facilitate group analysis, the Talairached functional images were spatially blurred using a 4-mm Gaussian full-width half-maximum filter to compensate for inter-subject anatomical variability. In all across-subject analyses, a activation volume and thresholding technique was used to correct for multiple comparisons in the group analysis. Appropriate activation volume and individual voxel p-value thresholds ($p=0.005$) were estimated by performing 5000 iterations in a Monte-Carlo simulation using the AlphaSim tool within AFNI (Cox, 1996). The location of activated regions in group statistical parametric maps was obtained using the Talairach atlas (Talairach and Tournoux, 1988) for cerebral activations and the Schmahmann atlas (Schmahmann, 2000) for activations in the cerebellum and its nuclei. Cortical activations were visualized using CARET (Van Essen et al., 2001); http://brainmap.wustl.edu/caret).

Changes in BOLD signal intensity (relative to rest) correlated with periods of ***CT*** or ***RT*** stabilization in many brain regions that contribute to control of the upper extremity (Table 1; Fig. 6A). We visualized the time series of BOLD activations for each ROI during stabilization against each load type for each subject. Two patterns of activation became evident. The first, an example of which is shown for an ROI spanning left primary motor and somatosensory cortices (Fig. 6B; M1/S1), was characterized by increases in percentage BOLD signal intensity change (PSC) throughout the ***RT*** stabilization periods and during the passive hand movements preceding and following ***CT*** stabilization. Motion sensitivity during active stabilization and passive movement might be expected from brain regions concerned with the estimation of - and on-line feedback correction for - performance errors (Marsden et al., 1972; Lee and Tatton, 1975; Evarts and Vaughn, 1978; Marsden et al., 1978; Strick, 1978; Horne and Butler, 1995; Scott, 2004). This idea is based on the assumption that passive movement of the wrist induces a discrepancy (error) between actual limb position and that expected given the recent history of motor output. The second pattern, an example is shown for the right middle frontal gyrus (Fig. 6B; BA 46), was characterized by a parallel increase in PSC during both stabilization conditions with no sensitivity to passive movement. This pattern might be expected from regions (i.e. prefrontal cortex, anterior cingulate cortex, rostral aspects of dorsal premotor and SMA cortices, and inferior aspects of posterior parietal cortex) involved in supervisory aspects of control such as evaluating the success of an ongoing task (Carter et al., 1998) as well as the resetting of behavioral goals when ongoing performance is deficient (Jahanshahi et al., 1995; Winstein et al., 1997; Jueptner and Weiller, 1998; Sakai et al., 1999). As shown for an ROI in the cerebellum (Fig 6B, CBLM), some regions exhibited an intermediate pattern (i.e. some sensitivity to stabilization type but little sensitivity to passive movement). To quantify these observations, we defined a 2-element feature vector $\Psi = \{\bar{S}, \Delta_M\}$ summarizing the average increase in PSC induced by passive movement in phase 2 ($\bar{S}$) and the difference in PSC between ***RT*** and ***CT*** trials during stabilization (Δ_M). The $\bar{S}$ feature was the average of 4 consecutive TR samples from each of the ***RT*** and ***CT*** trials, beginning 5 seconds (i.e. 2 TR) prior to the start of the stabilization period. The Δ_M feature was computed as the difference between the average ***RT*** and ***CT*** PSC time series during the middle 20 seconds (8 TR) of stabilization.

Using these features, we performed a k-means cluster analysis to identify ROIs demonstrating common patterns of sensitivity to trial type and/or passive movement. Two distinct groups were identified: ROIs that were sensitive to both trial type and passive movement (Cluster I; red regions in Fig. 6A), and those demonstrating increased BOLD activation over the duration of the trial with little sensitivity to passive movement (Cluster II; blue regions in Fig. 6A). Group separation and membership was visualized by plotting the coordinates of each ROI on the axes defined by the features of Ψ (Fig. 6C; Cluster I = red circles; Cluster II = blue squares). Regions showing significant sensitivity to passive movement ($\bar{S} \neq 0$; $p < 0.05$) are indicated by filled symbols. These include left M1/S1, SPL/IPL (BA 5 and 7), and SMA/CCZ. The left M1/S1, SPL/IPL (BA 5 and 7), and right STG (BA 39) were also significantly modulated by task type ($\Delta_M > 0$; $p < 0.05$). ROIs with membership in Cluster I were characterized by both a high sensitivity to trial type (being more active during RT trials) and a robust response to passive movement of the wrist. Such sensitivity to positioning errors is necessary for regions directly involved in the feedback control of movement kinematics (i.e. limb position, velocity and acceleration). Indeed, responsivity to passive movement has been considered a hallmark of brain regions participating in the optimal feedback control of movement (Scott, 2004). In contrast, Cluster II ROIs exhibited generally elevated BOLD activation during stabilization with little sensitivity to trial type or passive movement. This pattern of activity is expected from regions involved in supervisory aspects of control rather than in the moment-by-moment cancellation of position errors.

We performed a second BOLD regression analysis to identify brain regions involved in generating the discrete corrective movements observed behaviorally. We limited our investigation to the ***CT*** stabilization blocks because corrections were unambiguous and most often directed to decrease kinematic error. In particular, we wished to know whether the regions generating corrective movements might be a subset of the networks previously described or different networks. For this event-related analysis, we created input reference functions for each subject indicating the onset times of discrete corrective movements during ***CT*** stabilization. These time series had a value of 1 during each sampling instant (TR) wherein a discrete corrective movement occurred and 0 otherwise. Additional reference time series were included to mitigate effects of head motion and to model the average activity used to maintain limb position during CT stabilization. Regressors were convolved with a γ-variate function and the resulting functional images were pre-processed as described above. Voxel-wise, one-sided t-

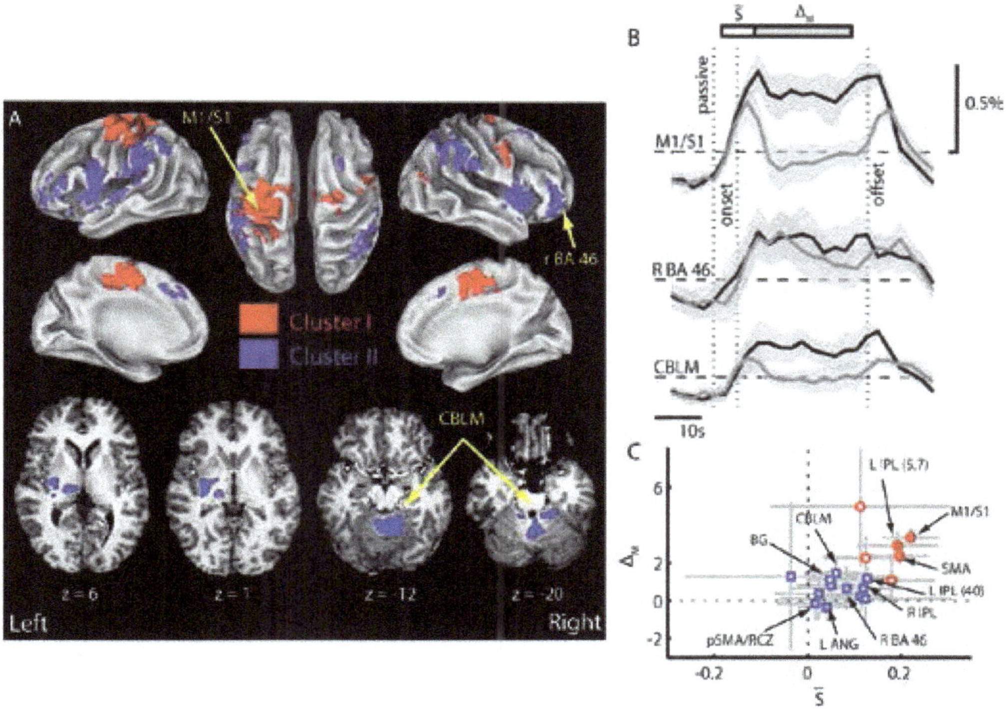

Figure 6. (A) Population maps showing significantly activated ROIs during periods of random ***RT*** or constant ***CT*** stabilization ($p < 0.05$; corrected for multiple comparisons). Cluster I ROIs are shown in red while Cluster II ROIs are shown in blue. Upper panels: activations mapped onto inflated representations of the cerebral hemispheres. Lower panels: activations in the basal ganglia, thalamus, cerebellar cortex (lobule IV-VI), and right dentate nucleus. (B) Percent signal change (PSC) of BOLD time series from ***RT*** (black) and ***CT*** (gray) stabilization periods. Shaded regions: ±2 SEM. Scale bars above the PSC plots indicate the time intervals used to calculate the components of $\Psi = \{\bar{S}, \Delta_v\}$. (C) Group membership for 18 ROIs was visualized by plotting the coordinates of each ROI within the plane defined by the features of Ψ (red: Cluster I; blue: Cluster II). Filled symbols: region where PSC differs significantly from resting baseline. Figure reproduced with permission from Suminski et al., 2007b.

tests found specific regions in Cluster I and Cluster II to be modulated discrete movement corrections. Interestingly, BOLD signal intensity *increased* with respect to baseline in a subset of regions in Cluster II, while a subset of regions in Cluster I exhibited BOLD signal *decreases* (Fig. 7; red and blue areas, respectively). These results highlight the manner in which Cluster I and II regions work together to maintain the position of the limb during stabilization against a deterministic perturbation: During CT trials, discrete corrective movements induce a persistent decrease in the magnitude of kinematic errors, thus reducing the need for feedback regulation of position and likely contributing to the inhibition of Cluster I ROIs. Conversely, we found the BOLD activity increased in a subset of Cluster II ROIs at the specific times when discrete movements were performed. Such behavior would be expected from brain regions involved in the resetting of behavioral goals (reference wrist angle) when performance is deficient.

		Tailarach Coordinates				
	Hem	X	Y	Z	Vol	Mean T
Cluster I						
Precentral Gyrus (BA 4,6)	L	-30.1	-19.4	51.3	14166	5.884
Medial Frontal Gyrus (BA 6)	B	-0.5	-11.6	48	7856	5.0334
Cingulate Gyrus (BA 24,31)						
Inferior/Superior Parietal Lobule (BA 5,7,40)	L	-30.3	-38.3	56.6	2630	4.7958
Precentral Gyrus (BA 6)	R	49.6	-2.4	39	957	4.5288
Precentral Gyrus (BA 6)	R	22.3	-15.4	61.2	866	4.2839
Middle Temporal Gyrus (BA 39)	R	52.6	-68.9	15.9	596	4.3556
Cluster II						
Cortical						
Insula (BA 13)	L	-47.5	0.2	8.3	8102	4.8657
Superior Temporal Gyrus (BA 22,41)						
Inferior Parietal Lobule (BA 40)	L	-50.9	-31.5	24.9	7477	4.9995
Insula (BA 13)	R	42.7	5.6	4.8	5633	5.0229
Superior Temporal Gyrus (BA 22)						
Inferior Parietal Lobule (BA 40)	R	53.4	-40.6	36.4	5125	4.3849
Supramarginal Gyrus						
Middle/Inferior Frontal Gyrus (BA 10,46)	R	39.2	38.5	3.5	2668	4.5259
Middle/Inferior Frontal Gyrus (BA 10,45,46)	L	-42	29.8	12.5	1334	4.3385
Inferior Parietal Lobule (BA 40)	L	-49.1	-53.3	39.9	1079	4.1923
Angular Gyrus						
Medial Frontal Gyrus (BA 6,8)	B	-3	25.4	41.5	1033	4.156
Cingulate Gyrus (BA 32)						
Superior Frontal Gyrus (BA 8)						
Superior Frontal Gyrus (BA 6)	R	22.1	13.3	51.6	687	4.5912
Middle Frontal Gyrus (BA 10)	L	-38.2	49.2	3.4	582	4.2741
Subcortical and Cerebellum						
Cerebellar Cortex Lobule IV, V, VI	B	5.9	-49.4	-14	9571	5.2885
Dentate	R					
Basal Ganglia and Thalamus	L	-19.7	-17	10.1	6684	5.025
L = Left; R = Right; B = Bilateral; BA = Broadman's Area						

Table 1. Brain regions exhibiting significant task-related activation during ***RT*** or ***CT*** trials.

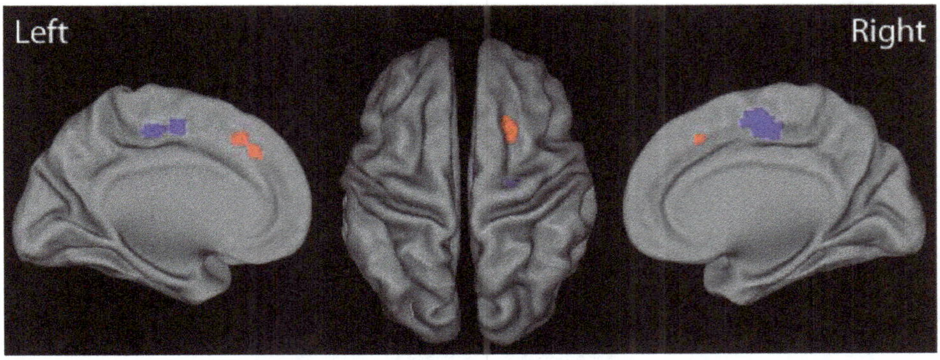

Figure 7. Activation maps showing regions where BOLD signal correlated with the generation of discrete corrective movements ($p < 0.05$, corrected for multiple comparisons). Increased BOLD activiy was observed in a subset of Cluster II regions [red: right pre-PMd, left medial frontal gyrus (BA 8) and rostral cingulate]. BOLD activaions decreased relative to resting state activity in Cluster I regions (blue: bilateral SMA and right PMd).

We performed a final set of multiple linear regression analyses to identify brain regions explicitly involved in the moment-by-moment and long-term evaluation and correction for kinematic and/or kinetic performance errors. We wished to know whether the activations identified in the preceding analyses were related to compensation for kinematic errors, generation of wrist torques, or both. Here, we performed four separate regressions using input reference functions corresponding to the magnitude of RMS wrist angle errors and RMS torque both on a trial-by-trial and TR-by-TR basis ($\mathbf{Error}_{Trial}$, $\mathbf{Error}_{TR}$, $\mathbf{Torque}_{Trial}$, and $\mathbf{Torque}_{TR}$). Each function was created from error or pressure data measured during the corresponding stabilization run within the MR-scanner. The value at each (TR) sampling instant for $\mathbf{Error}_{Trial}$ and $\mathbf{Torque}_{Trial}$ was set equal to the RMS error (or torque) value computed throughout the corresponding stabilization period (30 s integration window). The value at each (TR) sampling instant for $\mathbf{Error}_{TR}$ and $\mathbf{Torque}_{TR}$ (reference functions that varied on a moment-by-moment basis) was set equal to the RMS error (torque) value computed during that TR sampling period (2.5 s integration window). In all cases, the reference time series were convolved with a γ-variate function to model the temporal filtering properties of the hemodynamic response. Additional reference time series included head motion parameters and functions representing periods of ***RT*** and ***CT*** stabilization. The resulting functional images were processed as described above. Voxel-wise, one-sided t-tests were used to identify regions where BOLD signal covaried with $\mathbf{Error}_{Trial}$, $\mathbf{Error}_{TR}$, $\mathbf{Torque}_{Trial}$, or $\mathbf{Torque}_{TR}$.

Regions demonstrating increased sensitivity to errors that change on a moment-by-moment timescale ($\mathbf{Error}_{TR}$; Fig. 8 red) were predominantly members of Cluster I, while regions sensitive to kinematic errors on a much longer timescale ($\mathbf{Error}_{Trial}$; Fig. 8 blue) were more likely to be members of Cluster II (see also Table 2). Activation of the left IPL in the $\mathbf{Error}_{Trial}$ contrast was located more posterior to those activated regions of IPL in the $\mathbf{Error}_{TR}$ contrast. There were no overlapping activations in the $\mathbf{Error}_{Trial}$ and $\mathbf{Error}_{TR}$ contrasts. Importantly, no regions were found to be active in contrasts examining differences between either $\mathbf{Torque}_{Trial}$ or $\mathbf{Torque}_{TR}$ and resting baseline.

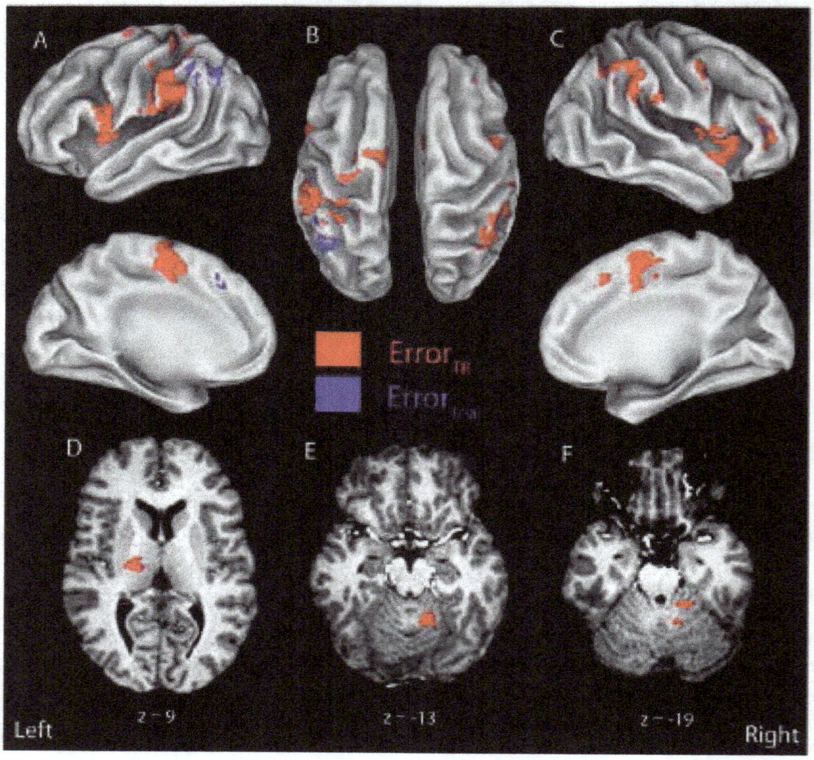

Figure 8. Activation maps showing regions wherein the BOLD response correlated with kinematic performance errors (i.e. state estimation errors) on both a moment-by-moment (***Error***$_{TR}$, red regions) and a trial-by-trial basis (***Error***$_{Trial}$, blue regions) ($p < 0.05$, corrected for multiple comparisons). Figure reproduced with permission from Suminski et al., 2007b.

	Tailarach Coordinates					
	Hem	**X**	**Y**	**Z**	**Vol**	**Mean T**
ErrorTR						
Cortical						
Inferior Parietal Lobule (BA 40)	L	51.3	29.9	28.4	3599	4.7941
Supramarginal Gyrus						
Postcentral Gyrus (BA 2)						
Insula (BA 13)						
Medial Frontal Gyrus (BA 6)	B	1.5	4.9	50	3056	4.7047
Superior Frontal Gyurs (BA 6)	L					
Cingulate Gyrus (BA 24)	R					

		Tailarach Coordinates				
	Hem	X	Y	Z	Vol	Mean T
Insula (BA 13)	R	-41	-8.3	2.9	2245	4.7498
Superior Temporal Gyrus (BA 22)						
Insula (BA 13)	L	47	-0.5	11.8	1986	4.9146
Superior Temporal Gyrus (BA 22)						
Inferior Parietal Lobule (BA 40)	R	-50.4	42	38.7	1706	4.2648
Supramarginal Gyrus						
Inferior Parietal Lobule (BA 5,40)	L	35.6	38.4	53.3	761	4.2931
Inferior Frontal Gyrus (BA 46)	R	-35.7	-34.5	14.9	756	5.0422
Middle Frontal Gyurs (BA 10)						
Precentral Gyrus (BA 6)	R	-46.3	2.3	43	247	4.7634
Precentral Gyrus (BA 44)	R	-53.7	-5.6	9.8	180	4.0774
Cingulate Gyrus (BA 32)	R	-8.6	-17.8	43.7	152	5.0572
Precentral Gyrus (BA 4)	L	28.5	21.6	63.2	115	3.9996
Subcortical and Cerebellum						
Basal Ganglia and Thalamus	L	18.8	14.4	7.1	1036	4.4593
Putamen						
Globus Pallidus (Medial/Lateral)						
Ventral Posterior Lateral						
Ventral Lateral						
Cerebellar Cortex Lobule IV, V, VI	R	-15.4	48.5	-16.1	871	4.2192
Dentate						
ErrorTrial						
Inferior Parietal Lobule (BA 40)	L	41.5	54.3	36.6	556	4.302
Supramarginal Gyrus						
Medial Frontal Gyrus (BA 8)	L	6.9	-20.3	43.6	45	3.9183
L = Left; R = Right; B = Bilateral; BA = Broadman's Area						

Table 2. Brain regions activated in the $Error_{TR}$ and $Error_{Trial}$ contrasts.

4. Summary and future directions

This chapter has described the development and validation of a novel, 1 DOF pneumatically actuated manipulandum. We demonstrated that the device was: 1) capable of generating computer controlled perturbations of movement and 2) compatible with the MR scanner such that performance of neither the device nor image quality was affected by robot operation. We then demonstrated device utility in a study of wrist posture stabilization against environmental perturbation. We provided behavioral evidence that subjects invoke three complementary compensatory responses when stabilizing the wrist in the absence of ongoing visual feedback of task performance. These compensatory responses include feedback regulation via spinal and long-loop reflexes, impedance modulation via antagonist muscle co-activation and feedforward, discrete corrective movements. Analysis of functional neuroimages obtained from the same subjects performing the same tasks revealed two distinct networks that were differentially excited by the task. The first (Cluster I) included a cerebello-thalamo-cortical network previously implicated in the online computation and feedback correction of errors (Marsden et al., 1972; Lee and Tatton, 1975; Evarts and Vaughn, 1978; Marsden et al., 1978; Strick, 1978; Horne and Butler, 1995). BOLD signal changes within these regions were correlated with moment-by-moment fluctuations in state estimation errors (Fig. 7, red regions; $\boldsymbol{Error}_{TR}$, 2.5 s integration period). That is, BOLD activity in these regions was elevated mainly during random torque perturbations and during passive movement of the hand, despite the absence of significant muscle activation during passive manipulation in the behavioral experiments and the production of the same average wrist torques in both tasks. A second network (Cluster II) exhibited similarly elevated BOLD activity during performance of both stabilization tasks. Brain regions demonstrating this pattern include the prefrontal cortex, rostral aspects of dorsal premotor and SMA cortices, and inferior aspects of posterior parietal cortex. These brain regions have previously been reported to contribute to the planning and execution of internally-generated, discrete motor actions (Jahanshahi et al., 1995; Winstein et al., 1997; Jueptner and Weiller, 1998; Sakai et al., 1999). Consistent with those reports, we found that BOLD activity increased within rostral PMd, SMA and cingulate cortex during time periods wherein subjects generated discrete corrective movements. Although discrete corrections were transient events, they gave rise to long-lasting performance improvements in most cases and so, they likely represent a resetting of the reference wrist angle when online (moment-by-moment) feedback control failed to satisfy subjective performance constraints. To do so, however, subjects first needed to determine when error had grown sufficiently large to warrant correction and then plan the direction and magnitude of corrective action. This type of supervisory role likely was supported by Cluster II ROIs demonstrating high sensitivity to state estimation errors over a longer, 30 s timeframe (Fig. 7, blue regions).

These results highlight the importance of both postural and movement trajectory control mechanisms in peripheral limb stabilization and suggest a possible neural basis for the distinct postural and trajectory (movement) control mechanisms recently isolated during point-to-point arm movements and movement sequences (Ghez et al., 2007; Scheidt and Ghez, 2007). Additional studies are needed to better understand how the brain combines the different control processes to minimize performance errors and how the brain uses information from multiple sensory feedback modalities to optimize limb stabilization and movement control. Such work will be greatly facilitated by the use of mechanically-active tools that apply physical perturbations to the limb while subjects undergo concurrent functional MR imaging.

Acknowledgements

This work was supported by NSF BES0238442, NIH NCRR M01-RR00058, 2 P01 MH51358, R01 HD053727 and by the Alvin W. and Marion Birnschein Foundation. We thank Kristine Mosier and Steve Rao for constructive feedback on an earlier version of this manuscript, Jeff Goldstein for crafting the manipulandum, Dr. N. Bansal for helpful suggestions regarding the statistical handling of the data, as well as Vanai Roopchansingh, Sally Durgerian, Matthew Verber and the MCW MRI technicians for assistance during FMRI data collection and analysis.

Author details

Aaron J. Suminski[1,2] and Robert A. Scheidt[1,3,4]

1 Biomedical Engineering, Marquette University, Milwaukee, WI, USA

2 Organismal Biology and Anatomy, University of Chicago, Chicago, IL, USA

3 Neurology, Medical College of Wisconsin, Milwaukee, WI, USA

4 Physical Medicine and Rehabilitation, Feinberg School of Medicine, Northwestern University, Chicago, IL, USA

References

[1] Carter CS, Braver TS, Barch DM, Botvinick MM, Noll D, Cohen JD (1998) Anterior cingulate cortex, error detection, and the online monitoring of performance. Science 280:747-749.

[2] Chinzei K, Kikinis R, Jolesz FA (1999) MR compatibility of mechatronic devices: design criteria. In: Medical Image Computing and Computer-Assisted Intervention Meeting - MICCAI'99., pp 1020-1030. Cambridge, UK.

[3] Cox RW (1996) AFNI: software for analysis and visualization of functional magnetic resonance neuroimages. Comput Biomed Res 29:162-173.

[4] Diedrichsen J, Shadmehr R (2005) Detecting and adjusting for artifacts in fMRI time series data. Neuroimage 27:624-634.

[5] Diedrichsen J, Hashambhoy Y, Rane T, Shadmehr R (2005) Neural correlates of reach errors. J Neurosci 25:9919-9931.

[6] Evarts EV, Tanji J (1976) Reflex and intended responses in motor cortex pyramidal tract neurons of monkey. J Neurophysiol 39:1069-1080.

[7] Evarts EV, Vaughn WJ (1978) Intended Arm Movements in Response to Externally Produced Arm Displacements in Man. In: Cerebral Motor Control in Man: Long Loop Mechanisms (Desmedt JE, ed), pp 178-192. Basel ; New York: Karger.

[8] Evarts EV, Fromm C (1981) Transcortical reflexes and servo control of movement. Can J Physiol Pharmacol 59:757-775.

[9] Fagg AH, Barto AG, Houk JC (1998) Learning to reach via corrective movements. In: Tenth Yale Workshop on Adaptive and Learning Systems, pp pp. 179-185. New Haven, CT.

[10] Flueckiger M, Bullo M, Chapuis D, Gassert R, Perriard Y (2005) fMRI compatible haptic interface actuated with traveling wave ultrasonic motor. In: IEEE Industry Applications Society Fortieth Annual Meeting pp 2075-2082 2073. Kowloon, Hong Kong.

[11] Ganesh G, Gassert R, Burdet E, Bleuler H (2004) Dynamics and control of an MRI compatible master-slave system with hydrostatic transmission. In: IEEE International Conference on Robotics and Automation, pp 1288-1294. New Orleans, LA.

[12] Gassert R, Burdet E, Chinzei K (2008) Opportunities and challenges in MR-compatible robotics: reviewing the history, mechatronic components, and future directions of this technology. IEEE Eng Med Biol Mag 27:15-22.

[13] Gassert R, Moser R, Burdet E, Bleuler H (2006) MRI/fMRI-compatible robotic system with force feedback for interaction with human motion. IEEE/ASME Transactions on Mechatronics 11:216-224.

[14] Ghez C, Scheidt R, Heijink H (2007) Different learned coordinate frames for planning trajectories and final positions in reaching. J Neurophysiol 98:3614-3626.

[15] Haacke EM, Brown RW, Thompson MR, Venkatesan R (1999) Magnetic resonance imaging : physical principles and sequence design. New York: Wiley.

[16] Haaland KY, Harrington DL (1989) Hemispheric control of the initial and corrective components of aiming movements. Neuropsychologia 27:961-969.

[17] Hidler J, Hodics T, Xu B, Dobkin B, Cohen LG (2006) MR compatible force sensing system for real-time monitoring of wrist moments during fMRI testing. J Neurosci Methods 155:300-307.

[18] Horne MK, Butler EG (1995) The role of the cerebello-thalamo-cortical pathway in skilled movement. Prog Neurobiol 46:199-213.

[19] Imamizu H, Miyauchi S, Tamada T, Sasaki Y, Takino R, Putz B, Yoshioka T, Kawato M (2000) Human cerebellar activity reflecting an acquired internal model of a new tool.[comment]. Nature 403:192-195.

[20] Jahanshahi M, Jenkins IH, Brown RG, Marsden CD, Passingham RE, Brooks DJ (1995) Self-initiated versus externally triggered movements. I. An investigation using

measurement of regional cerebral blood flow with PET and movement-related potentials in normal and Parkinson's disease subjects. Brain 118 (Pt 4):913-933.

[21] Jueptner M, Weiller C (1998) A review of differences between basal ganglia and cerebellar control of movements as revealed by functional imaging studies. Brain 121 (Pt 8):1437-1449.

[22] Kawato M, Kuroda T, Imamizu H, Nakano E, Miyauchi S, Yoshioka T (2003) Internal forward models in the cerebellum: fMRI study on grip force and load force coupling. Progress in Brain Research 142:171-188.

[23] Khanicheh A, Mintzopoulos D, Weinberg B, Tzika AA, Mavroidis C (2008) MR_CHIROD v.2: magnetic resonance compatible smart hand rehabilitation device for brain imaging. IEEE Trans Neural Syst Rehabil Eng 16:91-98.

[24] Khanicheh A, Muto A, Triantafyllou C, Weinberg B, Astrakas L, Tzika A, Mavroidis C (2005) MR compatible ERF driven hand rehabilitation device. In: IEEE 9th International Conference on Rehabilitation Robotics, pp 7-12. Chicago, IL.

[25] Lee RG, Tatton WG (1975) Motor responses to sudden limb displacements in primates with specific CNS lesions and in human patients with motor system disorders. Can J Neurol Sci 2:285-293.

[26] Marsden CD, Merton PA, Morton HB (1972) Servo action in human voluntary movement. Nature 238:140-143.

[27] Marsden CD, Merton PA, Morton HB, Adam JER, Hallett M (1978) Automatic and Voluntary Responses to Muscle Stretch in Man. In: Cerebral Motor Control in Man: Long Loop Mechanisms (Desmedt JE, ed), pp 167-177. Basel ; New York: Karger.

[28] Matthews PBC (1981) Muscle spindles their messages and their fusimotor supply. In: Sect, 1: The Nervous System (Brookhart JM, Mountcastle VB, Brooks VB, eds), pp 189-228. Bethesda: Am. Phisiol. Soc.

[29] Milner TE, Cloutier C (1993) Compensation for mechanically unstable loading in voluntary wrist movement. Experimental Brain Research 94:522-532.

[30] Peck KK, Sunderland A, Peters AM, Butterworth S, Clark P, Gowland PA (2001) Cerebral activation during a simple force production task: changes in the time course of the haemodynamic response. Neuroreport 12:2813-2816.

[31] Rao SM, Bandettini PA, Binder JR, Bobholz JA, Hammeke TA, Stein EA, Hyde JS (1996) Relationship between finger movement rate and functional magnetic resonance signal change in human primary motor cortex. J Cereb Blood Flow Metab 16:1250-1254.

[32] Riener R, Villgrattner T, Kleiser R, Nef T, Kollias S (2005) fMRI-Compatible Electromagnetic Haptic Interface. In: 27th Annual International Conference of the IEEE-EMBS, pp 7024-7027. Shanghi, China.

[33] Sakai K, Hikosaka O, Miyauchi S, Sasaki Y, Fujimaki N, Putz B (1999) Presupplementary motor area activation during sequence learning reflects visuo-motor association. J Neurosci 19:RC1.

[34] Scheidt RA, Ghez C (2007) Separate adaptive mechanisms for controlling trajectory and final position in reaching. J Neurophysiol 98:3600-3613.

[35] Schenck JF (1996) The role of magnetic susceptibility in magnetic resonance imaging: MRI magnetic compatibility of the first and second kinds. Medical Physics 23:815-850.

[36] Schmahmann JD (2000) MRI atlas of the human cerebellum. In. San Diego: Academic Press.

[37] Scott SH (2004) Optimal feedback control and the neural basis of volitional motor control. Nat Rev Neurosci 5:532-546.

[38] Sinkjaer T, Hayashi R (1989) Regulation of wrist stiffness by the stretch reflex. J Biomech 22:1133-1140.

[39] Sinkjaer T, Andersen JB, Ladouceur M, Christensen LO, Nielsen JB (2000) Major role for sensory feedback in soleus EMG activity in the stance phase of walking in man. J Physiol 523 Pt 3:817-827.

[40] Strick PL (1978) Cerebellar Involvement in 'Volitional' Muscle Responses to Load Changes. In: Cerebral Motor Control in Man: Long Loop Mechanisms (Desmedt JE, ed), pp 85-93. Basel ; New York: Karger.

[41] Suminski AJ, Ropella KM, Scheidt RA (2002) A pneumatically actuated manipulandum for neuromotor control research. In: IEEE EMBS Society Meeting, pp 2347-2348 vol.2343. Houston, TX.

[42] Suminski AJ, Zimbelman JL, Scheidt RA (2007a) Design and validation of a MR-compatible pneumatic manipulandum. J Neurosci Methods 163:255-266.

[43] Suminski AJ, Rao SM, Mosier KM, Scheidt RA (2007b) Neural and electromyographic correlates of wrist posture control. J Neurophysiol 97:1527-1545.

[44] Talairach J, Tournoux P (1988) Co-planar stereotaxic atlas of the human brain. Stuttgart/New York: Thieme.

[45] Thoroughman KA, Shadmehr R (1999) Electromyographic correlates of learning an internal model of reaching movements. J Neurosci 19:8573-8588.

[46] Todorov E, Jordan MI (2002) Optimal feedback control as a theory of motor coordination. Nat Neurosci 5:1226-1235.

[47] Vaillancourt DE, Thulborn KR, Corcos DM (2003) Neural basis for the processes that underlie visually guided and internally guided force control in humans. J Neurophysiol 90:3330-3340.

[48] Van Essen DC, Drury HA, Dickson J, Harwell J, Hanlon D, Anderson CH (2001) An integrated software suite for surface-based analyses of cerebral cortex. J Am Med Inform Assoc 8:443-459.

[49] Wann JP, Ibrahim SF (1992) Does limb proprioception drift? Exp Brain Res 91:162-166.

[50] Winstein CJ, Grafton ST, Pohl PS (1997) Motor task difficulty and brain activity: investigation of goal-directed reciprocal aiming using positron emission tomography. J Neurophysiol 77:1581-1594.

[51] Yu N, Hollnagel C, Blickenstorfer A, Kollias SS, Riener R (2008) Comparison of MRI-Compatible Mechatronic Systems With Hydrodynamic and Pneumatic Actuation. Mechatronics, IEEE/ASME Transactions on 13:268-277.

[52] Ziegler JG, Nichols NB (1942) Optimum settings for automatic controllers. ASME Trans 64:759-768.

6

Color Specificity in the Human V4 Complex – An fMRI Repetition Suppression Study

Tessa M. van Leeuwen, Karl Magnus Petersson, Oliver Langner, Mark Rijpkema and Peter Hagoort

1. Introduction

The hierarchy of color processing areas in the human brain starts from cone-opponent signals in the retina. Relayed by the lateral geniculate nucleus (LGN), color information arrives at the primary visual cortex (V1) and area V2, where color contrast is computed (Conway, 2009). Later visual area V4 and 'globs' of neurons in ventral occipital cortex (immediately anterior to V4) are deemed important for color constancy and for the luminance-invariant coding of individual hues. Not only electrophysiological data from non-human primate studies (Conway, Moeller, & Tsao, 2007; Kotake, Morimoto, Okazaki, Fujita, & Tamura, 2009; Kusunoki, Moutoussis, & Zeki, 2006; Matsumora, Koida, & Komatsu, 2008; Stoughton & Conway, 2008; Zeki, 1980), but also neuroimaging and lesion studies in humans implicate the 'V4 complex' in higher order color processing (Barbur & Spang, 2008; Bartels & Zeki, 2000; Bouvier & Engel, 2006; McKeefry & Zeki, 1997). It is known however, that V4 is not a color area per se, as it is also involved in shape and form processing (e.g. Schiller, 1995).

The posterior section of the human V4 complex (posterior fusiform gyrus) is referred to as V4; the anterior section (anterior fusiform gyrus) as V4α (Bartels & Zeki, 2000; McKeefry & Zeki, 1997). Other definitions have also been proposed for V4 (e.g. V8 (Hadjikhani, Liu, Dale, Cavanagh, & Tootell, 1998), VO1 (Brewer, Liu, Wade, & Wandell, 2005)). V4 is active in passive color tasks (Howard et al., 1998; McKeefry & Zeki, 1997; Sakai et al., 1995). Both subregions contribute to color constancy operations (Barbur & Spang, 2008; Bartels & Zeki, 2000). In tasks demanding active color manipulation, it is mainly V4α that is involved (Beauchamp, Haxby, Jennings, & DeYoe, 1999; Martin, Haxby, Lalonde, Wiggs, & Ungerleider, 1995; Morita et al., 2004; Simmons et al., 2007; Zeki & Marini, 1998). Murphey, Yoshor and Beauchamp (2008) have identified color-specific neurons in V4α in one patient, using electrophysiological methods. Altogether these findings suggest a functional distinction between V4 and V4α. Here, we investigate whether V4 and V4α exhibit different color selectivity properties.

We performed a functional magnetic resonance imaging (fMRI) experiment in which we applied repetition suppression. In repetition suppression, a stimulus is presented more than once (as in behavioral priming studies (e.g. Maccotta & Buckner, 2004). The process has been referred to as fMRI-adaptation (K. Grill-Spector & Malach, 2001), mnemonic filtering (Miller, Li, & Desimone, 1993); repetition suppression (Desimone, 1996); decremental responses (Brown & Xiang, 1998) and neural priming (Maccotta & Buckner, 2004). The blood-oxygen-level dependent (BOLD) response evoked by the second and later presentations of the stimulus is (in general) reduced compared to the response evoked by the first presentation (K Grill-Spector, Henson, & Martin, 2005; Henson, 2003). These priming-related repetition suppression effects can be elicited by different types of priming-paradigms, such as masked priming (Dehaene et al., 2001; Eddy, Schnyer, Schmid, & Holcomb, 2007), visual object priming (Cavina-Pratesi, Kentridge, Heywood, & Milner, 2010), and semantic priming (Luo et al., 2004). Depending on the type of stimulus that is processed, and on the stage of stimulus processing, different parts of the brain may show repetition suppression. Because repetition suppression would only occur in brain regions that are sensitive to the specific aspect of the stimulus that is being repeated, the technique allows for better spatial location determination than conventional fMRI studies. This can be illustrated by thinking about a paradigm in which familiar colored objects are visually presented to the participants (i.e. a red ball). Individually presented, these objects will activate all relevant brain areas that are involved in shape and color processing, as well as memory and semantic brain areas. However, when using the repetition suppression technique and showing a second stimulus in which for instance only the shape of the object is repeated, only shape areas will show a reduction in the BOLD response. In this way, repetition suppression may lead to enhanced precision in determining the location of relevant brain areas involved in specific processes of interest (K Grill-Spector, et al., 2005; K. Grill-Spector et al., 1999).

Here, we investigated the repetition of color. We hypothesized that in a collection of neurons with specific color selectivity, the repetition of the *same* color would reduce the BOLD response more than the presentation of two *different* colors: if the second color differs from the first color, this would recruit different neurons in case of very specific color selectivity of the neurons. Neurons with less specific color selectivity would respond to a wider range of colors and would not strictly require one particular color as input in order to become active (Conway, et al., 2007); hence, these neurons would show (some) repetition suppression not only when the same color, but also when two different colors are presented subsequently, because they would be (weakly) active for both presentations of colors.

We hypothesized that the color selectivity of neurons would increase when progressing from posterior (V4) to anterior (V4α) areas along the processing hierarchy.

Several fMRI studies have previously used repetition suppression to investigate color processing. Engel et al. (2005) deployed fMRI-adaptation to show repetition suppression effects for color in populations of both oriented and unoriented color-selective cells in visual cortex. Two other fMRI studies have aimed to identify regions in the ventral-occipital cortex that are selectively involved in color processing (and not texture or form processing) (Cant, Arnott, & Goodale, 2009; Cavina-Pratesi, et al., 2010). In both studies, 3D-objects were used of which the form, texture, and color could either stay identical from one stimulus presentation to the next (repetition suppression is expected), or be changed (no repetition suppression). Both studies found that the left anterior collateral sulcus, of which the stereotaxic coordinates correspond to left V4α, was more responsive when the color of the objects changed between subsequent stimulus presentations; in case of Cavina-Pratesi et al (2010), this effect was bilatereal, including also right anterior collateral sulcus. Cant et al. (2009) found additional, similar effects in right fusiform gyrus while Cavina-Pratesi et al. (2010) also found effects in left lingual gyrus. It should be noticed that in the study by Cant et al. (2009), the above mentioned regions were not solely selective to color as they also responded to changes in texture; it were primarily medial regions of the ventral stream along the fusiform gyrus that were showing selectivity to color changes. Taken together, these studies strongly suggest that (left) V4α contains neurons that are rather specifically tuned for color such that they reduce their activity when that same color is repeated. However, these studies yielded no clear evidence that the posterior fusiform gyrus (V4) exhibits similar color specificity, independent of texture information. In our study, we explicitly test whether area V4 shows similar repetition suppression effects for color as area V4α. We propose that neurons in V4α, situated later in the processing hierarchy, show greater specificity for color than neurons in V4 and that is why area V4α has been readily identified by repetition suppression paradigms and V4 has not been.

In our experiment we used simple patches of color (squares) that were always of the same form and texture, minimizing intrusion of these dimensions in the experiment. We applied a priming paradigm to obtain BOLD repetition suppression effects for color. The color of the prime square was either the *same* color (SC) as the target square, a *different* color (DC), or an *achromatic* color (AC) containing only grey values (r=g=b). In neurons with high color selectivity, the SC condition was hypothesized to reduce the BOLD response more than the DC condition. The achromatic color condition was included as a control condition for which we expected no or very little repetition suppression. We use an active task to engage the participants; the color of the target square had to be indicated with a button press and reaction times were analyzed. Because we wanted to investigate repetition suppression effects in both hemispheres and both sections of the V4-complex, we determined *a priori* regions of interest (ROIs) in anterior and posterior parts of the V4 complex to assess the effects in all of these regions (Figure 1). The ROIs were defined on the basis of findings from Bartels and Zeki (2000) and the coordinates of V4α corresponded to the reported effects by Cavina-Pratesi et al. (2010). We predicted that only in V4α, and not more posterior V4, the BOLD suppression effects would differ between repetitions of the same versus two different colors (SC and DC conditions).

2. Material and methods

2.1. Participants

Forty subjects aged 18-38 (mean age 26.2 years, *SD*=4.7 years, 4 males, 4 left-handed) participated. In both groups, 2 left handed individuals were present, making sure that any reaction time differences found between the groups were not influenced by handedness. All participants completed a pre-screening questionnaire to assess their medical history, handedness and MRI-compatibility. All had normal or corrected to normal vision and reported no color blindness, and were able to discriminate the stimulus colors. None reported a neurological or psychiatric disease. Informed consent was obtained (prior to scanning) after explanation of the experimental procedures. The study was approved by the local ethics committee, in accordance with the declaration of Helsinki. One participant was excluded prior to analysis after reassessment of her medical history, leaving 39 participants.

As the experiment was part of a larger study on synesthesia (van Leeuwen, Petersson, & Hagoort, 2010), 21 of the subjects were grapheme-color synesthetes (Hubbard & Ramachandran, 2005). The remaining 19 subjects were matched to the synesthetes on sex, age, handedness, and educational level. Differences between the two subgroups were not found and hence both groups were collapsed for this study.

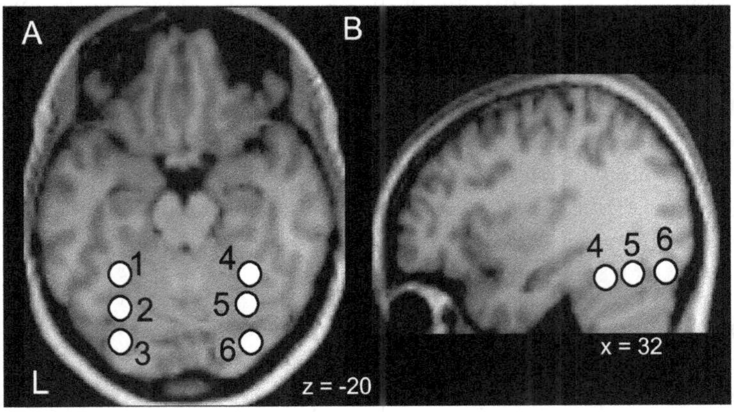

A) and B) Axial and sagittal brain slices, respectively, of template brain illustrating the position of the six ROIs in the V4 complex in the fusiform gyrus. See below for MNI coordinates (x,y,z) denoting the center of the 5 mm radius ROIs within different sections of the V4 complex. Coordinates are derived from Bartels and Zeki (2000, Table 1). 1. L V4α (-32,-50,-22); 2. L V4α/V4 (-30,-66,-22); 3. L V4 (-32,-82,-20); 4. R V4α (32,-50,-24); 5. V4α/V4 (30,-64,-22); 6. R V4 (32,-82,-20). L=left, R=right.

Figure 1. Location of regions of interest in the V4 complex.

2.2. Experimental design

We applied a priming paradigm to obtain BOLD repetition suppression effects for color. Both prime and target consisted of colored squares. The color of the prime was either the *same* color (SC) as the target, a *different* color (DC), or an *achromatic* color (AC). Different repetition suppression effects were predicted for each condition. In the SC trials (for instance a red square followed by another red square) we hypothesized that the repetition of the prime color in the target would lead to BOLD repetition suppression effects for the target square in neurons that are more selectively tuned for that color. The overlap between neuronal processing of the color of the prime and the color of the target would lead to fMRI adaptation effects, reducing the BOLD response (Henson, 2003). In the DC trials the color of the target differed from that of the prime (for instance a red square followed by a green square). We predicted that a repetition suppression effect in the DC condition would only occur if the different colors were (partly) processed by the same neuronal population; hence by neurons with a less specific color selectivity function (Conway, et al., 2007). In areas containing many neurons that exhibit specific color selectivity, DC trials would not lead to large repetition suppression effects; different neurons would code for the prime and target colors, inducing a relatively large BOLD response. We expected that only in V4α, and not in V4, the SC condition would lead to more BOLD suppression (and hence less activation) than the DC condition; this follows from our hypothesis that V4α contains neurons that are more specifically selective for color than neurons in V4.

We included the achromatic color condition as a control condition for which we expected no or very little repetition suppression. Here, the primes consisted of achromatic squares (grey values) while the targets were chromatic squares (for instance a grey square followed by a red square). In color sensitive regions (Beauchamp, et al., 1999; McKeefry & Zeki, 1997) and neurons (Conway, et al., 2007; Murphey, et al., 2008), the responses to achromatic stimuli are typically much weaker than responses to chromatic stimuli, although they may be higher than baseline. We therefore predicted that the responses to the achromatic primes would affect the responses to the chromatic targets relatively little; little or no repetition suppression would occur for the AC trials, resulting in a relatively strong BOLD response for the colored targets. For the SC and DC trials, we expected (some) repetition suppression to occur in all of the color-sensitive V4-complex. To assess the general responsiveness to color in the V4 complex we therefore compared the effects of the AC condition to the effects of the collapsed SC and DC conditions.

In addition to the color priming conditions, the design contained synesthetic priming conditions of which the trials were intermixed with the color priming trials. SC, DC, and AC manipulations were also present in the synesthetic priming, but the primes consisted of black graphemes (single letters, digits, or symbols) instead of squares. The synesthetic priming results will not be discussed in detail here and can be reviewed elsewhere (van Leeuwen, et al., 2010); synesthetic trials will be referred to as fillers.

During the experiment the participants indicated the color of the target square with a button press (one button for each color, hence a color decision was required): we used this active task because attention enhances the cortical responses to color (Chawla, Rees, & Friston, 1999;

Corbetta, Miezin, Dobmeyer, Shulman, & Petersen, 1991). On the basis of previous findings we expected faster reaction times for the same color trials, due to facilitating effects of the prime on target processing (DiPace, Marangolo, & Pizzamiglio, 1997; Marangolo, Dipace, & Pizzamiglio, 1993; Simon, 1988). Additionally, we expected the different color trials to cause reaction time interference (increased reaction times) due to the switch in color from prime to target; in case any facilitating processes already occurred for the prime, these would have to be overcome at the time of the response to the different target color. In the achromatic trials the achromatic prime was never informative of the target button to be pressed, because all the target colors were chromatic. We therefore expected that the reaction times for the different color trials would be slower than those for the achromatic trials due to more interference from chromatic color information from the prime.

2.3. Materials and apparatus

Color stimuli were derived from unique synesthetic hues of the synesthetic participants. The synesthetic colors were selected by the synesthetes prior to the practice session. After color selection, for each synesthete four letter and color pairs were chosen for which the letters elicited four clearly distinct and strong synesthetic colors. These synesthetically induced colors were used thoughout the experiment as primes and targets. Mainly the colors red, green, blue, and yellow were used. All colored squares had a size of 2.1º x 2.1º of visual angle and were presented using Presentation (version 10.2, *Neurobehavioral Systems Inc.*, www.neurobs.com). The background was light grey (full screen, 9.1 cd/m2). Stimuli were presented on a 44.5 x 33.5 cm display screen in the scanner tunnel, placed at a viewing distance of 60 cm (controlled by a Dell Pentium IV Windows XP computer, display mode 800 x 600 pixels at 60 Hz, projected by a EIKI X986 beamer).

All colors appeared equally often in both the SC and DC conditions, and equally often as prime and target stimuli. The mean luminance of the colored stimuli was 8.4 cd/m2 (*SD*=10.3 cd/m2). Black, dark grey, light grey, and white squares were used as achromatic primes in the AC trials and their mean luminance was 7.5 cd/m2 (*SD*=13.5 cd/m2), which did not differ significantly from that of the chromatic stimuli. Grey values (rgb) for the black, dark grey, light grey and white AC primes were (0,0,0), (80,80,80), (160,160,160), and (240,240,240), respectively. We used 4 different shades of achromatic squares because there were also 4 different colors present in the experiment. Hence also in the achromatic condition, we wanted to make use of 4 different prime stimuli to keep the same variation in the achromatic primes as in the colored primes. In other studies, for instance achromatic (=greyscale) Mondrian stimuli have been used as contrasts to colored Mondrian stimuli to map color areas (McKeefry & Zeki, 1997). Although the colored stimuli were used equally often in the SC and DC conditions (which constitutes our most important comparison), we wanted to avoid the possible confound of color luminance in our analyses. We therefore, for each trial, calculated the absolute difference in luminance between the stimuli and the background luminance. We modeled this luminance difference explicitly during analysis of the fMRI data by including it as a parametric modulation value with each trial, which could capture any effects that could solely be ascribed to variance in luminance.

2.4. Procedure

SC, DC, and AC trials appeared in a ratio of 1:2:1 (48:96:48), for a total of 192 trials (and 192 synaesthesia filler trials). The 1:2:1 ratio was chosen such that the expectancy of a same color trial matched the expectancy of any particular target color (25%) as closely as possible, to minimize behavioral strategy effects. The stimuli were divided into four identical runs, each containing 12 SC, 24 DC, and 12 AC trials for both the color priming and the filler trials, resulting in a total of 96 trials per run. Twenty-four null-events (20%, fixation only) were included in each run to avoid BOLD saturation. All stimuli were pseudo-randomized per run, with maximally 2 repetitions of prime type (SC, DC, or AC) and prime color, maximally 3 repetitions of the same target color, and maximally 5 repetitions of overall condition (color or filler).

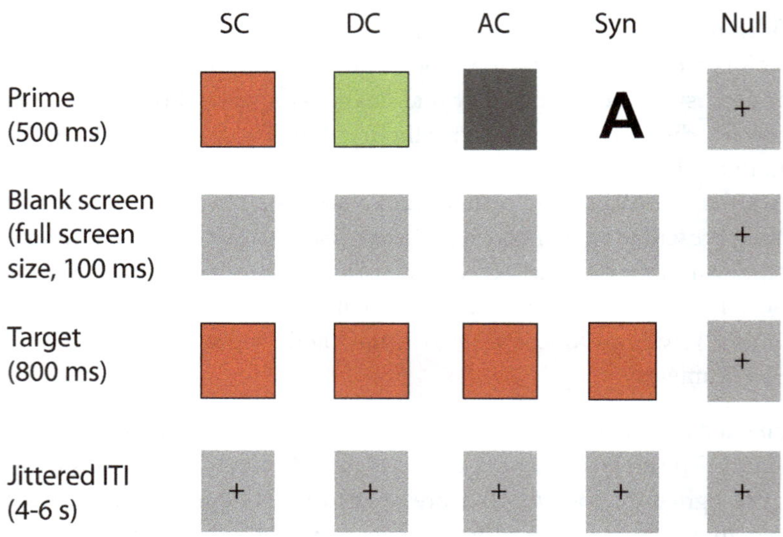

Figure 2. Experimental design. Each trial consisted of a prime stimulus followed by a blank screen, and a target stimulus (depicted from top to bottom). Prime and target stimuli were shown in the center of the screen and measured 2.1x2.1 degrees of visual angle only, surrounded by a grey background color. SC=same color, same color is repeated in prime and target (e.g. red (prime and target)); DC=different color, two different colors are used for prime and target (e.g. red for prime and green for target or green for prime and blue for target); AC=achromatic color, prime is always achromatic grey value (r=g=b) and target is in color. Syn, example of synaesthesia (filler) condition in which a letter was used as a prime; Null, depiction of null-event during which the fixation cross remained on the screen. In the synaesthesia (filler) condition, the letter could evoke synaesthesia in the target color (SCSyn), synaesthesia in a different color than the target (DCSyn) or evoke no synaesthesia (ACSyn); hence the same manipulations applied as in the color condition. The synaesthesia results are discussed elsewhere (van Leeuwen, et al., 2010). For number of trials and ratios see Section 2.4 Procedures.

Each trial consisted of a prime that was displayed for 500 ms, followed by a blank screen for 100 ms (light grey background color), and finally a target for 800 ms. During the jittered intertrial-interval of 4-6 seconds a fixation cross was displayed. Participants were instructed to indicate the color of the target squares fast but accurately by pressing one of four response buttons with the associated finger of their right hand. Each experimental color was assigned to one of the response buttons.

First, each participant completed 16 practice trials outside of the scanner containing exemplars of all conditions. Response devices were a normal keyboard for the practice session and an MR-scanner compatible Lumitouch response box for the fMRI session. After the practice trials the fMRI session began, starting with a 5 minute structural scan to familiarize participants with the scanner noise. Next, the participants completed the first two runs of the priming experiment (12 minutes each, 380 images), and were then allowed to take a break for 10 minutes outside of the scanner. The last two priming runs followed after the break. During scanning participants wore sound-attenuating headphones to protect their hearing from the scanner noise.

2.5. Image acquisition parameters

MR data were acquired with a 3.0 Tesla Siemens TrioTim MR scanner and an 8-channel head array (Invivo). A single shot gradient echo-planar imaging (EPI) sequence was used to acquire functional MR images (33 slices, TE=30 msec, TR=2090 msec, flip angle=80º, 224 mm FOV, 64 x 64 matrix, 3.5 x 3.5 mm voxel size, 3.0 mm slice thickness,.5 mm slice gap). Atlas-based registration (AutoAlign, Siemens (Van der Kouwe et al., 2005)) was applied for all EPI runs to ensure the same slice positions across all functional runs of one subject (also across the break). A high-resolution T1-weighted structural image was acquired for each subject (MPRAGE, TE=2.96 msec, TR=2300 msec, 256 mm FOV, 256 x 256 matrix, 1 mm3 resolution, acquisition time 5 minutes, accelerated with factor 2 by GRAPPA parallel imaging (Griswold et al., 2002)).

2.6. Data analysis

2.6.1. Behavioral data

The reaction time data were analyzed with a repeated measures ANOVA. Only correct trials were included. Reaction times that were more than two standard deviations away from the subject and condition mean were considered to be outliers and removed from the analysis. Mauchly's test of spericity was applied (as standardly implemented in SPSS) and in cases of non-sphericity, a Greenhouse-Geisser correction was used to adjust the degrees of freedom (uncorrected degrees of freedom are reported).

2.6.2. Imaging data

MR data were preprocessed and analyzed with SPM5 (Wellcome Department of Imaging Neuroscience, www.fil.ion.ucl.ac.uk/spm/software/spm5). Prior to analysis, the first five volumes of each subject were discarded to avoid transient T1 effects. To correct for head motion, the functional images of each subject were spatially realigned to the first image using a six parameter [translation in x, y, and z directions; rotations pitch, roll, and jaw] rigid body transformation for each image. Slice timing correction was applied and the images were normalized to the standard EPI template of SPM5 to allow for group inference. During normalization the images were resampled to a 2x2x2 mm resolution. Finally, all images were spatially filtered using a 10 mm FWHM isotropic Gaussian filter, as has been previously applied by others (van Leeuwen, et al., 2010; Van Wingen et al., 2008; Weiss, Zilles, & Fink, 2005; Wildgruber et al., 2005).

Statistical analyses were based on the General Linear Model (GLM) framework. For each subject, the design matrix was constructed and the BOLD signal was modeled by the canonical hemodynamic response function (HRF). A high-pass filter (128 sec cut-off) was used to remove low-frequency effects, and global scaling was applied to remove various global effects of no interest. The design matrix consisted of regressors modeling each of the six experimental conditions (SC, DC, and AC conditions for color and fillers) and one parametric modulation regressor for each of the six experimental regressors to model the luminance difference with the background. All events were modeled by the onset of the target squares. The six realignment parameters that were obtained during preprocessing were included in the model as covariates of no interest. Parameter estimates were obtained for each condition and each participant to generate relevant contrast images and allow for second-level random effects analysis. Coordinates are reported in MNI space (x, y, z).

2.7. Region of Interest analyses

To assess repetition suppression effects in anterior and posterior parts of the V4 complex, we determined regions of interest (ROIs) on the basis of a review by Bartels and Zeki (2000). In Table 1 of the review, the minimum and maximum extent (in x, y, and z directions) of V4 and V4α activations are listed. We determined two (left and right hemisphere) ROIs in the anterior part of V4α (y=-50), and two ROIs in the posterior part of V4 (y=-80), at intermediate x and z coordinate positions. We added two ROIs at the V4α/V4 border (y=-65) to complete our survey of the V4 complex. The center coordinates of each ROI were converted to MNI space (with tal2mni, derived from http://imaging.mrc-cbu.cam.ac.uk/imaging/MniTalairach) and ROIs (spheres with a 5 mm radius (10 mm diameter)) were subsequently created using MarsBaR (Brett, Anton, Valabregue, & Poline, 2002). Figure 1 shows the ROI positions on a template brain and the ROI center coordinates are listed in the figure legend.

To look at repetition suppression effects for color in the different ROIs, we extracted the mean values of the GLM parameter estimates for each priming condition (SC, DC, and AC) for each subject and for each selected ROI using MarsBaR (Brett, et al., 2002). First, we confirmed overall color sensitivity in the V4 complex (in the left and right hemisphere) by comparing the BOLD effects for the SC and DC conditions with the AC condition. We then tested the specific hypothesis that the SC trials would lead to less activation (due to more repetition suppression) than DC trials in V4α, but not in V4; leading to an interaction effect. The mean parameter estimates of the ROIs were therefore subjected to a repeated measures ANOVA with the within-subjects factors region (V4α and V4) and prime type (SC and DC), separately for each hemisphere.

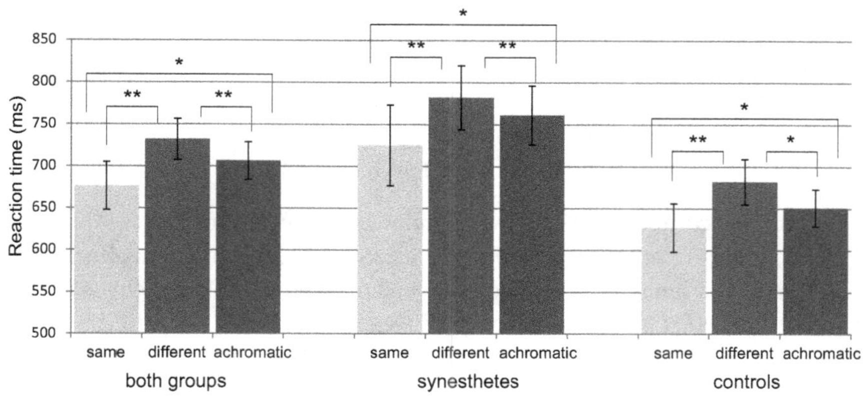

Figure 3. Behavioral effects of color priming. Mean reaction times in milliseconds for the same color (light grey bars), different color (dark grey bars) and achromatic color (near black bars) conditions. Error bars denote ± standard error of the mean. * (p<.05) and ** (p<.001) denote significant differences in reaction times of the repeated measures ANOVA with factor prime type (SC, DC, and AC), for both groups collapsed (N=38) depicted on the left. For illustrative purposes, the results per group are also depicted (synesthetes (N=19) in the middle and for controls (N=19) on the right. Here, * (p<.05) and ** (p<.001) denote the significance of the results of separate ANOVAs for each group.

3. Results

We excluded one participant from the analyses, due to an overall high error rate of 27.1% on the behavioral task (the average error rate of the remaining participants (N=38) was 3.9% (*SD*=4.3%)).

3.1. Behavioral data

We expected to see an effect of prime type (SC, DC, and AC) on the reaction times (RTs). Incorrect responses (for percentages see Figure 3) and outliers (5.8% total) were discarded. The average RTs are summarized in Figure 3, separated for the two subgroups of participants. Before looking at the within-subjects effects on the reaction times and error rates of the group of 38 participants, we verified there were no effects of subgroup (synesthetic and non-synesthetic). A main effect of subgroup was present in the reaction times ($F(1,36)=4.825$, $p<.05$); synesthetes showed longer reaction times overall. This was presumably caused by an increase in overall task difficulty for synesthetes due to the inclusion of the synesthetic priming condition. There was no subgroup x prime type interaction, indicating that the priming effects did not differ across subgroups. Therefore the RT data of all 38 participants were combined for further analyses and an ANOVA with only the factor prime type was run, including all 38 participants. For the error rates, no main effect of subgroup and no subgroup x prime type interaction were found. The average error rates across all participants were 4.3%, 4.6%, and 2.6% for the same, different, and achromatic color condition, respectively. A repeated measures ANOVA of the RTs with the within-subjects factor prime type revealed a significant effect of prime type ($F(2,74)=12.688$, $p<.001$). Planned comparisons showed that the RTs of the same color condition were much faster than the RTs of the different color condition ($F(1,37)=20.228$, $p<.001$, 56 msec faster) and also faster than the achromatic condition RTs ($F(1,37)=5.436$, $p<.05$, 30 msec faster). The RTs of the different color condition were also significantly slower than the RTs of the achromatic trials ($F(1,37)=13.959$, $p<.001$, 25 msec slower). The results are in line with previous findings on color priming (Marangolo, et al., 1993; Simon, 1988) and show that a repetition of the prime color in the target yields an RT advantage.

To check for speed-accuracy trade-offs, we calculated a repeated measures ANOVA with the within-subjects factor prime type for the error rates. We found a significant effect of prime type ($F(2,74)=6.829$, $p<.05$). Planned comparisons revealed an effect only for the AC condition in comparison to the SC ($F(1,37)=8.090$, $p<.01$) and DC conditions ($F(1,37)=13.228$, $p<.001$); there were less errors in the AC condition. SC and DC conditions did not differ in error rate ($F(1,37)=.306$, n.s.). The results indicate there was no speed-accuracy trade-off between the SC and the DC conditions, as there were no more errors in the SC condition.

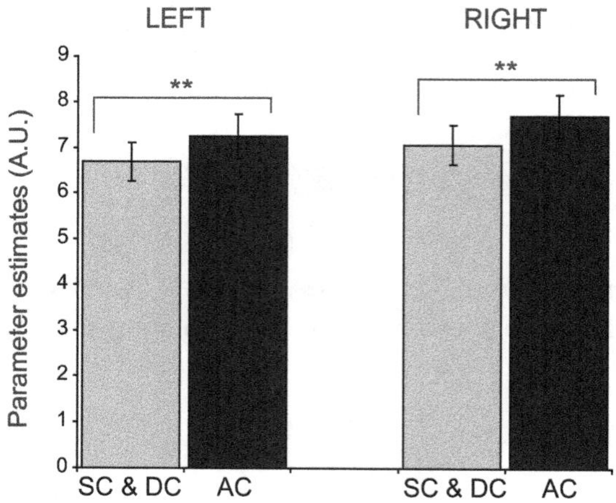

The difference between the AC trials (achromatic primes, no repetition suppression expected) and the collapsed SC and DC trials (colored primes, repetition suppression expected) in left and right hemisphere. A significant difference (**=p<.001) implies color sensitivity of the area. Mean parameter estimates (N=38) collapsed across the 3 ROIs are plotted. Error bars depict ± standard error of the mean.

Figure 4. Color sensitivity in the left and right V4 complex.

3.2. fMRI data

3.2.1. Region of Interest analyses

To look at repetition suppression effects for color in the different ROIs, we extracted the mean values of the parameter estimates for each priming condition (SC, DC, and AC) for each subject and for each selected ROI. First, we confirmed that color-induced repetition suppression was indeed occurring for the SC and DC conditions in the left and right V4 complex. We averaged the BOLD effects of these conditions for each participant and compared them to the effects of the AC condition (collapsed across the 3 ROIs within each hemisphere). In both the left and right hemisphere, there was a significantly reduced BOLD response for the averaged SC-DC conditions compared to the AC condition (left: $F(1,113)=13.634$, $p<.001$; right: $F(1,113)=22.563$, $p<.001$), which is illustrated in Figure 5.

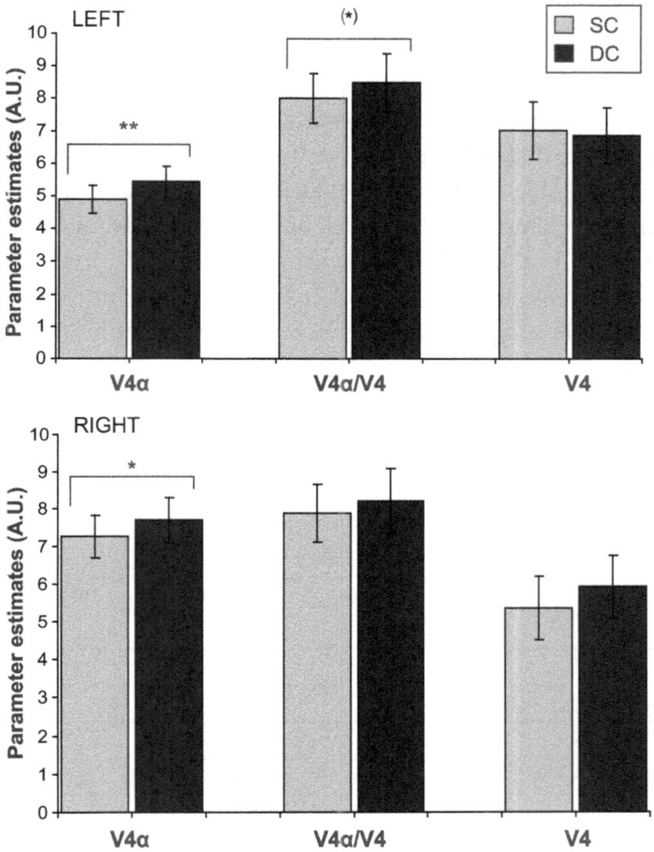

Mean parameter estimates (N=38) for each ROI are plotted for the SC and DC conditions. Error bars depict ± standard error of the mean. * (p<.05) and ** (p<.001) denote significant effects, (*) denotes a marginal effect.

Figure 5. Specificity of color selectivity in the V4 complex.

Next, in a repeated measures ANOVA with the factors region (V4α and V4) and prime type (SC and DC), we investigated a region by prime type interaction effect. In the left hemisphere, we found a significant interaction ($F(1,74)=4.123$, $p<.05$). There was no significant interaction in the right hemisphere ($F(1,74)=.089$, n.s.). Because we were interested in potential differences between the color selectivity properties of V4α and V4, we analyzed the ROIs in V4α and V4 separately. In left V4α, the SC condition showed a significantly lower BOLD effect than the DC condition ($F(1,37)=19.952$, $p<.001$), while in left V4, there was no effect of prime type ($F(1,37)=.256$, n.s.). The same pattern was found in the right hemisphere: right V4α

($F(1,37)=6.778$, $p<.05$), and right V4 ($F(1,37)=2.260$, n.s.). The mean BOLD effects for the SC and DC conditions of each ROI are summarized in Figure 5. A marginal difference between the SC and DC conditions is present at the V4α/V4 border in the left hemisphere ($F(1,37)=3.540$, $p<.068$). On the right, there are no effects at the V4α/V4 border ($F(1,37)=1.872$, n.s.).

3.2.2. *Whole brain analyses*

To illustrate the distribution of brain regions that showed an adaptation effect for color, the whole brain analysis of the contrast of AC trials compared to the averaged SC and DC conditions (overall effect of color-induced repetition suppression) is summarized in Figure 6A and Table 1. It can be seen that color-induced repetition suppression occurs in the bilateral V4 complex (fusiform gyrus, Figure 6A), as well as in the left cuneus and frontal regions. The effects in fusiform gyrus comprise V4α as well as more posterior V4. The comparison of the DC versus SC condition is also included (Figure 6B). This contrast was masked with brain regions that showed an overall adaptation effect for color, to exclude effects in areas that did not show an overall color adaptation effect. A significant effect in left fusiform gyrus was found, corresponding to the coordinates of area V4α, in line with previous repetition suppression studies (Cant, et al., 2009; Cavina-Pratesi, et al., 2010). In Figure 6C, the comparison of DC versus SC is shown for two representative individual subjects highlighting the anatomical position of the effects in fusiform gyrus. There were no significant whole brain effects of luminance.

Brain region	k	p	MNI coordinates (x, y, z)	T-value
AC > (SC & DC)				
L fusiform gyrus (BA 37/19)	1687	.000	-32, -50, -20	7.66
R fusiform gyrus (BA 37/19)	1805	.000	30, -52, -20	6.02
L cuneus/middle occ. gyrus (BA 18/19)	825	.001	-24, -82, 6	4.97
R cingulate gyrus (BA 31)	1170	.000	20, -40, 32	4.83
L medial frontal gyrus (BA 10)	312	.048	-14, 52, 8	4.53
L rolandic operculum	904	.000	-38, -16, 24	4.50
R medial frontal gyrus (BA 11)	495	.009	12, 56, -12	4.45
DC > SC*				
L fusiform gyrus (BA 37)	188	.017	-32, -48, -22	4.19
			-28, -56, -18	3.88
			-24, -66, -14	3.67

fMRI whole brain results of color priming (N=38, random effects analyses, whole brain threshold p<.001uncorrected, extent threshold 200 voxels). Cluster size (k), corrected P-values at cluster-level (p), MNI coordinates of local maxima and T-values are listed. Brodmann areas (BA) are in parentheses. R=right, L=left. *corrected for search volume (at whole brain threshold p<.001unc, extent threshold 100 voxels) with overall adaptation effect of AC > (SC & DC), to exclude effects in areas that did not show an overall color adaptation effect.

Table 1. Whole brain results of color priming

4. Discussion

Literature on color processing in human ventral occipital cortex suggests that a functional division exists between more anterior (V4α) and posterior (V4) sections of the human V4 complex. In this study, we show a functional segregation of V4α and V4 on the basis of the color adaptation properties of the neurons within the two sections. Our data suggest that in V4α, neurons are tuned for a smaller range of colors compared to neurons in V4. Although previous studies already reported repetition suppression for color in areas corresponding to left V4α (Cant, et al., 2009; Cavina-Pratesi, et al., 2010) which is similar to own our whole brain results, our region of interest approach made it possible to additionally assess repetition suppression in the right hemisphere and in the posterior V4 complex. We were able to show that repetition suppression also occurs in right hemisphere V4α but not in more posterior sections of the V4 complex. A stronger specificity for color in V4α is in line with the findings of Murphey et al. (2008), who identified color-selective neurons in V4α by means of electrophysiological recordings in a patient suffering from epilepsy. Electrical stimulation of the neurons that surrounded an inserted electrode led to the conscious perception of the same color for which these neurons were selective, suggesting rather color specific color selectivity in this area. Our results additionally demonstrate that this color specificity does not occur to the same degree in V4, an area where Murphey et al. (2008) did not record. Although our paradigm is not suitable to determine whether neurons in V4α are actually responsive to only *one* particular color, the localized effect that we see in V4α provides evidence for a functional subdivision between V4 and V4α.

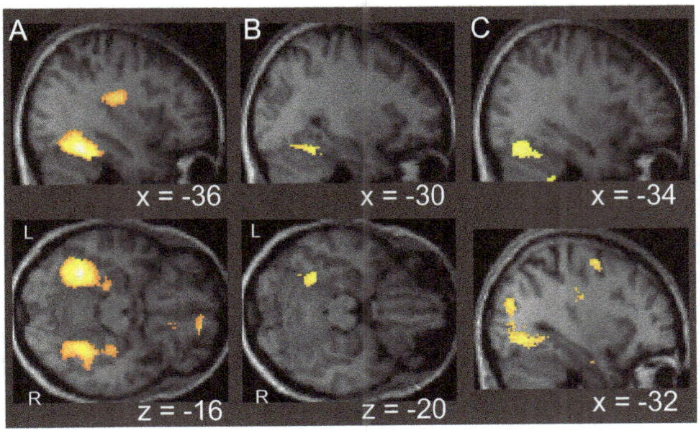

A) Sagittal (top) and axial (bottom) anatomical brain slices (template brain) with the group effects (N=38) of the contrast of the achromatic condition versus the averaged different color and same color conditions (AC > (DC & SC)). The position of the effects in left and right fusiform gyrus is shown (see Table 1). Random effects analyses, whole brain threshold p<.001unc, extent threshold 200 voxels. L=left, R=right. B) Sagittal (top) and axial (bottom) brain slices (template brain) with the group effect (N=38) of stronger adaptation for the same color condition than for the different color condition (DC > SC, also see Table 1). Random effects analyses, whole brain threshold p<.001unc, extent threshold 100 voxels, corrected for search volume with the contrast in A. C) Sagittal brain slices of two single participants with the same contrast as in B, showing individual activation patterns in left fusiform gyrus. Whole brain threshold p<.05unc, extent threshold 50 voxels.

Figure 6. Whole brain results of color priming.

Many studies report activity in area V4α when active color manipulations and tasks are involved, like color sequencing (Beauchamp, et al., 1999), object color (Martin, et al., 1995; Zeki & Marini, 1998) and color imagery (Howard, et al., 1998). A direct link between color awareness, perceptual knowledge about color, and specific color-selective neurons in the brain has been proposed (Barsalou, Simmons, Barbey, & Wilson, 2003; Goldberg, Perfetti, & Schneider, 2006; Simmons, et al., 2007). The findings of Murphey et al. (2008) in V4α strongly support this idea. Our data and set-up do not allow us to conclude that V4α is involved in color awareness or knowledge about color, but our results do suggest that the more narrow selectivity of color neurons in V4α may lie at the basis for the importance of this area in active color manipulations. Selective signaling for color is a requirement for the specific assignment of a color to an object or for making a decision about color identity; this process may take place in V4α.

It is unlikely that a lack of detection power caused the absence of color-specific BOLD reduction effects in area V4. First of all, the anatomical locations of all our ROIs were well within the extent of locations of visual areas as listed in Bartels and Zeki (2000). Also, data from a separate color viewing experiment in the same subjects indicate strong activation of overlapping fusiform areas (van Leeuwen, et al., 2010). It is therefore unlikely that a suboptimal location of the ROIs caused the absence of any effects. Furthermore, it was clear that V4 was engaged during our task. In the left hemisphere, there was no prime type effect in V4, but the overall BOLD response to the SC and DC conditions in V4 was actually higher than in V4α ($F(1,75)=12.775$, $p<.001$).

Importantly, the areas in which our ROIs were located were responsive to color overall (contrast of AC condition compared to average DC and SC conditions), as shown in Figure 4 and in the whole brain results (Figure 5 and Table 1). Our whole brain results show effects in bilateral fusiform gyrus which correspond very well to previous findings in the literature for the preference of chromatic over achromatic stimuli in ventral-occipital regions (e.g. Bartels & Zeki, 2000; Beauchamp, et al., 1999; Howard, et al., 1998; McKeefry & Zeki, 1997; Mullen, Dumoulin, McMahon, de Zubicaray, & Hess, 2007; Sakai, et al., 1995). In principle, we could have expected overall adaptation effects for color (AC > (DC & SC) in more visual regions than only V4 and middle occipital gyrus. However, our stimuli were specifically designed to induce effects in brain regions involved in higher-order color processing. The stimuli were rather small, and contained neither specific orientation, nor motion, nor texture, and the adaptation period was very brief; primary visual areas may not have been stimulated enough by our stimuli to show adaptation effects. Even though many visual regions are generally responsive to color, the above mentioned brain regions actually *prefer* chromatic stimuli over achromatic stimuli (e.g. Bartels & Zeki, 2000; Mullen, et al., 2007), which may explain why we find adaptation effects exactly in those regions.

It is also important to note that the pattern of brain activity in V4α was different from the pattern of behavioral priming in the reaction times. It is not the case that the repetition suppression effects in V4α are merely reflecting the behavioral task demands; the reaction times showed a clear interference effect for the different color trials (Figure 3), while the brain activity in bilateral V4α was strongest for the achromatic condition, as expected for the repetition suppression effect (see Figure 4 for the collapsed data). Also, when we included reaction times into our model as an additional regressor, the pattern of brain activity in visual areas did not change (data not shown). This evidence indicates that the effects of the reaction times were independent from the perceptual effects of stimulus repetition. Horner and Henson (2008) researched the effects of response learning and stimulus repetition in the brain, and found that perceptual repetition suppression in posterior brain areas is independent of the task that the subjects were performing. Our data support this finding.

In future studies, the challenge will be to learn more about the spatial organization of the human anterior color center. In macaque, Conway et al. (2007) have shown that color-biased cells in the inferior temporal cortex, anterior to area V4, are organized in 'globs' of luminance-invariant cells, and are alternated with 'interglob' regions that contain non-luminance-invariant neurons. Perhaps neurons in V4α are also organized in such a pattern. Kotake et al. (2009) and Conway and Tsao (2009) have demonstrated that in macaque area V4, neurons are spatially organized by color preference; a similar arrangement may be present in humans. A suggestion for future research would be to apply a repetition suppression paradigm in which the difference between the prime and target color was varied gradually, to investigate the spatial arrangement of perceptually similar colors. Another promising method are fMRI studies in which multi-voxel pattern analysis is applied (Haynes & Rees, 2006). With this method, Parkes, Marsman, Oxley, Goulermas and Wuerger (2009) have identified patches of cells with the same color preference in primary visual cortex of humans, and Seymour, Clifford, Logothetis and Bartels (2009) have shown that classification of voxels based solely on color preference is possible in all early visual areas except V5/MT+. Likewise, Brouwer and Heeger (2009) have successfully classified stimulus color in V1, V2, V3, V4, and VO1 (V4α is sometimes referred to as VO1 (Brewer, et al., 2005)). Voxels in fMRI contain a very large amount of neurons, which is why the classification results do not exclude a patch-like clustering of color responsive neurons in V4α. Importantly, Brouwer and Heeger (2009) also found that principal component scores (reflecting variation in the responses to different colors across voxels) in areas V4 and VO1 showed a progression through perceptual color space, which was not found for other color-responsive areas like V1. The results suggest a transformation in color processing from V1 to a more perceptual color representation in V4 and VO1, implying a spatial distribution of colors according to a perceptual similarity matrix.

5. Conclusion

To summarize, our results suggest that a functional division can be made between visual areas V4 and V4α within the human V4 complex, with more specific color selectivity taking place in V4α. This functional division may underlie the role of V4α in tasks that require active manipulation of color. Future studies will be able to reveal more details about the structural and functional organization of the human V4 complex; multi-voxel pattern analysis, high resolution (f)MRI, refined repetition suppression techniques, and studies combining color processing and behavior will be useful tools to advance our understanding of human color perception.

Acknowledgements

This work was supported by the Volkswagen-Foundation [grant number I/80 743].

Author details

Tessa M. van Leeuwen[1], Karl Magnus Petersson[1,2], Oliver Langner[1,3], Mark Rijpkema[1] and Peter Hagoort[1,2]

1 Donders Institute for Brain, Cognition and Behaviour, Radboud University Nijmegen, The Netherlands

2 Max Planck Institute for Psycholinguistics, Nijmegen, The Netherlands

3 Behavioural Science Institute, Radboud University Nijmegen, The Netherlands

References

[1] Barbur, J. L., & Spang, K. (2008). Colour constancy and conscious perception of changes of illuminant. *Neuropsychologia*, 46(3), 853-863.

[2] Barsalou, L. W., Simmons, W. K., Barbey, A. K., & Wilson, C. D. (2003). Grounding conceptual knowledge in modality-specific systems. *Trends in Cognitive Sciences*, 7(2), 84-91.

[3] Bartels, A., & Zeki, S. (2000). The architecture of the colour centre in the human visual brain: new results and a review. *European Journal of Neuroscience*, 12(1), 172-190.

[4] Beauchamp, M. S., Haxby, J. V., Jennings, J. E., & DeYoe, E. A. (1999). An fMRI version of the Farnsworth-Munsell 100-Hue test reveals multiple color-selective areas in human ventral occipitotemporal cortex. *Cerebral Cortex*, 9(3), 257-263.

[5] Bouvier, S. E., & Engel, S. A. (2006). Behavioral deficits and cortical damage loci in cerebral achromatopsia. *Cerebral Cortex*, 16(2), 183-191.

[6] Brett, M., Anton, J.-L., Valabregue, R., & Poline, J.-B. (2002). Region of interest analysis using an SPM toolbox [Abstract]. *8th International Conference on Functional Mapping of the Human Brain, Sendai, Japan*.

[7] Brewer, A. A., Liu, J., Wade, A. R., & Wandell, B. A. (2005). Visual field maps and stimulus selectivity in human ventral occipital cortex. [10.1038/nn1507]. *Nature Neuroscience*, 8(8), 1102-1109.

[8] Brouwer, G. J., & Heeger, D. J. (2009). Decoding and Reconstructing Color from Responses in Human Visual Cortex. *Journal of Neuroscience,* 29(44), 13992-14003.

[9] Brown, M. W., & Xiang, J. Z. (1998). Recognition memory: Neuronal substrates of the judgement of prior occurrence. [Review]. *Progress in Neurobiology,* 55(2), 149-189.

[10] Cant, J., Arnott, S., & Goodale, M. (2009). fMR-adaptation reveals separate processing regions for the perception of form and texture in the human ventral stream. *Experimental Brain Research,* 192(3), 391-405-405.

[11] Cavina-Pratesi, C., Kentridge, R. W., Heywood, C. A., & Milner, A. D. (2010). Separate Processing of Texture and Form in the Ventral Stream: Evidence from fMRI and Visual Agnosia. *Cerebral Cortex,* 20(2), 433-446.

[12] Chawla, D., Rees, G., & Friston, K. J. (1999). The physiological basis of attentional modulation in extrastriate visual areas. *Nature Neuroscience,* 2(7), 671-676.

[13] Conway, B. R. (2009). Color vision, cones, and color-coding in the cortex. *Neuroscientist,* 15(3), 274-290.

[14] Conway, B. R., Moeller, S., & Tsao, D. Y. (2007). Specialized color modules in macaque extrastriate cortex. *Neuron,* 56(3), 560-573.

[15] Conway, B. R., & Tsao, D. Y. (2009). Color-tuned neurons are spatially clustered according to color preference within alert macaque posterior inferior temporal cortex. *Proceedings of the National Academy of Sciences of the United States of America,* 106(42), 18034-18039.

[16] Corbetta, M., Miezin, F., Dobmeyer, S., Shulman, G., & Petersen, S. (1991). Selective and divided attention during visual discriminations of shape, color, and speed: functional anatomy by positron emission tomography. *Journal of Neuroscience,* 11(8), 2383-2402.

[17] Dehaene, S., Naccache, L., Cohen, L., Le Bihan, D., Mangin, J. F., Poline, J. B., et al. (2001). Cerebral mechanisms of word masking and unconscious repetition priming. [Article]. *Nature Neuroscience,* 4(7), 752-758.

[18] Desimone, R. (1996). Neural mechanisms for visual memory and their role in attention. [Article; Proceedings Paper]. *Proceedings of the National Academy of Sciences of the United States of America,* 93(24), 13494-13499.

[19] DiPace, E., Marangolo, P., & Pizzamiglio, L. (1997). Response bias in color priming. *Acta Psychologica,* 95(1), 3-14.

[20] Eddy, M. D., Schnyer, D., Schmid, A., & Holcomb, P. J. (2007). Spatial dynamics of masked picture repetition effects. [Article]. *NeuroImage,* 34(4), 1723-1732.

[21] Engel, S. A. (2005). Adaptation of oriented and unoriented color-selective neurons in human visual areas. *Neuron,* 45(4), 613-623.

[22] Goldberg, R. F., Perfetti, C. A., & Schneider, W. (2006). Perceptual knowledge retrieval activates sensory brain regions. *Journal of Neuroscience*, 26(18), 4917-4921.

[23] Grill-Spector, K., Henson, R. N. A., & Martin, A. (2005). Repetition and the brain: neural models of stimulus-specific effects. *Trends in Cognitive Sciences*, 10(1), 15-23.

[24] Grill-Spector, K., Kushnir, T., Edelman, S., Avidan, G., Itzchak, Y., & Malach, R. (1999). Differential processing of objects under various viewing conditions in the human lateral occipital complex. [Article]. *Neuron*, 24(1), 187-203.

[25] Grill-Spector, K., & Malach, R. (2001). fMR-adaptation: a tool for studying the functional properties of human cortical neurons. [Article]. *Acta Psychologica*, 107(1-3), 293-321.

[26] Griswold, M. A., Jakob, P. M., Heidemann, R. M., Nittka, M., Jellus, V., Wang, J., et al. (2002). Generalized autocalibrating partially parallel acquisitions (GRAPPA). *Magnetic Resonance in Medicine*, 47(6), 1202-1210.

[27] Hadjikhani, N., Liu, A. K., Dale, A. M., Cavanagh, P., & Tootell, R. B. H. (1998). Retinotopy and color sensitivity in human visual cortical area V8. [10.1038/681]. *Nature Neuroscience*, 1(3), 235-241.

[28] Haynes, J.-D., & Rees, G. (2006). Decoding mental states from brain activity in humans. *Nature Reviews Neuroscience*, 7, 523-534.

[29] Henson, R. N. A. (2003). Neuroimaging studies of priming. *Progress in Neurobiology*, 70, 53-81.

[30] Horner, A. J., & Henson, R. N. (2008). Priming, response learning and repetition suppression. *Neuropsychologia*, 46(7), 1979-1991.

[31] Howard, R. J., ffytche, D. H., Barnes, J., McKeefry, D., Ha, Y., Woodruff, P. W., et al. (1998). The functional anatomy of imagining and perceiving colour. *Neuroreport*, 9(6), 1019-1023.

[32] Hubbard, E. M., & Ramachandran, V. S. (2005). Neurocognitive mechanisms of synesthesia. *Neuron*, 48, 509–520.

[33] Kotake, Y., Morimoto, H., Okazaki, Y., Fujita, I., & Tamura, H. (2009). Organization of color-selective neurons in macaque visual area V4. *Journal of Neurophysiology*, 102(1), 15-27.

[34] Kusunoki, M., Moutoussis, K., & Zeki, S. (2006). Effect of background colors on the tuning of color-selective cells in monkey area V4. *Journal of Neurophysiology*, 95(5), 3047-3059.

[35] Luo, Q., Peng, D. L., Jin, Z., Xu, D., Xiao, L. H., & Ding, G. S. (2004). Emotional valence of words modulates the subliminal repetition priming effect in the left fusiform gyrus: an event-related fMRI study. [Article]. *NeuroImage*, 21(1), 414-421.

[36] Maccotta, L., & Buckner, R. L. (2004). Evidence for neural effects of repetition that directly correlate with behavioral priming. [Article]. *Journal of Cognitive Neuroscience,* 16(9), 1625-1632.

[37] Marangolo, P., Dipace, E., & Pizzamiglio, L. (1993). Priming effect in a color discrimination task. *Perceptual and Motor Skills,* 77(1), 259-269.

[38] Martin, A., Haxby, J. V., Lalonde, F. M., Wiggs, C. L., & Ungerleider, L. G. (1995). Discrete cortical regions associated with knowledge of color and knowledge of action. *Science,* 270(5233), 102-105.

[39] Matsumora, T., Koida, K., & Komatsu, H. (2008). Relationship between color discrimination and neural responses in the inferior temporal cortex of the monkey. *Journal of Neurophysiology,* 100(6), 3361-3374.

[40] McKeefry, D., & Zeki, S. (1997). The position and topography of the human colour centre as revealed by functional magnetic resonance imaging. *Brain,* 120(12), 2229-2242.

[41] Miller, E., Li, L., & Desimone, R. (1993). Activity of neurons in anterior inferior temporal cortex during a short- term memory task. *The Journal of Neuroscience,* 13(4), 1460-1478.

[42] Morita, T., Kochiyama, T., Okada, T., Yonekura, Y., Matsumura, M., & Sadato, N. (2004). The neural substrates of conscious color perception demonstrated using fMRI. *Neuroimage,* 21(4), 1665-1673.

[43] Mullen, K. T., Dumoulin, S. O., McMahon, K. L., de Zubicaray, G. I., & Hess, R. F. (2007). Selectivity of human retinotopic visual cortex to S-cone-opponent, L/M-cone-opponent and achromatic stimulation. [Article]. *European Journal of Neuroscience,* 25(2), 491-502.

[44] Murphey, D. K., Yoshor, D., & Beauchamp, M. S. (2008). Perception matches selectivity in the human anterior color center. *Current Biology,* 18(3), 216-220.

[45] Parkes, L. M., Marsman, J. B. C., Oxley, D. C., Goulermas, J. Y., & Wuerger, S. M. (2009). Multivoxel fMRI analysis of color tuning in human primary visual cortex. *Journal of Vision,* 9(1), 13.

[46] Sakai, K., Watanabe, E., Onodera, Y., Uchida, I., Kato, H., Yamamoto, E., et al. (1995). Functional mapping of the human color-center with echo-planar magnetic-resonance-imaging. *Proceedings of the Royal Society B-Biological Sciences,* 261(1360), 89-98.

[47] Schiller, P. H. (1995). Effect of lesions in visual cortical area V4 on the recognition of transformed objects. [10.1038/376342a0]. *Nature,* 376(6538), 342-344.

[48] Seymour, K., Clifford, C. W. G., Logothetis, N. K., & Bartels, A. (2009). The coding of color, motion, and their conjunction in the human visual cortex. *Current Biology,* 19(3), 177-183.

[49] Simmons, W. K., Ramjee, V., Beauchamp, M. S., McRae, K., Martin, A., & Barsalou, L. W. (2007). A common neural substrate for perceiving and knowing about color. *Neuropsychologia,* 45(12), 2802-2810.

[50] Simon, J. R. (1988). A priming effect in a choice reaction-time task. *Acta Psychologica,* 69(1), 45-60.

[51] Stoughton, C. M., & Conway, B. R. (2008). Neural basis for unique hues. *Current Biology,* 18(16), R698-R699.

[52] Van der Kouwe, A. J., Benner, T., Fischl, B., Schmitt, F., Salat, D. H., Harder, M., et al. (2005). On-line automatic slice positioning for brain MR imaging. *NeuroImage,* 27(1), 222-230.

[53] van Leeuwen, T. M., Petersson, K. M., & Hagoort, P. (2010). Synaesthetic Colour in the Brain: Beyond Colour Areas. A Functional Magnetic Resonance Imaging Study of Synaesthetes and Matched Controls. *PLoS ONE,* 5(8), e12074.

[54] Van Wingen, G. A., Van Broekhoven, F., Verkes, R. J., Petersson, K. M., Backstrom, T., Buitelaar, J. K., et al. (2008). Progesterone selectively increases amygdala reactivity in women. [Article]. *Molecular Psychiatry,* 13(3), 325-333.

[55] Weiss, P. H., Zilles, K., & Fink, G. R. (2005). When visual perception causes feeling: enhanced cross-modal processing in grapheme-color synesthesia. *NeuroImage,* 28(4), 859-868.

[56] Wildgruber, D., Riecker, A., Hertrich, I., Erb, M., Grodd, W., Ethofer, T., et al. (2005). Identification of emotional intonation evaluated by fMRI. *NeuroImage,* 24, 1233-1241.

[57] Zeki, S. (1980). The representation of colors in the cerebral cortex. *Nature,* 284(5755), 412-418.

[58] Zeki, S., & Marini, L. (1998). Three cortical stages of colour processing in the human brain. Brain, 121, 1669-1685.

7

A Systematic Approach to Visual System Rehabilitation—Population Receptive Field Analysis and Real-time Functional Magnetic Resonance Imaging Neurofeedback Methods

T. Dorina Papageorgiou, Amalia Papanikolaou and Stelios M. Smirnakis

1. Introduction: Is visual rehabilitation inside a cortical scotoma possible, in principle?

Visual information transmission flows from the retinal ganglion cells to the lateral geniculate nucleus and then to the primary visual cortex (V1), the chief cortical relay of visual information to "higher" extrastriate areas. Beyond area V1, visual processing is distributed across multiple interconnected brain areas, the precise role of which and their interactions are not yet, completely understood. To add to the dynamic complexity of the system, feedback from higher areas and modulation by top-down processes, such as attention, are often critical in the formation of visual percepts (Deco and Lee; 2004; Olhausen, 2003; Kastner and Ungerleider, 2000; Mumford, 1994; Hubel and Weisel, 1977).

Impairment of visual function can occur at any point along the visual pathway from the eye to the cortex. We focus our discussion here on lesions of the primary visual cortex (area V1), which result in dense contralateral visual field defects known as "scotomas". Scotomas resulting from area V1 lesions often involve the contralateral half of the visual field resulting in hemianopia, or a contralateral visual field quadrant resulting in quadrantanopia. V1 lesions are the most prevalent injury of the visual cortex, often occurring as a result of posterior cerebral artery (PCA) stroke, hemorrhage, or traumatic brain injury (TBI) (Pambakian and Kennard, 1997; Zhang et al., 2006; Ajina and Kennard, 2012). Twenty to thirty percent of stroke survivors experience visual disability (Taylor, 1997; Gilhotra et al., 2002; Giorgi et al., 2009), while the incidence of significant visual perceptual impairment in TBI victims exceeds 50% in some studies (McKenna et al., 2006; Lew et al., 2007; Elisevich et al., 1984). The loss of visual perception inside a large scotoma can significantly affect the patient's ability to perform daily tasks, navigate in unknown environments, and function independently (Ajina and Kennard, 2012; Rizzo and Robin, 1996; Riggs, et al., 2007). Visual rehabilitation is clearly necessary for the quality of life of these patients. The literature describing visual rehabilitation efforts is extensive and doing justice to it goes well beyond the scope of this chapter. We should mention at the outset that we do not discuss here, the large literature on practicing eye movement strategies or, using prisms to remap the unseen onto the seen part of the visual field. Instead, we focus on novel approaches that aim to enhance perception inside the visual field scotoma.

To date, no established method exists to rehabilitate visual perception in adult patients with lesions of the primary visual cortex. The lack of effective methods for rehabilitation has led to the general perception that the adult visual cortex has decreased capacity to compensate after injury. This engenders diminished hope that successful strategies can be established to promote the recovery of visual perception after cortical injury. This is partly justified, as several attempts claiming to have achieved significant results have failed. The most notable recent example is an effort by Nova Vision claiming that a rehabilitative paradigm based on a "saccade-to-target" task could significantly shrink dense visual field scotomas (Kasten et al.; 1998, 1999; 2000, 2001, 2006; Poggel et al., 2001, 2004, 2006; Sabel et al., 2000, 2004; Werth and Moehrenschlager, 1999; Zihl and VonCramon, 1979; Zihl and Von Carmon, 1985; Jobke et al., 2009). Although early psychophysical training methods and Nova Vision studies were seen as promising (Kerkhoff et al., 1992; Kerkhoff et al., 1994; Julkunen, 2003; Kasten et al., 1995; 1998a, b, 1999; 2000, 2001; Poggel et al., 2001, 2004, 2006; Sabel et al., 2000, 2004; Werth and Moehrenschlager, 1999; Zihl and VonCramon, 1979; Zihl, 1990), later studies implementing rigorous eye movement controls failed to find a reduction of the visual field scotoma in patients with V1 lesions (Reinhard et al., 2005; Horton, 2005a; Horton, 2005b; Pleger et al., 2003).

Although these efforts are disappointing, the rehabilitation of scotomas resulting from V1 injuries is not altogether a cause without hope (Kasten et al., 1998; Huxlin et al., 2009; Schmid et al., 2010; Poggel et al., 2010; Sahraie et al., 2010; Schmid et al., 2009; Alexander and Cowey, 2009). On one hand, patchy injuries to area V1 or its inputs in the optic radiation seem to be amenable to rehabilitation, as training can help recruit and strengthen surviving connections. In support of this, Sabel and colleagues (Kasten et al., 1999) showed that ~74% of patients with partial optic nerve involvement showed significant recovery with training, compared to 29% of patients with post-chiasmatic lesions. This is likely the result of increased recruitment of partially lesioned fiber pathways or islands of residual vision (Fendrich et al., 1992). On the other hand, recent evidence suggests that even when lesions to area V1 or its proximal inputs are dense, it may be possible to some extent to functionally bypass the area of the injury.

First, there exist anatomical pathways that bypass the area of V1 injury (fig. 1). One such pathway projects from the retina to the koniocellular (intercalated) layers of the lateral geniculate nucleus directly, or to the superior colliculus and from there to extrastriate cortex. This pathway originates in the retinal Pγ class of ganglion cells, which comprises ~10% of the total ganglion cell number, is particularly dense near the fovea (Henry and Reid, 2000), and is known to survive retrograde degeneration following V1 lesions (Cowey and Stoerig, 1989). Another V1-bypassing pathway projects from the retina to the pulvinar directly or via the superior colliculus and from there to the extrastriate visual areas. Notably, although parvocellular and magnocellular projections to the lateral geniculate nucleus and beyond markedly atrophy following striate cortical lesions (Vanburen, 1963; Mihailovic et alo., 1971), superior collicular (Dineen et al., 1982) and pulvinar (Cowey, 1974) projections remain unchanged.

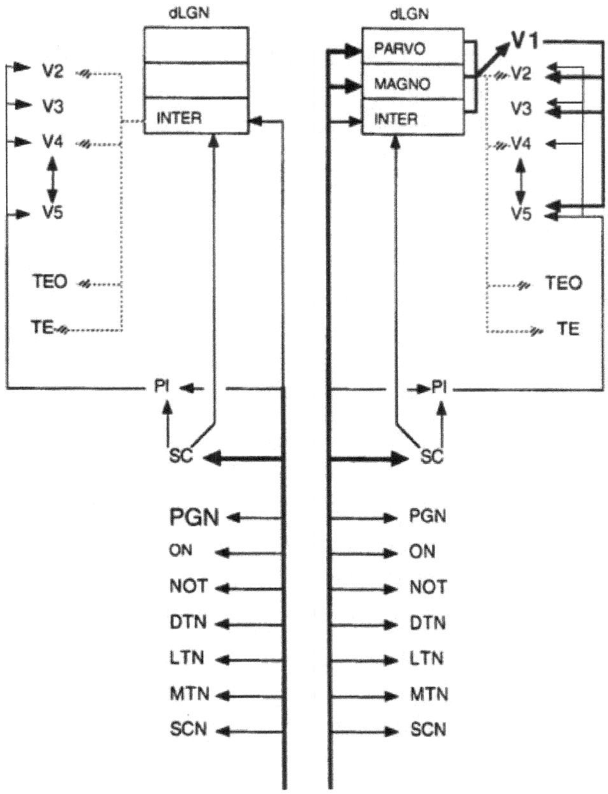

Figure 1. Overview of relevant anatomical visual pathways (Modified with permission from Stoerig and Cowey, 1997): Possible extra-geniculostriate pathways contributing to blindsight behavior, and residual extrastriate cortex activity, adapted from Stoerig and Cowey (Stoerig and Cowey, 1997). This diagram shows known retinofugal inputs, and some of the subsequent projections. On the right, the pathways are shown with intact V1. On the left V1 has been lesioned. Two pathways stand out as potentially mediating the residual activity observed in extrastriate cortex (Rodman et al., 1989; Schmid et al., 2009; Schmid et al., 2010), as well as related aspects of blindsight behavior: **1)** The koniocellular pathway (dotted lines) from the K (intercalated) layers of the thalamus directly to areas V2, V3, V4, V5/MT. This pathway originates in the retinal Pγ class of ganglion cells, comprising ~10% of total ganglion cells, survives retrograde degeneration following V1 lesions, and is particularly dense near the fovea (Cowey and Stoerig, 1989; Henry and Reid, 2000). This pathway receives both direct retinal and superior collicular input. **2)** The projection from the inferior pulvinar to V2, V3, V4, V5/MT, which also receives direct input from the retina, as well as input from the retinotectal (superior colliculus) pathway. PGN: pre-geniculate nucleus, ON: olivary nucleus, NOT: nucleus of optic tract, MTN, LTN, DTN: medial, lateral, dorsal terminal accessory optic nuclei, SCN: suprachiasmatic nucleus, SC: superior colliculus, PI: inferior pulvinar.

Second, these pathways have been shown to be functional under certain conditions. Lesions of area V1 or its post-chiasmatic afferents deprive the extrastriate visual cortex of its main input and result in a dense contralateral visual field scotoma inside which conscious visual perception is thought to be irreversibly lost (Cowey and Stoerig, 1991; Stoerig and Barth, 2001). Remarkably, despite the absence of a conscious visual percept, a capacity to process certain attributes of the visual stimulus persists inside the scotoma, the phenomenon known as "blindsight" (Kluver, 1936; Poppel et al., 1973; Weiskrantz, 1974). The blindsight phenomenon implies that at least some extra-geniculo-striate retinofugal pathways (Cowey, 2010; Schmid et al., 2010; Weiskrantz, 2004; Schoenfeld et al, 2002; Moore et al., 2001; Goebel et al., 2001; Stoerig and Cowey, 1997; Moore et al., 1995; Cowey and Stoerig, 1991; Girard et al., 1991; Pasik and Pasik, 1971) can functionally bypass area V1. This is corroborated by experiments in humans and primates, which have directly demonstrated that extrastriate areas can be modulated by the visual stimulus in the absence of V1 input (Rodman et al., 1989; Baseler et al., 1999; Goebel et al., 2001; Schmid et al., 2009; Schmid et al., 2010). For example, Rodman and Gross demonstrated that area V5/MT can be directly activated through the pathway bypassing area V1 via the superior colliculus (Rodman et al., 1989; Rodman et al., 1990), while Schmid et al. (Schmid et al., 2009; Schmid et al., 2010) demonstrated that early extrastriate areas V2, V3 can be visually modulated by the LGN in the absence of V1 input. Schmid et al. further demonstrated that transiently inactivating LGN in V1 lesioned animals both abolishes visual modulation in areas V2, V3 and returns the monkey's blindsight performance to chance. Unfortunately the V1-bypassing pathways that mediate the blindsight phenomenon are by themselves weak and of limited practical value. The potential of these pathways to induce recovery remains unrealized. This underscores the need to examine the mechanisms underlying the recovery reported in recent studies (Huxlin et al., 2008; Huxlin et al., 2009; Sahraie et al., 2006) in order to understand how to develop effective rehabilitative paradigms. It remains to be examined whether novel neuro-rehabilitative training algorithms may be able to strengthen V1-bypassing pathways enough to derive practical benefit.

Third, training can improve performance inside the scotoma of subjects with area V1 lesions. Behavioral training in healthy subjects can improve visual performance by inducing plastic changes in the physiology of visual networks (Karni and Sagi, 1991; Liu et al., 2000; Yang and Maunsell, 2004; Ahissar and Hochstein, 1997). Perceptual learning is retinotopically specific, suggesting it involves a use-dependent synaptic enhancement induced by pre-and postsynaptic activity (Brown et al., 1988). Studies in humans (Pleger et al., 2003; Taub et al., 2002; Weiller, C. 1998; Lindberg et al., 2003, Takeuchi et al., 2005) and animals (Rudolph et al., 1994; Rudolph and Pasternak, 1999; Rudolph and Delay, 1993, Fabre-Thorpe et al., 1994; Friel et al., 2000; Huxlin and Pasternak, 2004) with V1 lesions, as well as behavioral studies of "blindsight" (Chokron et al., 2008; Stoerig and Cowey, 1997; Sahraie et al., 2006; Overgaard, 2011), suggest that visual performance in the scotoma can also improve with training (Raninen et al., 2007; Henriksson et al., 2007). More recently, following their work on cats (Huxlin et al., 2006), Huxlin et al. trained subjects with V1+ lesions to perform a two-alternative forced choice random dot kinematogram (RDK) direction of motion discrimination task in their blind hemifield (Huxlin et al., 2009). *Remarkably, direction of motion discrimination thresholds recovered from chance to normal at trained locations (Huxlin et al., 2009).* Eye movements were strictly controlled, and there were no obvious artifacts that could confound the findings. Recovery was retinotopically specific but could be extended by training consecutively adjacent locations that lay progressively deeper inside the scotoma, inducing recovery up to ~20^0 from the scotoma border in one subject. Furthermore, recovery in this task appeared to carry some practical significance, as the subjects' ability to dodge basketballs "thrown" at them from the blind hemifield in a virtual reality environment, improved (Iorizzo et al., 2011). These findings sparked renewed interest in studying visual rehabilitation strategies. This is encouraging but it is necessary to note that visual rehabilitation results appear more variable across the literature (see table 1, in a recent review by Sabel et al. (Sabel et al., 2011), and (Horton, 2005a; Horton, 2005b) for a critical review of the field). Three important questions remain to be answered regarding scotomas resulting from V1 lesions: i) can visual rehabilitative training result in improved visual performance of practical significance? ii) what is the underlying mechanism of recovery? and 3) what is the optimal method for visual rehabilitative training?

In summary, even though visual rehabilitation following area V1+ lesions is a difficult problem, it is not a hopeless endeavor. Anatomical pathways bypassing the area of the lesion exist, and they have been demonstrated to be functional in certain situations. Although early trials have been inconclusive, a recent report by Huxlin et al. (Huxlin et al., 2009), suggests that some recovery is possible, at least in the domain of visual motion perception. Further studies are needed to 1) independently corroborate the results of Huxlin et al. (Huxlin et al., 2009), 2) to understand what visual attributes and what types of lesions are amenable to recovery, and 3) to study the mechanism of recovery. *It is important to note that we do not expect even successful rehabilitation methods to restore vision to pre-lesion levels.* For one, the quality of the restored visual percept will most likely, differ from normal. The reason is that, following V1 lesions, the magnocellular and parvocellular pathways largely degenerate (fig. 1), shifting the balance towards the koniocellular pathway, which is spared. Nevertheless, visual rehabilitation could succeed, by training patients to use the qualitatively and quantitatively different form of visual perception mediated by appropriately strengthened V1-bypassing pathways. The hope is that such an approach will be possible, and may confer considerable practical significance.

2. Using fMRI to functionally characterize and classify cortical lesions and corresponding scotomas

In order to design effective visual rehabilitation strategies for cortical scotomas we have to grapple with the issue of lesion variability. Cortical lesions differ from individual to individual, and this impacts whether or not the resulting scotoma is amenable to rehabilitation. Consequently, some patients show good recovery following visual rehabilitative training (Kasten et al., 1998; Huxlin, 2009) and others no recovery at all (Reinhard et al., 2005; Horton et al., 2005a; Horton et al., 2005b; and our personal observation). It remains unclear what criteria one may use to select patients more likely to recover. Scotomas are mapped using visual field perimetry to determine the part of the visual field where visual perception is impaired. A problem faced in studies of visual rehabilitation is that patients often have heterogeneous lesions, even though the extent and density of their perceptual visual scotomas, measured by perimetry, match. Conversely, the anatomical characterization of the lesion is not always a reliable indication of the properties or, the extent of the resulting scotoma. Consequently, neither visual field perimetry maps nor, purely anatomical information are sufficient indicators of the capacity for rehabilitation.

A measure of the ability of visual stimuli presented inside the scotoma to elicit perceptually sub-threshold activity in spared visual cortex would add valuable information. Functional magnetic resonance imaging (fMRI) can be used to identify which sectors of the visual field scotoma remain able to transmit visual information to spared regions of the visual cortex (fig. 3), downstream from the lesion. This can help to classify functionally different types of lesions that yield similar scotomas, and to identify regions of the scotoma that elicit different patterns of functional activation and may therefore, have different capacity for rehabilitation. The underlying hypothesis is that sectors of the scotoma that can still convey visual information to higher areas, bypassing the cortical lesion, will be more amenable to rehabilitation. Moreover, the extrastriate areas that get activated may reveal clues about the attributes of the visual stimulus that will be more amenable to rehabilitation.

We propose to apply state-of-the-art fMRI methods to characterize voxel by voxel how population receptive fields (Wandell et al., 2007; Dumoulin and Wandell, 2008; Amano et al., 2009; Lee et al., 2013) in spared visual areas are organized to cover the visual field following cortical visual pathway injuries (see figs. 2, and 3) (Baseler et al., 2011). The population receptive field (pRF) of a voxel refers to the region of visual space that elicits a visually-induced modulation of the BOLD (Blood-Oxygen-Level-Dependent) signal in that voxel. Various pRF models have been proposed in the literature (Dumoulin and Wandell, 2008; Zuiderbaan et al., 2012; Lee et al., 2013). The simplest and most commonly used model is a circularly symmetric 2D Gaussian with center (x,y) and radius (σ) (Dumoulin and Wandell, 2008). The BOLD time series predicted by this model is derived by convolving the pRF model with the stimulus sequence and the BOLD hemodynamic response function (HRF; Boynton et al., 1996; Worsley et al., 2002). The pRF's parameters are then estimated by fitting the BOLD signal predicted by the model to the actual BOLD signal measurement obtained from each voxel.

Early methods of retinotopic mapping, such as ring and wedge stimuli (DeYoe et al., 1996; Dougherty et al., 2003; Engel et al., 1994; Sereno et al., 1995), as well as moving bar stimuli (Wandell et al., 2007), which traverse the visual field in different directions can usually provide robust pRF estimates (see fig. 2) rendering them useful for studying cortical reorganization. One limitation of direct-fit pRF estimation methods is that these can result in estimation biases at the scotoma border (Lee et al., 2013). Recently, a 2-step pRF estimation method based on first estimating the pRF topography, thresholding it, and then fitting an appropriate pRF model has been introduced to largely circumvent this problem (Lee et al., 2013). This is the preferred method to use near the scotoma border.

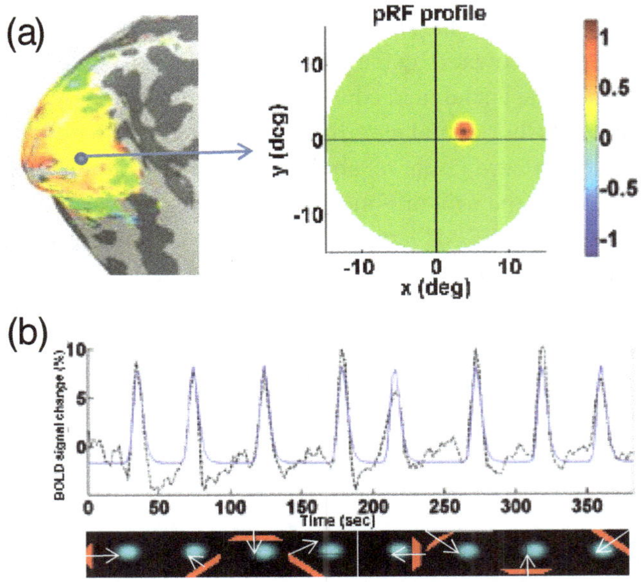

Figure 2. The populat on receptive field (pRF) model. This model estimates the region of the visual field that elicits a response in a small region (voxel) of the visual cortex. One implementation of the pRF model is a circularly symmetric Gaussian receptive field in visual space whose center and radius are estimated by fitting the BOLD signal responses to the estimated responses elicited by convolving the model with the moving bar stimulus and the hemodynamic response. (**a**) shows the estimated position and size of the pRF in the visual field of a voxel located in V1. (**b**) shows the BOLD time-series (dashed line) and the model prediction (solid line) from the same voxel. The model explains a large amount of variance in the time course data. Below, we illustrate the position and direction of motion of the stimulus bar that elicited the peaks in the BOLD signal.

2.1. Visual field coverage maps can potentially help to guide rehabilitation strategies

Population receptive field analysis can help measure the residual capacity of each area to process visual information following V1+ injuries. Plotting the pRF maps from all voxels in a given area together as a color map reveals the "visual field coverage map" of that area. This represents the part of the visual field that can visually modulate the area. Note that visual field coverage maps of extrastriate areas often overlap with the area of the dense perceptual scotoma, measured by visual field perimetry. This is illustrated in the second panel of figure 3 for area hV5/MT+, an area important for visual motion perception (Zeki et al., 2004; ffytche et al., 2000; Zeki and ffytche et al., 1998). Note that the pRF maps of many area hV5/MT+ voxels lie inside the perceptual scotoma (left upper quadrant in fig. 3). In fact, in this specific case (fig. 3), they cover the whole extent of the scotoma. This implies that hV5/MT+ is activated by visual stimuli presented in the left upper quadrant even though the subject does not perceive these stimuli. This suggests that there is a functional V1-bypassing pathway to area hV5/MT+ that may be able to promote recovery, if harnessed appropriately. Therefore, a promising rehabilitation strategy would be to find ways to strengthen this pathway. It is likely, that it will be easier to rehabilitate visual motion perception inside parts of the scotoma that are covered by the pRF maps of area hV5/MT+. It is also, likely that rehabilitation will be even easier in parts of the scotoma that are also covered by the pRF maps of spared, earlier, visual areas. The third panel of fig. 3 illustrates the visual field coverage map of the spared portion of area V1. Note, that this extends above the horizontal meridian to partly overlap with the area of the scotoma. This defines two regions where visual rehabilitation may be different, according to the above hypothesis. The region of the scotoma indicated by the green arrow is represented in the coverage maps of both area hV5/MT+ and the spared area V1, and is expected to have higher potential for rehabilitation. The region of the scotoma indicated by the blue arrow is represented only in the coverage map of area hV5/MT+ and is expected to present a more difficult challenge for rehabilitation. Visual field coverage maps (Amano et al., 2009) obtained by fMRI are an important adjunct to perimetric maps as they often provide complementary information (personal observation) and will likely be useful in tailoring therapy to appropriate visual field locations.

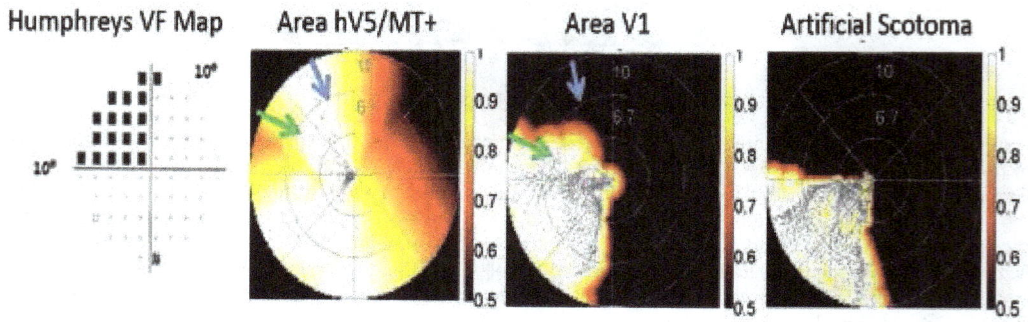

Figure 3. Visual Field Coverage Maps of spared visual areas with significant overlap with the region of the scotoma, define visual field locations that may be more amenable to rehabilitation. *Humphreys VF Map panel:* Humphreys 10-2 visual field map, illustrating that the subject had a dense left upper quadrantanopia. *Area hV5/MT+ panel:* The visual field coverage map (Amano et al., 2009) of the right hV5/MT+ shows visual field locations that evoke significant activity from hV5/MT+ of the lesioned hemisphere. At each visual field location, the highest pRF value of all pRFs that cover this location is plotted. PRF normalization limits the range of values between 0-1. Large values indicate significant visual modulation. Note, that although the subject is blind in the left upper quadrant, the subject's hV5/MT+ responds to stimuli presented in the left upper quadrant. A potential advantage of using visual field coverage maps is that therapy can be individualized to each patient's appropriate visual field locations, which are not necessarily predictable from perimetric maps. *Area V1 Panel:* Visual field coverage map of the *spared* right area V1 extends above the left horizontal meridian into the dense area of the scotoma seen in the Humphreys map. This activity may be induced in orthotopic voxels that survive and are partially active following the V1 lesion (Kasten et al., 1998), or in anatomically ectopic V1 voxels that belong to the upper occipital lobe, which would ordinarily have had receptive fields in the left lower visual field quadrant. Note, that this area does not cover the entire quadrant, as is the case of the coverage map in area hV5/MT+. This mismatch will likely have implications for rehabilitation. *For example, it may be easier to rehabilitate regions of the scotoma where the visual field coverage maps of spared V1 and hV5/MT+ are congruent (green arrow), as opposed to incongruent (blue arrow). Control with AS (artificial scotoma) Panel:* Visual field coverage map from the entire area V1 of a normal subject with an "artificial scotoma" simulating left upper quadrantanopia. By artificial scotoma we mean an area of the stimulus being excluded, in order to simulate the patient's scotoma. Note, that the visual field coverage map in this control case is as expected, i.e. it does not encroach into the left upper quadrant.

2.2. Quantitative pRF measurements provide a useful biomarker for gauging the effect of rehabilitation strategies

Fig. 4 illustrates that pRF measurements in area hV5/MT+ ipsilateral to a chronic V1+ lesion differ from those in the normal hemisphere. Specifically, pRFs in hV5/MT+ voxels of the lesioned hemisphere are smaller on average, and pRF-centers cluster near the vertical meridian (x=0; fig. 4C). Training may further change the pRF topography. Changes in the pRF topography before and after training can be a potentially useful biomarker for evaluating different rehabilitation paradigms before perceptual recovery becomes evident. Applying this approach systematically can help to formulate new hypotheses guiding future rehabilitation attempts. For example, one hypothesis is that following visual motion rehabilitation training the sensitivity to motion stimuli of the human motion selective area complex (hV5/MT+) will increase, and this increase will correlate with behavioral recovery. Alternatively, attentional networks or, other "higher" areas that receive input from hV5/MT+ may reorganize to process visual motion information more effectively. Analyzing pRF maps obtained from visually responsive areas before and after training, will allow us to investigate the above hypotheses and to adopt appropriate rehabilitation strategies.

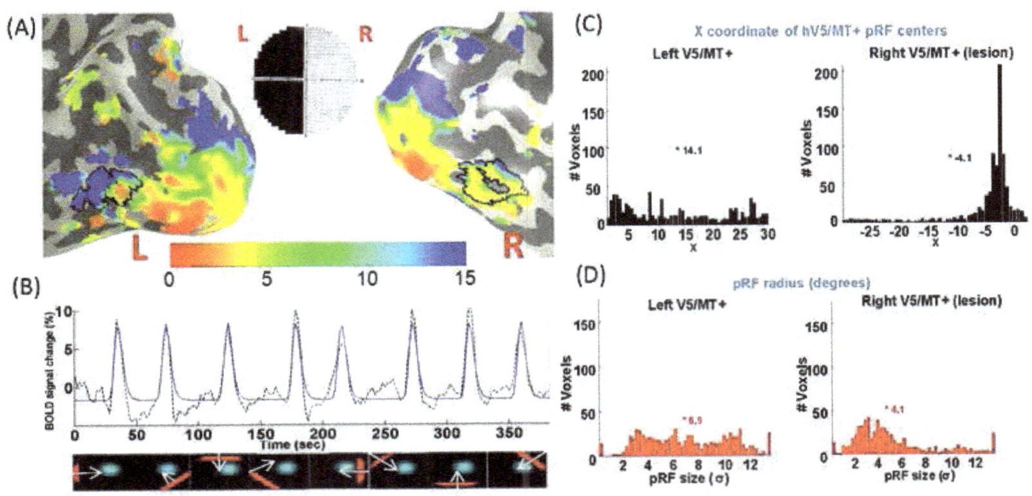

Figure 4. *hV5/MT+* pRF mapping in a hemianopic patient: (A) Inflated occipital lobe of the normal (left) and lesioned (right) hemisphere with hV5/MT+ outlined on the eccentricity map. Mid-inset is a 30-2 Humphrey perimeter showing dense left hemianopia. (B) Illustrates the method used to calculate pRF parameters (same as in fig. 2). The pRF model parameters are optimized to fit the BOLD signal voxel by voxel. Note the close fit between the BOLD time-series (dashed line) and the pRF model prediction (solid line). The position and direction of motion of the stimulus bar that elicited each response is illustrated (bottom). (C) The X coordinate of the pRF centers in hV5/MT+ of the normal (left) hemisphere is evenly distributed while in the lesioned (right) hemisphere it clusters near the vertical meridian (x=0). Note however, that the pRF centers still lie within the scotoma (negative X values). (D): Distribution of pRF radii of hV5/MT+ voxels in the intact (left) and in the lesioned (right) hemisphere. The distribution of pRF radii shifts to smaller values in area hV5/MT+ of the lesioned hemisphere. This may be because ipsilesional hV5/MT+ voxels are driven by a V1-bypassing pathway that drives visual periphery less effectively.

In summary, pRF measurements:

1. Classify subregions of the perimetric scotoma depending on how they are covered by spared visual areas; different regions will likely have different potential for rehabilitation.
2. Allow us to study the mechanism by which rehabilitation strategies improve visual performance.
3. Serve as quantitative biomarkers for evaluating the effects of training before perceptual recovery becomes evident, accelerating the pursuit of a rational strategy for visual rehabilitation.

Other methods of analysis can be applied here, but we do not have the space to do them justice. We mention briefly the promise of recent developments in effective connectivity analysis (Fuji et al., 2009; Stilla et al., 2008; Hinrichs et al., 2006) and diffusion tensor imaging (Wedeen et al., 2012; Yeatman et al., 2012; Van den Stock et al., 2011; Sherbondy et al., 2008; Fields, 2008; Okada et al., 2007; Schoth et al., 2006; Kikuta et al., 2006; Dougherty et al., 2005; Taoka et al., 2005; de Gelder et al., 2005; Reinges et al., 2004; Morris et al., 2001) for studying inter-area pathways that survive post-lesion, and whether they can get stronger by training. Population receptive field and effective connectivity analysis can be used to explore visual system reorganization and recovery following injury, and to generate concrete hypotheses on how to enhance and accelerate recovery of visual function by the application of cutting-edge rehabilitative strategies.

3. How to approach visual rehabilitation?

To date, we have little understanding of how the visual cortex reorganizes after injury, and no proven effective treatment strategies to rehabilitate the recovery of visual perception in the affected portion of the visual field in V1-lesioned patients. Understanding how to manipulate the brain's capacity for plasticity is an important step in the long-term effort to design treatments aiming to enhance the ability of the nervous system to recover after injury. To make progress along this front we need to: i) study the mechanisms by which the adult brain adapts and reorganizes after injury; and ii) devise approaches that will allow us to manipulate the process of reorganization to induce visual recovery.

The network of visual areas can be viewed as a heavily interconnected circuit subject to a series of hierarchy rules. Early areas usually process sensory information initially, by passing it on to higher areas, and in turn, extract "higher" order features and control the flow of information through feedback loops. Increased performance following training can therefore be the result of changes that occur in early areas (Schoups et al., 2001; Yotsumoto et al., 2008; Censor and Sagi, 2009; Karni and Sagi, 2008), or the result of changes that occur in "higher" visual areas and attentional networks (Law and Gold, 2008; Yang and Maunsell, 2004; Lewis et al., 2009). Area V1 injuries, interrupt the cardinal feed-forward pathway but, as discussed above, visually driven information can still activate surviving extrastriate areas through bypassing routes (Cowey, 1974; Dineen et al., 1982; Rodman et al., 1989; Cowey and Stoerig, 1997; Baseler et al.,

1999; Goebel et al., 2001; Schmid et al., 2009; Schmid et al., 2010). The pattern of activity elicited in surviving visual areas interacts with higher "centers" in frontal, parietal and temporal lobes but, in the absence of V1 input, fails to generate a strong visual percept. We suggest here two general, non-mutually exclusive approaches to visual rehabilitation:

"Bottom-up" approach: Visual rehabilitation strengthens V1-bypassing pathways to increase the response elicited in surviving extrastriate areas.

"Top-down" approach: Visual rehabilitation reorganizes higher "centers" to learn to process the changed patterns of activity elicited in extrastriate areas by V1-bypassing inputs.

Non-invasive approaches to visual rehabilitation aim to enhance these pathways by recruiting the mechanisms of plasticity the brain uses for learning. Various behavioral approaches have been used. They usually involve performing a visual task that directs attention to a sub-threshold stimulus, requires a choice, and then provides feedback about correct and incorrect choices (see fig. 5). Although such methods are effective for perceptual learning in general (Yotsumoto et al., 2008; Law and Gold, 2008; Yang and Maunsell, 2004), in the domain of rehabilitation of a dense perceptual scotoma results have been at best variable (Huxlin et al., 2009; Raninen et al., 2007 Sahraie, et al., 2006; Reinhard et al., 2005; Horton et al., 2005a; Horton et al., 2005b; Pleger et al., 2003). The most notable exception has been a recent well-controlled report by Huxlin and co-workers (Huxlin et al., 2009), which demonstrated strong recovery of direction of visual motion perception inside the scotoma of 5 hemianopic subjects (Huxlin et al., 2009; Huxlin, 2006). Two other groups independently, Sahraie et al. and Raninen et al., report that visual sensitivity can improve with training in humans with homonymous scotomas (Sahraie, 2006; Henriksson et al., 2007; Raninen et al., 2007). Encouraging results were also obtained by Pleger and co-workers, who showed that visual cortex reorganization was possible via daily visual stimulation training over a period of 6 months in 3 subjects with partial cortical blindness (Pleger et al., 2003). Although these are encouraging reports, the issue remains far from settled (Horton et al., 2005a; Horton et al., 2005b). Additional studies corroborating recent results and probing the mechanism of recovery are clearly needed to guide the implementation of new, more effective, rehabilitation strategies. In what follows, we discuss the promise and challenges of a new visual rehabilitation approach, which aims to use "real time" fMRI neurofeedback to train subjects to promote plasticity in V1-bypassing pathways relevant to recovery.

4. Introduction to real-time functional magnetic resonance imaging neurofeedback approaches

Less than two decades ago, the real-time functional magnetic resonance (rt-fMRI) method has been introduced (Cox, 1995) in the field of neuro-rehabilitation, which extracts the BOLD (Blood-Oxygen-Level-Dependent) signal from the subject's brain in real-time and uses it to provide feedback to the subject. Since the BOLD signal reflects neural activity this approach is called real-time fMRI neurofeedback (rt-fMRI nFb). Multiple studies have shown that rt-fMRI nFb, can train subjects to modulate the magnitude and spatial extent of the activity elicited in various cortical and subcortical areas (Berman et al., 2011; Bray et al., 2007; Caria et al., 2007; Caria et al., 2010; Chiew et al., 2012; deCharms et al., 2004; deCharms et al., 2005; Frank et al., 2012; Haller et al., 2010; Hamilton et al., 2011; Hinds et al., 2011; Johnson et al., 2012; Johnson et al., 2011; Johnson et al; 2010; Lee et al., 2012; Li et al., 2012; McCaig et al., 2011; Papageorgiou et al., 2009a; Papageorgiou et al., 2009b; Papageorgiou et al., 2013; Posse et al., 2003; Rota et al., 2009; Ruiz et al., 2013; Scharnowski et al., 2012; Shibata et al., 2011; Subramanian et al., 2011; Sulzer et al., 2013; Veit et al., 2012; Weiskopf et al., 2007; Weiskopf et al., 2004; Weiskopf et al., 2003; Yoo and Jolesz, 2002; Yoo et al., 2008; Zotev et al., 2011). The goal of this approach is to train subjects to control the pattern of their brain activity in a way that promotes a desired behavior. It can also be used to boost the neural capacity for learning and plasticity (Shibata et al., 2012; Scharnowski et al., 2012; Shibata et al., 2011; Weiskopf et al., 2004; deCharms et al., 2004; deCharms et al., 2005). If this is applied effectively, it could serve as a useful tool to promote neuro-rehabilitation.

The ability of rt-fMRI nFb to induce a behavioral change was first shown by Weiskopf et al. (Weiskopf et al., 2003) and deCharms et al. (deCharms et al., 2005). In the deCharms et al. study, chronic-pain patients were coached to decrease their pain by learning to control the BOLD signal intensity of the rostral Anterior Cingulate Cortex (rACC), a region known to be involved in pain perception (Apkarian et al., 2005; Peyron et al., 2000). After training, subjects were able to voluntarily increase or decrease the rACC BOLD signal intensity, and this correlated with an increased or decreased level of pain, respectively; i.e., a 50% decrease in the rACC activity of chronic pain subjects corresponded approximately to a 64% decrease in their pain. This effect was specific to rtfMRI nFb training applied to rACC; i.e., no effect was seen after similar training conducted without rtfMRI NFb or, after sham rtfMRI nFb training derived from the activity of another subject's rACC.

Similar results have been obtained in other cortical and subcortical domains (Posse et al., 2003; Lee et al., 2011; Hamilton et al., 2011; Ruiz et al., 2013). A recent study showed that healthy volunteers were able to volitionally regulate the activity of their insula when given rt-fMRI nFb (Lee et al., 2011). Posse and his team (Posse et al., 2003) trained subjects to upregulate their amygdala, an area whose level of activity is associated with sad affect and depression (Wang et al., 2012; Anand et al., 2007; Liu et al., 2011). Amygdala upregulation induced by rt-fMRI feedback was positively correlated with self-ratings of sadness across repeated fMRI sessions (Posse et al., 2003). Conversely, Hamilton et al. used rt-fMRI nFb to train subjects to downregulate subgenual ACC and posterior cingulate cortex, resulting in positive mood induction (Hamilton et al., 2011). Sham rt-fMRI nFb showed no effect. Ruiz et al. showed that schizophrenic patients can be trained by rt-fMRI nFb to voluntarily control their anterior insula bilaterally (Ruiz et al., 2013). The effect of bilateral anterior insula activation is reflected on their ability to recognize face emotion, a known deficit in schizophrenia. These findings collectively, suggest that: 1) rt- fMRI nFb can be used to train subjects to voluntarily control specific areas; 2) changes in the activity of certain areas can be associated with significant behavioral changes; 3) rt-fMRI nFb training can achieve stronger behavioral results than similar training without nFb; and 4) rt-fMRI training can induce plastic changes that can outlast the period of the training inside the magnet and even induce visual perceptual learning (Shibata et al. 2011).

Shibata et al. in a seminal study used rt-fMRI nFb to induce perceptual learning (Shibata et al., 2011). Rt-fMRI nFb methods were used to enable subjects to induce activity patterns in their early visual cortex corresponding to one particular orientation. Initially, the subjects performed an orientation discrimination task and a decoder of area V1/V2 activity was constructed to classify a pattern of the measured fMRI signals into one of three orientations. Once the decoder was constructed, each subject participated in a 5 to 10-day rt-fMRI nFb stage, during which they learned to induce patterns of activity in areas V1/V2 corresponding to the target orientation. During this stage, subjects were instructed to maximize the signal delivered to them via feedback, but were not told how to induce the desired patterns of activity that would result in increased activity. Subjects did not know what was to be learned. Using this strategy they were able to induce visual perceptual learning specific to the target orientation in areas V1/V2. Learning occurred as a function of the subject's ability to elicit the particular pattern of activation corresponding to the target orientation in early visual areas. Remarkably, subjects were able to generate this pattern simply by being given the instruction to maximize feedback, without being aware that the pattern to be elicited had anything to do with orientation. This demonstrated that the rt-fMRI nFb method can be used to induce highly specific activity patterns within a brain region and that repeatedly eliciting the desired pattern of activity is sufficient to induce plasticity in early visual areas. These findings suggest that rt-fMRI nFb training can be used to induce plasticity in a highly selective manner in the visual system.

The studies described above (Ruiz et al., 2013; Linden et al., 2012; Subramanian et al., 2011; Shibata et al., 2011; Lee et al., 2011; Hamilton et al., 2011; deCharms et al., 2004; Posse et al., 2003) show that manipulating the activity in select brain areas can induce plasticity. Modified paradigms can also be designed to increase plasticity along specific pathways, by co-activating input and recipient neuronal populations. For example, a projection from area A to recipient area B in the brain can increase or, decrease in strength, depending on the relative activity between input projections from A and recipient neurons in B. Rt-fMRI nFb does not have the temporal resolution necessary to precisely implement Hebbian mechanisms of plasticity. Nevertheless it can be used to train the subject to voluntarily manipulate the activity level of select neuronal populations in area B while their input from A is presented. The hypothesis is that "top-down" activation of area B enhanced by nFb judiciously paired with "bottom-up" presentation of inputs that activate A, can act together to increase the strength of the projection A->B. Below, we discuss an example outlining how this proposal might work for the rehabilitation of visual motion perception following area V1 lesions (see also fig. 5).

Area hV5/MT+ is associated with global coherent visual motion perception. The goal is to use rt-fMRI nFb methods to strengthen the neural pathways bypassing the V1 lesion and project to area hV5/MT+ in order to improve visual motion perception of random dot kinematogram (RDK) stimuli (see fig. 5). The first step is to train the subject to voluntarily upregulate their hV5/MT+ activity. To do this we ask the subject to practice mental imagery of fully coherent visual motion stimuli in their blind hemifield, moving in the direction of the anticipated stimulus. During mental imagery, the subject receives rt-fMRI nFb proportional to the activity

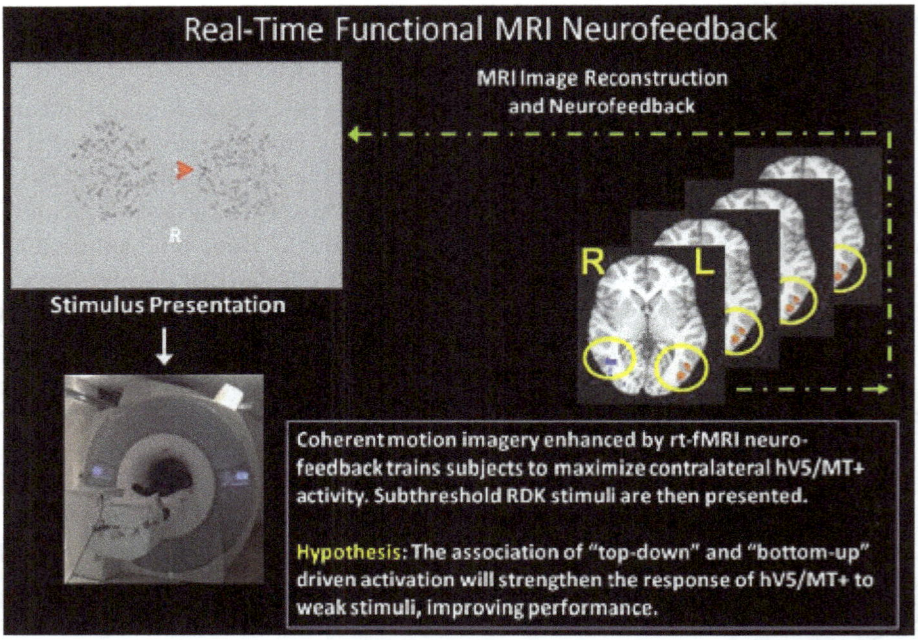

Figure 5. Rt-fMRI nFb paradigm for rehabiliating visual motion perception. The subject lies supine inside the scanner, while s/he is presented with a 0% coherent RDK stimulus. Brain volumes are acquired every 2sec (TR). hV5/MT+ (circled) is selected as our ROI. Turbo Brain Voyager software (Brain Innovation) is used to deliver nFb. The BOLD signal in hV5/MT+ is estimated in real time (every TR), normalized, and "fed" back, via the length of a horizontal arrow at fixation, to train the subject to upregulate area hV5/MT+. Subjects are instructed to attend to the RDK they are cued towards, either right (R) or left (L) and imagine that it is coherent (when in fact it is not). This increases the level of activity in the contralateral hV5/MT+ : (i) superimposing coherent motion via imagery on the right RDK increases left hV5/MT+ activity, which is color-coded in red; (ii) superimposing coherent motion via imagery on the left RDK increases right hV5/MT+ activity, which is color-coded in blue. The subject uses the length of the arrow to determine how successful their strategy is and try harder, if needed. *When the rt-fMRI nFb driven, "top-down," hV5/MT+ activation crosses a threshold, sub-threshold RDK stimuli are presented. The association of "top-down" and "bottom-up" activation will engage Hebbian-like learning mechanisms aiming to strengthen the response of hV5/MT+ to sub-threshold stimuli.* The hypothesis is that once these pathways are strengthened, the presentation of sub-threshold stimuli will elicit enough activity in area hV5/MT+ to improve performance in the direction of motion discrimination task. We note that *hV5/MT+ can be upregulated via rt-fMRI nFb enhanced imagery even when it has lost its V1 input.* Once the subject learns how to upregulate hV5/MT+ inside the magnet over the period of training, we hypothesize that s/he will also be able to transfer this learned voluntary ability during training outside the MRI environment.

in their hV5/MT+ via a visual interface at fixation (red arrow in fig. 5). Subjects are trained to maximize ipsi-lesional hV5/MT+ activity using the imagery task. This nFb mediated, "top-down" increase in hV5/MT+ activity will then be paired with the presentation of visual motion stimuli that are invisible (sub-threshold) to subjects with V1+ lesions. We hypothesize that, by repeatedly presenting sub-threshold visual motion stimuli while hV5/MT+ is activated in a "top-down" fashion by nFb, we will engage Hebbian-like association learning mechanisms (Hebb, 1946; Rebesco and Miller, 2011; Gallistel and Matzel, 2013). These mechanisms will promote plasticity in the surviving, V1-bypassing pathways that get activated by the stimulus presentation and project to area hV5/MT+. In other words, we hypothesize that after nFb training, regions of area hV5/MT+ deprived of V1 input will respond more strongly to visual stimuli presented inside the scotoma, improving performance. If successful, this strategy will induce a "neural bypass" of V1 function with respect to visual motion perception.

One advantage that rt-fMRI nFb methods have over behavioral feedback approaches is that specific brain pathways or areas can be selectively trained. It is then, feasible to train targeted components of the neural circuit that are likely to contribute to recovery. One example is strengthening neural pathways that bypass the region of an injury to promote recovery. Thus far, we have been discussing a univariate rt-fMRI nFb approach, where the nFb provided is proportional to the activity of a specific region of interest (in the above example, area hV5/MT +) or, pattern of activity (Shibata et al., 2011). An alternative to the univariate nFb method is the multivariate classification approach (Papageorgiou et al., 2013; Papageorgiou et al., 2009; LaConte et al., 2007; Mourao-Miranda et al., 2005). In this approach, a classification algorithm, usually, the support vector machine (Vapnik, 1995) is trained on a set of relevant data in order to identify the brain networks that are involved in a specific computation (task). This is akin to the localizer that is used to identify the region of interest in the univariate approach. In fact, in the case of presentation of RDK stimuli, the multivariate SVM approach picks out chiefly area hV5/MT+, as expected (see fig. 6 below). However, in other cases, this approach may reveal different patterns of activity than expected, helping to formulate new hypotheses about the networks that might contribute to rehabilitation. Once the parameters of the classification algorithm are trained, the algorithm can be used to provide neuro-feedback to the subject in separate sessions. This approach may be effective in cases where the pathways that need to be modulated to induce recovery are not known a-priori.

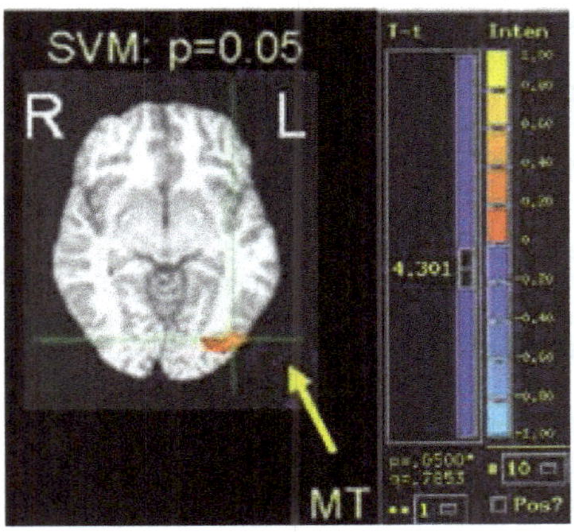

Figure 6. The support vector machine (SVM) algorithm defines area hV5/MT+ when it is trained on coherent motion RDKs. Subjects are fixating while two RDKs are presented simultaneously on symmetric locations in the right (red color-coded activation) and left (blue color-coded activation) visual hemi-fields. The RDK presented in the left visual field was always kept at 0% coherence (no global motion direction), while the RDK in the right visual field alternated between 0% coherence and 100% coherence. A support vector machine algorithm was trained on the whole brain to classify when the coherent RDK (right visual field/red-color coded activation) was presented. The color map indicates the region that was important in classifying the presentation of a 100% coherent vs a 0% coherent RDK in the right visual field. As expected, the area corresponds to area hV5/MT+. Three subjects tested gave consistent results (3dANOVA2 performed in AFNI, p=0.05).

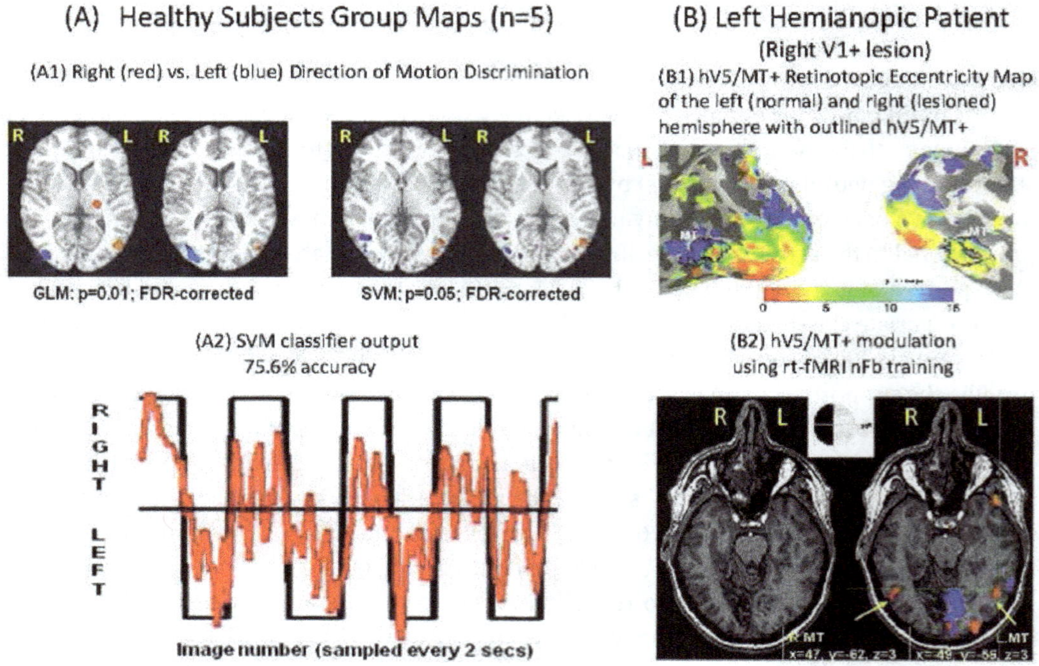

Figure 7. Rt-fMRI nFb can be used to selectively upregulate hV5/MT+ in a top-down manner during an imagery task. In the absence of a coherent moving stimulus, subjects (n=5) were able to use imagery of coherent motion to selectively upregulate hV5/MT+ via rt-fMRI nFb training. (**A**) Non-coherent RDKs were presented symmetrically in the L and the R hemifield and subjects were cued to imagine that the Left or the Right RDK contained coherent motion. The level of contralateral hV5/MT+ activity was delivered via the length of an arrow at the fixation point. (**A1**) Red/blue regions correspond to voxels upregulated when the subject is instructed to imagine coherent motion in the right/left visual field, respectively. Similar results are obtained when using a standard GLM (left panel), versus plotting the weight vector of the support vector machine (SVM) algorithm that classifies whether subjects imagined coherent motion to the left versus the right hemifield (right panel). The regions identified correspond to area hV5/MT+ in both hemispheres (color red, blue). *Therefore,subjects can be trained via rt-fMRI nFb to modulate theirhV5/MT+ activity even in the absence of a coherentlymoving stimulus;* (**A2**) Output (red curve) of a support vector machine classifier indicating the side of the visual field where the subject imagined coherent motion. The correct choice indicated by the black curve; the prediction of the classifier by the red curve. Positive values indicate the subject was instructed to imagine coherent motion on the right, negative on the left. Note that area hV5/MT+ activity can predict the subject's perceptual state. (**B1**) Eccentricity maps of a subject with left hemianopia illustrating that area hV5/MT+ (outlined) of the lesioned (right) hemisphrere can be visually driven. Only the posterior lateral aspect of the two inflated hemispheres is presented. (**B2**) Illustrates that *hV5/MT+ can also be upregulated via rt-fMRI nFb training in a V1+ lesioned patient.* **Left Panel:** Right (R) PCA lesion, resulting in left (L) hemianopia (inset). **Right Panel:** Red color-coded areas represent the activity elicited by the subject's coherent motion imagery in the left (hemianopic) visual field, while blue color-coded area represents non-coherent motion presentation, as generated by GLM. Left hemianopic visual field imagery of coherent motion activated hV5/MT+ bilaterally. Preliminary data for implementing the proposal we outlined above are encouraging as they suggest that ipsilesional hV5/MT+ activity: (1) conveys information about the stimulus (**B1**), and (2) can be upregulated using rt-fmri nFb imagery in V1+ lesioned patients (**B2**).

In summary, emerging strategies based on rt-fMRI nFb hold considerable promise, as: 1) they can be used to enhance plasticity in a number of systems (Berman et al., 2011; Bray et al., 2007; Caria et al., 2010; deCharms et al., 2004; Haller et al., 2010; Johnson et al., 2012; Johnston et al., 2010; Lee et al., 2012; Li et al., 2012; McCaig et al., 2011; Papageorgiou et al., 2013; Posse et al., 2003; Ruiz et al., 2013; Subramanian et al., 2011; Sulzer et al., 2013; Veit al., 2012; Yoo and Jolesz, 2002; Yoo et al., 2008; Zotev et al., 2011) including in the visual system of healthy participants (Scharnowski et al., 2012; Shibata et al., 2011); 2) they may be in some cases superior to normal behavioral methods (deCharms et al., 2005); 3) they can be tailored to induce perceptual learning (plasticity) in a highly specific fashion (Shibata et al., 2011); 4) their multivariate variant can be used to identify pathways relevant to recovery; and 5) induced learning effects are reported to persist outside the magnet, after the end of training (Ruiz et al., 2013; Sulzer et al., 2013). In the long-term, rtfMRI nFb methods promise to induce cortical plasticity that is efficient, robust and specific for each patient. Lessons learned are likely to apply beyond the visual system to disorders of motor function, cognition, speech, language and emotion.

5. Challenges and future considerations using rt-fMRI nFb for visual rehabilitation

Many challenges need to be overcome in order to study the efficacy of rt-fMRI nFb methods in visual rehabilitation. Primarily, we need to develop effective rt-fMRI nFb paradigms in subjects with V1 lesions. The challenge is to implement rt-fMRI nFb training protocols to strengthen specific pathways that are hypothesized to play a role in rehabilitating performance. It is important to understand which pathways are more amenable to rehabilitation and what is the best rt-fMRI nFb paradigm to use. This requires elucidating which factors are "necessary and sufficient variables for learning" (Weiskopf, 2012). The answers to these questions will in general depend on the specifics of the injury that requires rehabilitation, as well as on other factors such as the subject's motivation.

Quantifying the degree of induced reorganization using population receptive field (pRF) methods is complementary to behavioral performance measures and represents a valuable neuroimaging biomarker for studying the mechanism of recovery induced by nFb rehabilitation methods. Information obtained will then, allow us to refine future rehabilitative approaches. Several different pathways may be able to contribute to recovery. For example, in the case of the visual motion rehabilitation example, the focus was on strengthening "bottom-up" pathways to enhance the response of the ipsilesional area hV5/MT+ to the visual motion stimulus. One can hypothesize other strategies that focus instead on reorganizing higher areas, such as frontal eye fields (FEF), supplementary eye fields (SEF) areas involved in the generation of visual motion percepts downstream of hV5/MT+ by "reading out" the weak activity that persists in extrastriate cortex following V1+ lesions. Or, one can focus on strategies that reorganize attentional networks, such as middle frontal gyrus (mFG), intraparietal sulcus (IPS), superior parietal lobule (SPL), and anterior cingulate cortex (ACC) that enhance the weakened responses elicited in surviving areas following V1+ lesions.

There are important technical challenges. The criticism is often mounted that rt-fMRI nFb approaches are impractical because they require large amounts of magnet time. Although this have some truth in it, preliminary studies reveal that time spent inside the magnet is much less than what pure behavioral methods, require. Deciding how many rt-fMRI nFb sessions are needed to induce plasticity is a question that still needs to be answered. Preliminary evidence suggests that as few as 5-10 sessions can be sufficient to induce a strong perceptual learning effect in normal subjects (Shibata et al., 2011), but this will need to be validated in the case of patients with V1 lesions. Healthy participants and patients undergoing rt-fMRI nFb training sessions inside the magnet can learn to voluntarily elicit the desired pattern of activity. Subjects could then, gradually learn to implement this process outside the magnet, transferring their experience from rt-fMRI nFb sessions to ordinary behavioral sessions. We do not have adequate evidence yet, to determine under what conditions training accomplished inside the rt-fMRI environment can be transferred outside the magnet, but there is reason to be hopeful (Ruiz et al., 2013; Sulzer et al., 2013). The clinical applicability of rt-fMRI nFb training will become significantly broader if it becomes feasible to decouple the patient's training sessions from the rt-fMRI nFb environment. Another important question is how long the effects of rt-fMRI nFb training are expected to last and whether this depends on the number of rt-fMRI nFb sessions used for training. Here too, there is reason for optimism given the results of Shibata et al. who managed to induce perceptual learning within 5 sessions of rtfMRI nFb (Shibata et al., 2011).

Many important challenges remain. However, it is now possible to mount a systematic approach to visual rehabilitation using novel rt-fMRI nFb methods guided by pRF analysis of spared visual areas. This approach promises to teach us a lot about the visual system's capacity for plasticity after injury, and offers hope that effective, and robust visual rehabilitation methods, such as the novel rt- fMRI nFb approach will be used in the field of visual neuro-rehabilitation.

6. Conclusion

Rehabilitating visual loss that occurs as a result of primary visual cortex injury is a difficult problem. To date, we have little understanding of the plasticity mechanisms operating in the adult visual system following V1 injury. Consequently, no reliable method exists to effectively rehabilitate V1-lesioned patients who experience loss of visual perception in the contralateral hemifield (Horton, 2005a; Horton, 2005b; Pambakian and Kennard, 1997). Interestingly, recent results have shown that visually driven activity persists in extrastriate cortex following chronic area V1+ lesions (Schmid, 2010; Schmid, 2009; Rodman, 1989; Rodman, 1990; Baseler, 1999), and that it is possible in some cases to rehabilitate visual motion perception (Das, 2010; Huxlin, 2009; Raninen et al., 2007; Henriksson et al., 2007; Sahraie et al., 2010). This confirms the existence of functional pathways that bypass the V1+ lesion, providing direct input to spared extrastriate cortex. Such pathways are generally too weak to result in practical benefit. However, appropriate training strategies may be able to strengthen them sufficiently to induce recovery.

Real-time fMRI neuro-feedback strategies allow subjects to voluntarily modulate activity in certain brain areas or, neural pathways. These methods can be harnessed and used to promote plasticity (Shibata et al., 2011). For example, we hypothesize that rt-fMRI nFb may be used to strengthen pathways that bypass the region of V1 injury to transmit visual motion information to area hV5/MT+. One paradigm that could, in theory, be used to accomplish this is the following: Subjects are trained by rt-fMRI nFb to voluntarily upregulate their hV5/MT+ activity. Whenever hV5/MT+ activity crosses a pre-set threshold, sub-threshold visual stimuli are presented. Repeated pairing of the "top-down" nFb-driven activation with the "bottom-up" stimulus-driven activation will engage Hebbian-like association learning mechanisms, strengthening the response of hV5/MT+ to visual motion stimuli. Visual motion stimuli that were previously sub-threshold may then, rise above threshold following training, improving performance.

Rehabilitating dense visual field scotomas requires adopting a systematic approach. Changes brought about by new rehabilitation strategies should be mapped and their mechanism studied. We have presented evidence that pRF analysis is an excellent tool for this purpose, quantifying changes and providing rich data for formulating hypotheses about what regions of the visual field may be more amenable to rehabilitation and what pathways contribute to recovery.

We conclude that, even though rt-fMRI nFb methods are currently in their infancy, they hold considerable promise for inducing plasticity in targeted pathways promoting successful rehabilitation. Although here, we have focused on the visual system, principles discussed apply to the neuro-rehabilitation of several other domains of brain function, such as motor control, language, speech (Papageorgiou et al., 2009a; Papageorgiou et al., 2009b; Papageorgiou et al., 2013), emotion and cognition.

Acknowledgements

Part of the work that is presented here was supported by: (i) a McNair Foundation award, a McNair Medical Institute (MMI) award and a Fight for Sight Grant to T.D. Papageorgiou; and (ii) an NEI RO1 (EY019272), DoD (W81XWH-08-2-0146), and an HHMI Early Career Award to S. M. Smirnakis.

Author details

T. Dorina Papageorgiou[1], Amalia Papanikolaou[2] and Stelios M. Smirnakis[1,2]

1 Departments of Neuroscience and Neurology, Baylor College of Medicine, Houston, Texas, USA

2 Departments of MaxPlanck Institute for Biological Cybernetics, Tuebingen, Germany

References

[1] Ahissar, M. and S. Hochstein (1997). "Task difficulty and the specificity of perceptual learning." Nature 387(6631): 401-6.

[2] Ajina, S. and C. Kennard (2012). "Rehabilitation of damage to the visual brain." Rev Neurol (Paris) 168(10): 754-61.

[3] Alexander, I. and A. Cowey (2009). "The cortical basis of global motion detection in blindsight." Exp Brain Res 192(3): 407-11.

[4] Amano, K., B. A. Wandell, et al. (2009). "Visual field maps, population receptive field sizes, and visual field coverage in the human MT+ complex." J Neurophysiol 102(5): 2704-18.

[5] Anand, A., Y. Li, et al. (2007). "Reciprocal effects of antidepressant treatment on activity and connectivity of the mood regulating circuit: an FMRI study." J Neuropsychiatry Clin Neurosci 19(3): 274-82.

[6] Apkarian, A. V., M. C. Bushnell, et al. (2005). "Human brain mechanisms of pain perception and regulation in health and disease." Eur J Pain 9(4): 463-84.

[7] Baseler, H. A., A. Gouws, et al. (2011). "Large-scale remapping of visual cortex is absent in adult humans with macular degeneration." Nat Neurosci 14(5): 649-55.

[8] Baseler, H. A., A. B. Morland, et al. (1999). "Topographic organization of human visual areas in the absence of input from primary cortex." J Neurosci 19(7): 2619-27.

[9] Berman, B. D., S. G. Horovitz, et al. (2012). "Self-modulation of primary motor cortex activity with motor and motor imagery tasks using real-time fMRI-based neurofeedback." Neuroimage 59(2): 917-25.

[10] Boynton, G. M., S. A. Engel, et al. (1996). "Linear systems analysis of functional magnetic resonance imaging in human V1." J Neurosci 16(13): 4207-21.

[11] Bray, S., S. Shimojo, et al. (2007). "Direct instrumental conditioning of neural activity using functional magnetic resonance imaging-derived reward feedback." J Neurosci 27(28): 7498-507.

[12] Brown, T. H., P. F. Chapman, et al. (1988). "Long-term synaptic potentiation." Science 242(4879): 724-8.

[13] Caria, A., R. Sitaram, et al. (2010). "Volitional control of anterior insula activity modulates the response to aversive stimuli. A real-time functional magnetic resonance imaging study." Biol Psychiatry 68(5): 425-32.

[14] Caria, A., R. Veit, et al. (2007). "Regulation of anterior insular cortex activity using real-time fMRI." Neuroimage 35(3): 1238-46.

[15] Censor, N. and D. Sagi (2009). "Global resistance to local perceptual adaptation in texture discrimination." Vision Res 49(21): 2550-6.

[16] Chiew, M., S. M. LaConte, et al. (2012). "Investigation of fMRI neurofeedback of differential primary motor cortex activity using kinesthetic motor imagery." Neuroimage 61(1): 21-31.

[17] Chokron, S., C. Perez, et al. (2008). "From blindsight to sight: cognitive rehabilitation of visual field defects." Restor Neurol Neurosci 26(4-5): 305-20.

[18] Corbetta, M. and G. L. Shulman (2002). "Control of goal-directed and stimulus-driven attention in the brain." Nat Rev Neurosci 3(3): 201-15.

[19] Cowey, A. (2010). "Visual system: how does blindsight arise?" Curr Biol 20(17): R702-4.

[20] Cowey, A. (1974). "Atrophy of retinal ganglion cells after removal of striate cortex in a rhesus monkey." Perception 3(3): 257-60.

[21] Cowey, A. and P. Stoerig (1997). Blindsight in man and monkey. Brain 120(Pt 3): 535-59.

[22] Cowey, A. and P. Stoerig (1989). "Projection patterns of surviving neurons in the dorsal lateral geniculate nucleus following discrete lesions of striate cortex: implications for residual vision." Exp Brain Res 75(3): 631-8.

[23] Cowey, A. and P. Stoerig (1991). "The neurobiology of blindsight." Trends Neurosci 14(4): 140-5.

[24] Cox, R. W. (1996). "AFNI: software for analysis and visualization of functional magnetic resonance neuroimages." Comput Biomed Res 29(3): 162-73.

[25] Das, A. and K. R. Huxlin (2010). "New approaches to visual rehabilitation for cortical blindness: outcomes and putative mechanisms." Neuroscientist 16(4): 374-87.

[26] de Gelder, B., J. S. Morris, et al. (2005). "Unconscious fear influences emotional awareness of faces and voices." Proc Natl Acad Sci U S A 102(51): 18682-7.

[27] deCharms, R. C., K. Christoff, et al. (2004). "Learned regulation of spatially localized brain activation using real-time fMRI." Neuroimage 21(1): 436-43.

[28] deCharms, R. C., F. Maeda, et al. (2005). "Control over brain activation and pain learned by using real-time functional MRI." Proc Natl Acad Sci U S A 102(51): 18626-31.

[29] Deco, G. and T. S. Lee (2004). "The role of early visual cortex in visual integration: a neural model of recurrent interaction." Eur J Neurosci 20(4): 1089-100.

[30] DeYoe, E. A., G. J. Carman, et al. (1996). "Mapping striate and extrastriate visual areas in human cerebral cortex." Proc Natl Acad Sci U S A 93(6): 2382-6.

[31] Dineen, J., A. Hendrickson, et al. (1982). "Alterations of retinal inputs following striate cortex removal in adult monkey." Exp Brain Res 47(3): 446-56.

[32] Dougherty, R. F., M. Ben-Shachar, et al. (2005). "Functional organization of human occipital-callosal fiber tracts." Proc Natl Acad Sci U S A 102(20): 7350-5.

[33] Dougherty RF, V.M. Koch, et al. (2003). "Visual field representations and locations of visual areas V1/2/3 in human visual cortex." J Vis. 3(10):586-98.

[34] Dumoulin, S. O. and B. A. Wandell (2008). "Population receptive field estimates in human visual cortex." Neuroimage 39(2): 647-60.

[35] Elisevich, K. V., R. M. Ford, et al. (1984). "Visual abnormalities with multiple trauma." Surg Neurol 22(6): 565-75.

[36] Engel, S. A., D. E. Rumelhart, et al. (1994). "fMRI of human visual cortex." Nature 369(6481): 525.

[37] Fabre-Thorpe, M., F. Levesque, et al. (1994). "Preservation of pointing accuracy toward moving targets after extensive visual cortical ablations in cats." Cortex 30(4): 585-601.

[38] Fendrich, R., C. M. Wessinger, et al. (1992). "Residual vision in a scotoma: implications for blindsight." Science 258(5087): 1489-91.

[39] ffytche, D.H., A. Howseman, et al. (2000). Human area V5 and motion in the ipsilateral visual field. Eur J Neurosci. 12(8):3015-25.

[40] Fields, R. D. (2008). "White matter in learning, cognition and psychiatric disorders." Trends Neurosci 31(7): 361-70.

[41] Frank, S., S. Lee, et al. (2012). "The obese brain athlete: self-regulation of the anterior insula in adiposity." PLoS One 7(8): e42570.

[42] Friel, K. M., A. A. Heddings, et al. (2000). "Effects of postlesion experience on behavioral recovery and neurophysiologic reorganization after cortical injury in primates." Neurorehabil Neural Repair 14(3): 187-98.

[43] Fujii, T., H. C. Tanabe, et al. (2009). "An investigation of cross-modal plasticity of effective connectivity in the blind by dynamic causal modeling of functional MRI data." Neurosci Res 65(2): 175-86.

[44] Gall, C., B. Steger, et al. (2013). "Evaluation of two treatment outcome prediction models for restoration of visual fields in patients with postchiasmatic visual pathway lesions." Neuropsychologia.

[45] Gallistel, C. R. and L. D. Matzel (2013). "The neuroscience of learning: beyond the Hebbian synapse." Annu Rev Psychol 64: 169-200.

[46] Gilhotra, J. S., P. Mitchell, et al. (2002). "Homonymous visual field defects and stroke in an older population." Stroke 33(10): 2417-20.

[47] Giorgi, R. G., R. L. Woods, et al. (2009). "Clinical and laboratory evaluation of peripheral prism glasses for hemianopia." Optom Vis Sci 86(5): 492-502.

[48] Girard, P., P. A. Salin, et al. (1991). "Visual activity in areas V3a and V3 during reversible inactivation of area V1 in the macaque monkey." J Neurophysiol 66(5): 1493-503.

[49] Goebel, R., L. Muckli, et al. (2001). "Sustained extrastriate cortical activation without visual awareness revealed by fMRI studies of hemianopic patients." Vision Res 41(10-11): 1459-74.

[50] Haller, S., N. Birbaumer, et al. (2010). "Real-time fMRI feedback training may improve chronic tinnitus." Eur Radiol 20(3): 696-703.

[51] Hamilton, J. P., G. H. Glover, et al. (2011). "Modulation of subgenual anterior cingulate cortex activity with real-time neurofeedback." Hum Brain Mapp 32(1): 22-31.

[52] Hebb, D.O. (1949). Distinction in coherent neural network between resting and working brain states. The organization of behavior. New York: Wiley & Sons.

[53] Henriksson, L., A. Raninen, et al. (2007). "Training-induced cortical representation of a hemianopic hemifield." J Neurol Neurosurg Psychiatry 78(1): 74-81.

[54] Henry, S.H. R.C. Reid (2000). The koniocellular pathway in primate vision. Annual Review of Neuroscience 23: 127-153.

[55] Hinds, O., S. Ghosh, et al. (2011). "Computing moment-to-moment BOLD activation for real-time neurofeedback." Neuroimage 54(1): 361-8.

[56] Hinrichs, H., H. J. Heinze, et al. (2006). "Causal visual interactions as revealed by an information theoretic measure and fMRI." Neuroimage 31(3): 1051-60.

[57] Hopfinger, J. B., M. H. Buonocore, et al. (2000). "The neural mechanisms of top-down attentional control." Nat Neurosci 3(3): 284-91.

[58] Horton, J. C. (2005a). "Disappointing results from Nova Vision's visual restoration therapy." Br J Ophthalmol 89(1): 1-2.

[59] Horton, J. C. (2005b). "Vision restoration therapy: confounded by eye movements." Br J Ophthalmol 89(7): 792-4.

[60] Hua, T., P. Bao, et al. (2010). "Perceptual learning improves contrast sensitivity of V1 neurons in cats." Curr Biol 20(10): 887-94.

[61] Hubel, D. H. and Wiesel, T. N. (1977). Ferrier Lecture: Functional Architecture of Macaque Monkey Visual Cortex, Proceedings of the Royal Society of London. Series B, Biological Sciences, Vol. 198, No. 1130 (May 19, 1977), pp. 1-59 Published by: The Royal Society Stable URL: http://www.jstor.org/stable/77245.

[62] Huxlin, K. R., J. M. Williams, et al. (2008a). "A neurochemical signature of visual recovery after extrastriate cortical damage in the adult cat." J Comp Neurol 508(1): 45-61.

[63] Huxlin, K. R. (2008b). "Perceptual plasticity in damaged adult visual systems." Vision Res 48(20): 2154-66.

[64] Huxlin, K. R., T. Martin, et al. (2009). "Perceptual relearning of complex visual motion after V1 damage in humans." J Neurosci 29(13): 3981-91.

[65] Huxlin, K. R. and T. Pasternak (2004). "Training-induced recovery of visual motion perception after extrastriate cortical damage in the adult cat." Cereb Cortex 14(1): 81-90.

[66] Huxlin, K. Plasticity of Visual Perception After Permanent Damage to the Adult Visual Cortex. in "Visual Field restoration Therapy Symposium"— Nanos Annual Meeting. 2006. Tuscon, AZ.

[67] Iorizzo, D. B., M. E. Riley, et al. (2011). "Differential impact of partial cortical blindness on gaze strategies when sitting and walking - an immersive virtual reality study." Vision Res 51(10): 1173-84.

[68] Jobke, S., E. Kasten, et al. (2009). "Vision restoration through extrastriate stimulation in patients with visual field defects: a double-blind and randomized experimental study." Neurorehabil Neural Repair 23(3): 246-55.

[69] Johnson, K. A., K. Hartwell, et al. (2012). "Intermittent "real-time" fMRI feedback is superior to continuous presentation for a motor imagery task: a pilot study." J Neuroimaging 22(1): 58-66.

[70] Johnston, S., D. E. Linden, et al. (2011). "Upregulation of emotion areas through neurofeedback with a focus on positive mood." Cogn Affect Behav Neurosci 11(1): 44-51.

[71] Johnston, S. J., S. G. Boehm, et al. (2010). "Neurofeedback: A promising tool for the self-regulation of emotion networks." Neuroimage 49(1): 1066-72.

[72] Julkunen, L., O. Tenovuo, et al. (2003). "Rehabilitation of chronic post-stroke visual field defect with computer-assisted training: a clinical and neurophysiological study." Restor Neurol Neurosci 21(1-2): 19-28.

[73] Karni, A. and D. Sagi (1991). "Where practice makes perfect in texture discrimination: evidence for primary visual cortex plasticity." Proc Natl Acad Sci U S A 88(11): 4966-70.

[74] Kasten, E., U. Bunzenthal, et al. (2007). "Vision restoration therapy does not benefit from costimulation: A pilot study." J Clin Exp Neuropsychol 29(6): 569-84.

[75] Kasten, E., U. Bunzenthal, et al. (2006). "Visual field recovery after vision restoration therapy (VRT) is independent of eye movements: an eye tracker study." Behav Brain Res 175(1): 18-26.

[76] Kasten, E., E. Muller-Oehring, et al. (2001). "Stability of visual field enlargements following computer-based restitution training -- results of a follow-up." J Clin Exp Neuropsychol 23(3): 297-305.

[77] Kasten, E., D. A. Poggel, et al. (1999). "Restoration of vision II: residual functions and training-induced visual field enlargement in brain-damaged patients." Restor Neurol Neurosci 15(2-3): 273-87.

[78] Kasten, E., D. A. Poggel, et al. (2000). "Computer-based training of stimulus detection improves color and simple pattern recognition in the defective field of hemianopic subjects." J Cogn Neurosci 12(6): 1001-12.

[79] Kasten, E. and B. A. Sabel (1995). "Visual field enlargement after computer training in brain-damaged patients with homonymous deficits: an open pilot trial." Restor Neurol Neurosci 8(3): 113-27.

[80] Kasten, E., S. Wuest, et al. (1998a). "Residual vision in transition zones in patients with cerebral blindness." J Clin Exp Neuropsychol 20(5): 581-98.

[81] Kasten, E., S. Wust, et al. (1998b). "Computer-based training for the treatment of partial blindness." Nat Med 4(9): 1083-7.

[82] Kastner, S. and L. G. Ungerleider (2000). "Mechanisms of visual attention in the human cortex." Annu Rev Neurosci 23: 315-41.

[83] Kerkhoff, G., U. Munssinger, et al. (1992). "Rehabilitation of homonymous scotomata in patients with postgeniculate damage of the visual system: saccadic compensation training." Restor Neurol Neurosci 4(4): 245-54.

[84] Kerkhoff, G., U. Munssinger, et al. (1994). "Neurovisual rehabilitation in cerebral blindness." Arch Neurol 51(5): 474-81.

[85] Kikuta, K., Y. Takagi, et al. (2006). "Early experience with 3-T magnetic resonance tractography in the surgery of cerebral arteriovenous malformations in and around the visual pathway." Neurosurgery 58(2): 331-7; discussion 331-7.

[86] Kluver, H. (1936). An analysis of the effects of the removal of the occipital lobes in monkeys, J Psychol, 2: 49-61.

[87] LaConte, S. M., S. J. Peltier, et al. (2007). "Real-time fMRI using brain-state classification." Hum Brain Mapp 28(10): 1033-44.

[88] Law, C. T. and J. I. Gold (2008). "Neural correlates of perceptual learning in a sensory-motor, but not a sensory, cortical area." Nat Neurosci 11(4): 505-13.

[89] Lee, S., A. Papanikolaou, et al. (2013). "A new method for estimating population receptive field topography in visual cortex." Neuroimage 81: 144-57.

[90] Lee, S., S. Ruiz, et al. (2011). "Detection of cerebral reorganization induced by real-time fMRI feedback training of insula activation: a multivariate investigation." Neurorehabil Neural Repair 25(3): 259-67.

[91] Lew, H. L., J. H. Poole, et al. (2007). "Program development and defining characteristics of returning military in a VA Polytrauma Network Site." J Rehabil Res Dev 44(7): 1027-34.

[92] Lewis, C. M., A. Baldassarre, et al. (2009). "Learning sculpts the spontaneous activity of the resting human brain." Proc Natl Acad Sci U S A 106(41): 17558-63.

[93] Li, X., K. J. Hartwell, et al. (2012). "Volitional reduction of anterior cingulate cortex activity produces decreased cue craving in smoking cessation: a preliminary real-time fMRI study." Addict Biol 18(4): 739-48.

[94] Lindberg, P., H. Forssberg, et al. (2003). "[Rehabilitation after stroke. Imaging techniques show how the cortical reorganization is affected by training]." Lakartidningen 100(51-52): 4289-92.

[95] Linden DE, Habes I, et al. (2012). Real-time self-regulation of emotion networks in patients with depression. PLoS One 7(6):e38115.

[96] Liu, Z. and D. Weinshall (2000). "Mechanisms of generalization in perceptual learning." Vision Res 40(1): 97-109.

[97] Liu X, Zhu XH, Chen W. (2011). Distinction in coherent neural network between resting and working brain states. Brain Connect 1(5):377-88. doi: 10.1089/brain.2011.0044.

[98] Marshall, R. S., J. J. Ferrera, et al. (2008). "Brain activity associated with stimulation therapy of the visual borderzone in hemianopic stroke patients." Neurorehabil Neural Repair 22(2): 136-44.

[99] McCaig, R. G., M. Dixon, et al. (2011). "Improved modulation of rostrolateral prefrontal cortex using real-time fMRI training and meta-cognitive awareness." Neuroimage 55(3): 1298-305.

[100] McKenna, K., D. M. Cooke, et al. (2006). "The incidence of visual perceptual impairment in patients with severe traumatic brain injury." Brain Inj 20(5): 507-18.

[101] Mihailovic LT, Cupic D, Dekleva N. (1971). Changes in the numbers of neurons and glial cells in the lateral geniculate nucleus of the monkey during retrograde cell degeneration. J Comp Neurol 142: 223-9.

[102] Moore, T., H. R. Rodman, et al. (2001). "Direction of motion discrimination after early lesions of striate cortex (V1) of the macaque monkey." Proc Natl Acad Sci U S A 98(1): 325-30.

[103] Moore, T., H. R. Rodman, et al. (1995). "Localization of visual stimuli after striate cortex damage in monkeys: parallels with human blindsight." Proc Natl Acad Sci U S A 92(18): 8215-8.

[104] Morris, J. S., B. DeGelder, et al. (2001). "Differential extrageniculostriate and amygdala responses to presentation of emotional faces in a cortically blind field." Brain 124(Pt 6): 1241-52.

[105] Mourao-Miranda, J., A. L. Bokde, et al. (2005). "Classifying brain states and determining the discriminating activation patterns: Support Vector Machine on functional MRI data." Neuroimage 28(4): 980-95.

[106] Mumford, D. (1994). Neuronal architectures for pattern theoretic problems. In: Large Scale Neuronal Theories of the Brain, Koch C, Davis, JL, eds., MIT Press, pp. 125-152.

[107] Okada, T., Y. Miki, et al. (2007). "Diffusion tensor fiber tractography for arteriovenous malformations: quantitative analyses to evaluate the corticospinal tract and optic radiation." AJNR Am J Neuroradiol 28(6): 1107-13.

[108] Olshausen, B.A. Principles of Image Representation in Visual Cortex. In: The Visual Neurosciences, L.M. Chalupa, J.S. Werner, Eds. MIT Press, 2003: 1603-1615.

[109] Overgaard, M. (2011). "Visual experience and blindsight: a methodological review." Exp Brain Res 209(4): 473-9.

[110] Pambakian, A.L. and C. Kennard (1997). Can visual function be restored in patients with homonymous hemianopia? Br J Ophthalmol (4): p. 324-8.

[111] Papageorgiou, T. D., W. A. Curtis, et al. (2009a). "Neurofeedback of two motor functions using supervised learning-based real-time functional magnetic resonance imaging." Conf Proc IEEE Eng Med Biol Soc 2009: 5377-80.

[112] Papageorgiou, T.D., M. McHenry, J.L. Lisinski, J.P. White, and S.M. LaConte (2009b). Speech rate control using supervised learning-based rea-time fMRI. 15th Annual Meeting of the Organization for Human Brain Mapping, San Franscisco. Neuroimage, 47: p. 97.

[113] Papageorgiou, T.D., LaConte, S.M., Lisinski, J.L., Peng, X., and Smirnakis, S.M, Classification Accuracy and Spatial Networks on Motion Coherence using Real-time fMRI. Hum Brain Mapp, Barcelona, 2010.

[114] Papageorgiou, T. D., J. M. Lisinski, et al. (2013). "Brain-computer interfaces increase whole-brain signal to noise." Proc Natl Acad Sci U S A 110(33): 13630-5.

[115] Pasik, T. and P. Pasik (1971). "The visual world of monkeys deprived of striate cortex: effective stimulus parameters and the importance of the accessory optic system." Vision Res Suppl 3: 419-35.

[116] Pessoa, L., S. Kastner, et al. (2003). "Neuroimaging studies of attention: from modulation of sensory processing to top-down control." J Neurosci 23(10): 3990-8.

[117] Peyron, R., B. Laurent, et al. (2000). "Functional imaging of brain responses to pain. A review and meta-analysis (2000)." Neurophysiol Clin 30(5): 263-88.

[118] Pleger, B., A. F. Foerster, et al. (2003). "Functional magnetic resonance imaging mirrors recovery of visual perception after repetitive tachistoscopic stimulation in patients with partial cortical blindness." Neurosci Lett 335(3): 192-6.

[119] Plow, E. B., S. N. Obretenova, et al. (2011). "Combining visual rehabilitative training and noninvasive brain stimulation to enhance visual function in patients with hemianopia: a comparative case study." PM R 3(9): 825-35.

[120] Poggel, D. A., E. Kasten, et al. (2006). "Improving residual vision by attentional cueing in patients with brain lesions." Brain Res 1097(1): 142-8.

[121] Poggel, D. A., E. Kasten, et al. (2001). "Unusual spontaneous and training induced visual field recovery in a patient with a gunshot lesion." J Neurol Neurosurg Psychiatry 70(2): 236-9.

[122] Poggel, D. A., E. Kasten, et al. (2004). "Attentional cueing improves vision restoration therapy in patients with visual field defects." Neurology 63(11): 2069-76.

[123] Poggel, D. A., I. Mueller, et al. (2010). "Subjective and objective outcome measures of computer-based vision restoration training." NeuroRehabilitation 27(2): 173-87.

[124] Poppel, E., R. Held, et al. (1973). "Leter: Residual visual function after brain wounds involving the central visual pathways in man." Nature 243(5405): 295-6.

[125] Posse, S., D. Fitzgerald, et al. (2003). "Real-time fMRI of temporolimbic regions detects amygdala activation during single-trial self-induced sadness." Neuroimage 18(3): 760-8.

[126] Raninen, A., S. Vanni, et al. (2007). "Temporal sensitivity in a hemianopic visual field can be improved by long-term training using flicker stimulation." J Neurol Neurosurg Psychiatry 78(1): 66-73.

[127] Rebesco, J. M. and L. E. Miller (2011). "Stimulus-driven changes in sensorimotor behavior and neuronal functional connectivity application to brain-machine interfaces and neurorehabilitation." Prog Brain Res 192: 83-102.

[128] Reinges, M. H., T. Krings, et al. (2004). "Functional and diffusion-weighted magnetic resonance imaging for visualization of the postthalamic visual fiber tracts and the visual cortex." Minim Invasive Neurosurg 47(3): 160-4.

[129] Reinhard, J., A. Schreiber, et al. (2005). "Does visual restitution training change absolute homonymous visual field defects? A fundus controlled study." Br J Ophthalmol 89(1): 30-5.

[130] Riggs, R. V., K. Andrews, et al. (2007). "Visual deficit interventions in adult stroke and brain injury: a systematic review." Am J Phys Med Rehabil 86(10): 853-60.

[131] Rizzo, M. and D. A. Robin (1996). "Bilateral effects of unilateral visual cortex lesions in human." Brain 119 (Pt 3): 951-63.

[132] Rodman, H. R., C. G. Gross, et al. (1989). "Afferent basis of visual response properties in area MT of the macaque. I. Effects of striate cortex removal." J Neurosci 9(6): 2033-50.

[133] Rodman, H. R., C. G. Gross, et al. (1990). "Afferent basis of visual response properties in area MT of the macaque. II. Effects of superior colliculus removal." J Neurosci 10(4): 1154-64.

[134] Rota, G., R. Sitaram, et al. (2009). "Self-regulation of regional cortical activity using real-time fMRI: the right inferior frontal gyrus and linguistic processing." Hum Brain Mapp 30(5): 1605-14.

[135] Rudolph, K. and T. Pasternak (1999). "Transient and permanent deficits in motion perception after lesions of cortical areas MT and MST in the macaque monkey." Cereb Cortex 9(1): 90-100.

[136] Rudolph, K. K., V. P. Ferrera, et al. (1994). "A reduction in the number of directionally selective neurons extends the spatial limit for global motion perception." Vision Res 34(24): 3241-51.

[137] Rudolph, T. M. and E. R. Delay (1993). "Recovery of a temporally based visual discrimination after visual cortex lesion in the rat." Behav Brain Res 53(1-2): 189-99.

[138] Ruiz, S., K. Buyukturkoglu, et al. (2013). "Real-time fMRI brain computer interfaces: Self-regulation of single brain regions to networks." Biol Psychol.

[139] Sabel, B. A., P. Henrich-Noack, et al. (2011). "Vision restoration after brain and retina damage: the "residual vision activation theory"." Prog Brain Res 192: 199-262.

[140] Sabel, B. A. and E. Kasten (2000). "Restoration of vision by training of residual functions." Curr Opin Ophthalmol 11(6): 430-6.

[141] Sabel, B. A., S. Kenkel, et al. (2004). "Vision restoration therapy (VRT) efficacy as assessed by comparative perimetric analysis and subjective questionnaires." Restor Neurol Neurosci 22(6): 399-420.

[142] Sahraie, A., M. J. Macleod, et al. (2010). "Improved detection following Neuro-Eye Therapy in patients with post-geniculate brain damage." Exp Brain Res 206(1): 25-34.

[143] Sahraie, A., C. T. Trevethan, et al. (2006). "Increased sensitivity after repeated stimulation of residual spatial channels in blindsight." Proc Natl Acad Sci U S A 103(40): 14971-6.

[144] Schmid, M. C., S. W. Mrowka, et al. (2010). "Blindsight depends on the lateral geniculate nucleus." Nature 466(7304): 373-7.

[145] Schmid, M. C., T. Panagiotaropoulos, et al. (2009). "Visually driven activation in macaque areas V2 and V3 without input from the primary visual cortex." PLoS One 4(5): e5527.

[146] Schoenfeld, M. A., H. J. Heinze, et al. (2002). "Unmasking motion-processing activity in human brain area V5/MT+ mediated by pathways that bypass primary visual cortex." Neuroimage 17(2): 769-79.

[147] Schoth, F., U. Burgel, et al. (2006). "Diffusion tensor imaging in acquired blind humans." Neurosci Lett 398(3): 178-82.

[148] Schoups, A., R. Vogels, et al. (2001). "Practising orientation identification improves orientation coding in V1 neurons." Nature 412(6846): 549-53.

[149] Sereno, M. I., A. M. Dale, et al. (1995). "Borders of multiple visual areas in humans revealed by functional magnetic resonance imaging." Science 268(5212): 889-93.

[150] Scharnowski, F., C. Hutton, et al. (2012). "Improving visual perception through neurofeedback." J Neurosci 32(49): 17830-41.

[151] Sherbondy, A. J., R. F. Dougherty, et al. (2008). "Identifying the human optic radiation using diffusion imaging and fiber tractography." J Vis 8(10): 12 1-11.

[152] Shibata K, L.H. Chang, (2012). Decoding reveals plasticity in V3A as a result of motion perceptual learning. PLoS One. 7(8):e44003.

[153] Shibata, K., T. Watanabe, et al. (2011). "Perceptual learning incepted by decoded fMRI neurofeedback without stimulus presentation." Science 334(6061): 1413-5.

[154] Stilla, R., R. Hanna, et al. (2008). "Neural processing underlying tactile microspatial discrimination in the blind: a functional magnetic resonance imaging study." J Vis 8(10): 13 1-19.

[155] Stoerig, P. and E. Barth (2001). "Low-level phenomenal vision despite unilateral destruction of primary visual cortex." Conscious Cogn 10(4): 574-87.

[156] Subramanian, L., J. V. Hindle, et al. (2011). "Real-time functional magnetic resonance imaging neurofeedback for treatment of Parkinson's disease." J Neurosci 31(45): 16309-17.

[157] Sulzer, J., R. Sitaram, et al. (2013). "Neurofeedback-mediated self-regulation of the dopaminergic midbrain." Neuroimage 83C: 817-825.

[158] Stoerig, P. and A. Cowey (1997). "Blindsight in man and monkey." Brain 120 (Pt 3): 535-59.

[159] Takeuchi, N., T. Chuma, et al. (2005). "Repetitive transcranial magnetic stimulation of contralesional primary motor cortex improves hand function after stroke." Stroke 36(12): 2681-6.

[160] Taoka, T., M. Sakamoto, et al. (2005). "Diffusion tensor imaging in cases with visual field defect after anterior temporal lobectomy." AJNR Am J Neuroradiol 26(4): 797-803.

[161] Taub, E., G. Uswatte, et al. (2002). "New treatments in neurorehabilitation founded on basic research." Nat Rev Neurosci 3(3): 228-36.

[162] Taylor, T. N. (1997). "The medical economics of stroke." Drugs 54 Suppl 3: 51-7; discussion 57-8.

[163] Van den Stock, J., M. Tamietto, et al. (2011). "Cortico-subcortical visual, somatosensory, and motor activations for perceiving dynamic whole-body emotional expressions with and without striate cortex (V1)." Proc Natl Acad Sci U S A 108(39): 16188-93.

[164] Vanburen, J. M. (1963). "Trans-Synaptic Retrograde Degeneration in the Visual System of Primates." J Neurol Neurosurg Psychiatry 26: 402-9.

[165] Vapnik, N. (1995). The nature of statistical learning theory. Springer.

[166] Veit, R., V. Singh, et al. (2012). "Using real-time fMRI to learn voluntary regulation of the anterior insula in the presence of threat-related stimuli." Soc Cogn Affect Neurosci 7(6): 623-34.

[167] Wandell, B. A., S. O. Dumoulin, et al. (2007). "Visual field maps in human cortex." Neuron 56(2): 366-83.

[168] Wang, L., W. Dai, et al. (2012). "Amplitude of low-frequency oscillations in first-episode, treatment-naive patients with major depressive disorder: a resting-state functional MRI study." PLoS One 7(10): e48658.

[169] Wedeen, V. J., D. L. Rosene, et al. (2012). "The geometric structure of the brain fiber pathways." Science 335(6076): 1628-34.

[170] Weiller, C. (1998). "Imaging recovery from stroke." Exp Brain Res 123(1-2): 13-7.

[171] Weiskopf, N. (2012). "Real-time fMRI and its application to neurofeedback." Neuroimage 62(2): 682-92.

[172] Weiskopf, N., R. Sitaram, et al. (2007). "Real-time functional magnetic resonance imaging: methods and applications." Magn Reson Imaging 25(6): 989-1003.

[173] Weiskopf, N., F. Sharnowski, et al., (2004). Self-regulation of local brain activity using real-time functional magnetic resonance imaging (fMRI). J Physiol Paris, 98(4-6): p. 357-73.

[174] Weiskopf, N., R. Veit, et al. (2003). "Physiological self-regulation of regional brain activity using real-time functional magnetic resonance imaging (fMRI): methodology and exemplary data." Neuroimage 19(3): 577-86.

[175] Weiskrantz, L. (2004). "Roots of blindsight." Prog Brain Res 144: 229-41.

[176] Weiskrantz, L., E. K. Warrington, et al. (1974). "Visual capacity in the hemianopic field following a restricted occipital ablation." Brain 97(4): 709-28.

[177] Werth, R. and M. Moehrenschlager (1999). "The development of visual functions in cerebrally blind children during a systematic visual field training." Restor Neurol Neurosci 15(2-3): 229-41.

[178] Worsley, K. J., C. H. Liao, et al. (2002). "A general statistical analysis for fMRI data." Neuroimage 15(1): 1-15.

[179] Yang, T. and J. H. Maunsell (2004). "The effect of perceptual learning on neuronal responses in monkey visual area V4." J Neurosci 24(7): 1617-26.

[180] Yeatman, J. D., R. F. Dougherty, et al. (2012). "Tract profiles of white matter properties: automating fiber-tract quantification." PLoS One 7(11): e49790.

[181] Yoo, S. S. and F. A. Jolesz (2002). "Functional MRI for neurofeedback: feasibility study on a hand motor task." Neuroreport 13(11): 1377-81.

[182] Yoo, S. S., J. H. Lee, et al. (2008). "Neurofeedback fMRI-mediated learning and consolidation of regional brain activation during motor imagery." Int J Imaging Syst Technol 18(1): 69-78.

[183] Yotsumoto, Y., T. Watanabe, et al. (2008). "Different dynamics of performance and brain activation in the time course of perceptual learning." Neuron 57(6): 827-33.

[184] Zeki, S. (2004) Thirty years of a very special visual area, area V5. J. Physiol. 557, 1–2.

[185] Zeki S., and D.H. ffytche (1998). The Riddoch syndrome: insights into the neurobiology of conscious vision. Brain 121(Pt 1):25-45.

[186] Zhang, X., S. Kedar, et al. (2006). "Natural history of homonymous hemianopia." Neurology 66(6): 901-5.

[187] Zihl, J. and D. von Cramon (1979). "Restitution of visual function in patients with cerebral blindness." J Neurol Neurosurg Psychiatry 42(4): 312-22.

[188] Zihl, J. and D. von Cramon (1985). "Visual field recovery from scotoma in patients with postgeniculate damage. A review of 55 cases." Brain 108 (Pt 2): 335-65.

[189] Zotev, V., F. Krueger, et al. (2011). "Self-regulation of amygdala activation using real-time FMRI neurofeedback." PLoS One 6(9): e24522.

[190] Zuiderbaan, W., B. M. Harvey, et al. (2012). "Modeling center-surround configurations in population receptive fields using fMRI." J Vis 12(3): 10.

8

Learning-Based Cross-Modal Plasticity in the Human Brain: Insights from Visual Deprivation fMRI

Lora Likova

1. Introduction

Neuroimaging, and functional Magnetic Resonance Imaging (fMRI) in particular, has brought dramatic changes in all fields of brain studies, one of the notable fields under intensive development being that of brain plasticity. To overcome the artificiality of typical experimental paradigms, this chapter presents a set of interrelated investigations focused on the reorganization of working memory and sensorimotor mechanisms as a result of training in a complex 'real-life' paradigm. The novel paradigm that I have introduced is based on the spatiomotor task of drawing, because drawing – from artistic to technical – is a 'real-life' task that uniquely incorporates diverse aspects of perceptual, cognitive and motor skills, thus activating the full *perception-cognition-action 'loop'*. It is important to recognize that drawing engages a wide range of spatial manipulation abilities (e.g., spatio-constructional decisions, coordinate transformations, geometric understanding and visualization), together with diverse mental representations of space, conceptual knowledge, motor planning and control mechanisms, working and long-term memory, attentional mechanisms, as well as, empathy, emotions and forms of embodied cognition (Grossi and Trojano, 1999, for review; Trojano et al., 2009; Likova, 2012a; 2013). Furthermore, the development of a novel training method in non-visual forms of drawing, the Cognitive-Kinesthetic Drawing Method (Likova, 2010a), makes it possible to use drawing for studying training-based cross-modal reorganization in visual areas activated by non-visual tasks.

A further advanced aspect of the studies is that they were run across subject populations with diverse levels of visual experience, ranging from sighted (under blindfolded conditions), through late-onset blind with past visual experience, to congenitally blind who have never had any visual input to stimulate the visual system.

A problem, specific to the studies on brain plasticity in the blind, is that usually such studies do not include training, but simply compare activation in the blind to that in the sighted. The studies in this chapter have taken a different , *training-based* approach, which allows us to go beyond a mere task/activation correlation to *causal* inferences and also to investigate the *evolution* of plastic changes *within the same* brain. Again, this was possible thanks to our novel Cognitive-Kinesthetic Method for teaching people to draw without vision, coupled with a novel *memory paradigm* based on drawing. The pre/post-training brain changes were assessed by fMRI; the respective behavioral changes were evaluated by pre/post-training comparisons of the drawing performance. Cross-group analyses between the diverse subject populations allowed us to evaluate novel hypotheses on cross-modal brain plasticity, and moreover, suggested a need for re-conceptualization of basic principles of the functional architecture of the brain.

1.1. The novel approach

Conceptual Framework

1. *Space transcends any specific sensory modality.* As emphasized by the phenomenon of drawing by the blind (e.g., Kennedy, 1993, 2000, 2003, 2006; Ponchilla, 2008; Likova, 2010 a,b; 2012a,b; 2013), space and spatial structure are not represented solely by the visual modality. The visual system may be the modality best suited to process spatial information, but it is not the only one. Thus, when deprived of visual input, the brain is capable of employing the 'free' visual resources in the most relevant way. (As there is an ambiguity in the use of the term 'spatial', particularly in the working memory and imagery literature, we note that when used in this paper, 'spatial' refers to the perception of any spatial structure – 2D or 3D, static or dynamic – *independently* of the sensory modality exploring it. For example, a face can be recognized by exploring its spatial structure with the hands, or a geometric function can be 'seen' by audio-graphics, etc.) Our view is that *drawing* deals with spatial structures in this general sense, and consequently it has the advantage that can readily be 'translated' from a visual into a tactile form.

2. *Closing the perception-cognition-action loop is a powerful amplifier for learning* , so the *task* selection is critical. *Drawing* is a complex task precisely orchestrating multiple brain mechanisms, thus our hypothesis is that, consequently, it is suitable for an integrative, perception-cognition-action paradigm.

3. *Training in highly engaging unfamiliar tasks* that provide fun and inspiring outcomes is a fruitful paradigm for driving brain reorganization and assessing its earlier stages. *Drawing* is such a task, particularly when studied under the unusual circumstances of visual deprivation.

4. *Tasks demanding detailed re-expression of memory representations force the development of precise and robust memory. Drawing* from memory demands such explicit *re-expression* through the motor loop, and consequently it demands 'high-resolution' internal representations to be communicated back through the drawing act.

5. *A direct memory 'readout' would be a big advantage for memory-studying paradigms. Drawing* from memory provides such direct memory 'readout' in the form of the drawn image, as it ensures an explicit expression of the remembered information by externalization of the mental representation that guides the drawing hand.

Drawing as a Novel Memory Paradigm Incorporating the Framework Principles

Since drawing uniquely incorporates the principles in our conceptual framework outlined above, we used drawing to develop a paradigm for both *studying* and *training* memory (e.g., Likova, 2010b; 2012a,b). We hypothesized that *memory-guided* drawing, in particular, has a powerful potential for training because it forces the learners not to just passively explore the stimuli, but to develop detailed and stable *memory* representations (*Drawing/Memory Hypothesis*). Furthermore, we conceptualized that, as our novel paradigm can be adapted from the visual to the tactile modality, it can become an effective tool for studying *learning-based cross-modal brain reorganization.*

The Need for the Cognitive-Kinesthetic Training Method

The visual appreciation of line drawings (e.g., Fig. 1) seems such an effortless process that we may not be aware of the invisible work of powerful high-level cognitive mechanisms that provide the artist with the ability to transform a 3D object into its 2D projection by abstracting just the right contours into a line drawing, and we may not appreciate how our brains make the 'inverse transformation' to the immediate understanding of what such 2D drawings represent.

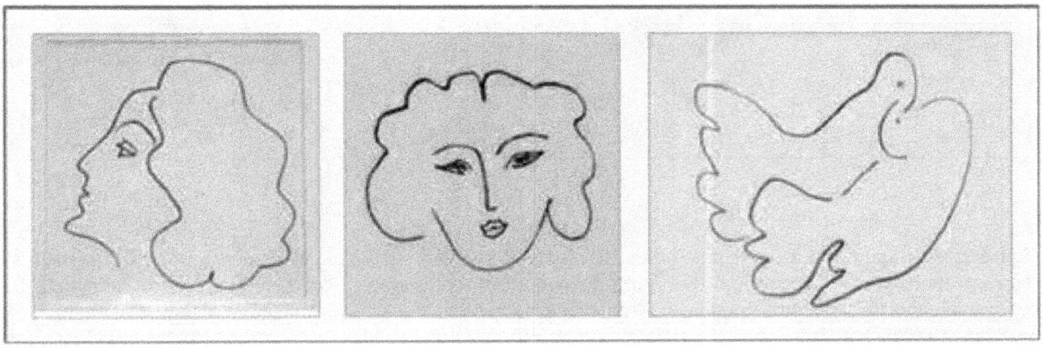

Figure 1. Matisse: Lithographes No. 54: ' *Marie'* (left), No. 35: ' *Ma Maîtresse'* (center), No. 45: ' *Les Colombes Amoureuses'* (right), from the illustrations for Ronsard's *'Florilège des Amours'* (1948).

It came as a surprise, therefore, to find that, when exposed for the first time to 2D raised-line drawings, many blind participants had tremendous difficulty in the tactile recognition and comprehension of the depicted 3D objects. This 'negative' finding, however, provided us with the opportunity to employ a learning paradigm *in adults* , thus enabling for the first time the investigations of the developmental process of key cognitive components important in drawing, such as *spatial memory.*

The inherently visual nature of drawing, however, is an obvious barrier for the implementation of the drawing-based memory paradigm to research and rehabilitation of people with blindness or profound visual impairment. This issue was successfully overcome by implementing the C-K method that I have conceptualized and developed for training freehand drawing without vision, guided solely by *non-visually acquired* memory. This unique method has already shown that it can enhance detailed working memory, and in particular, the generation and maintenance of robust spatial-memory representations (Likova, 2012a,b; 2013), which are crucial for replacing the *'eye-hand'* coordination (lost under blindness) by *'non-visual memory-hand'* coordination (Fig. 2). Moreover, I have proposed that an effective approach to blindness requires wide-spectrum blindness rehabilitation through a unified, single task, and have shown that the C-K method is highly promising to fulfill that demand.

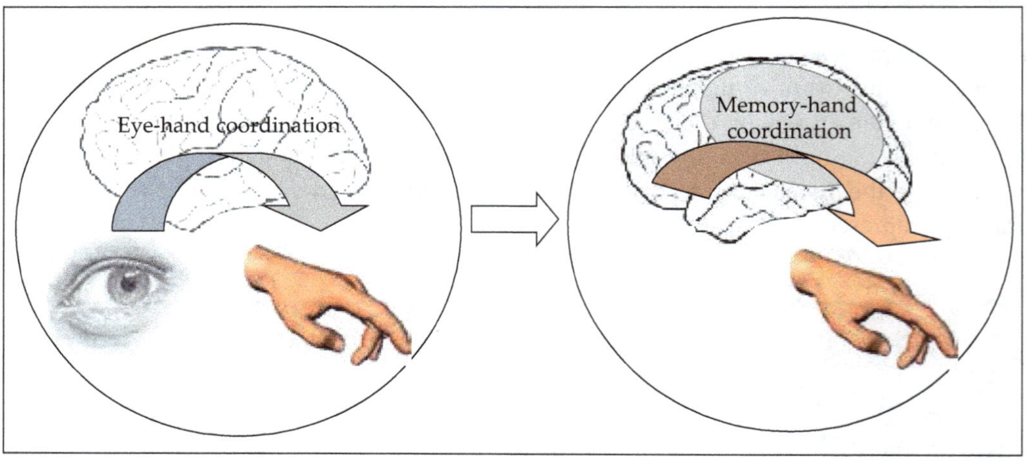

Figure 2. Illustration of our conceptualization that targeted training for development of robust nonvisual memory representations for spatiomotor coordination is needed when the 'eye-hand' coordination is lost or impaired. This conceptualization underlies the Cognitive-Kinesthetic Drawing Method and its rehabilitation potential.

The Cognitive-Kinesthetic training proved to be very effective in the successful training even of people who are totally blind. In only a week of 1 - 1.5 hour/day training sessions, the participants learn to draw complex structures, such as faces and objects (Fig. 3A).

Moreover, to provide for pre/post training comparisons of brain activation, we have developed an innovative fMRI platform, which includes an MRI-compatible multisensory drawing tablet, with a stylus incorporating a fiber-optic motion-capture system to record the drawing movements to 1 mm accuracy. The C-K Method, with the technological advances of the innovative experimental platform, allowed us to run the first neuroimaging studies on *learning* to draw and on *cross-modal memory reorganization*.

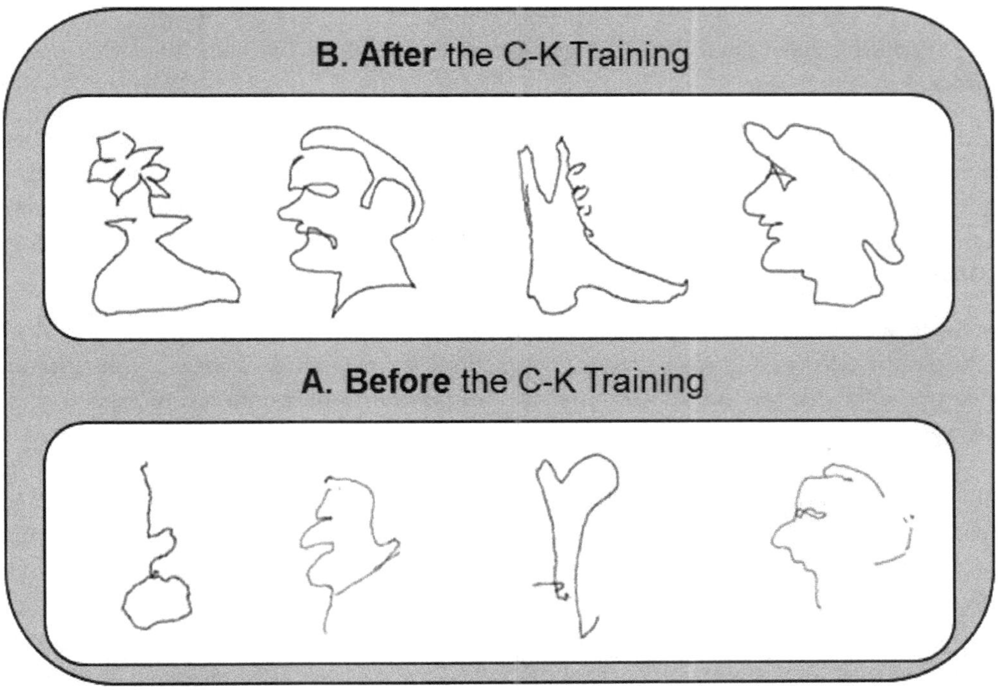

Figure 3. Examples of drawings from different totally blind participants recorded by our motion-capture system in the fMRI scanner. A. Bottom row: The same faces and objects drawn by the same subjects before the training.B.Top row:Blind subjects drawings after a week of the Cognitive-Kinesthetic training.

1.2. The working memory 'Sketchpad' puzzle

More than a century ago, Helmholtz (1871) had pointed out that artists possess not only advanced observational capabilities, but also an enhanced *memory* of the observed images. While the first part of this statement is often cited in vision science, the memory-related aspect has been widely neglected. Our recent results, however, come fully in support of Helmholtz' observation, and are consistent with the *Drawing/Memory Hypothesis* that we propose.

Freehand memory-guided drawing, in particular, challenges the neural system to provide encoding, retrieval and effective 'projection' of memory representations back onto some form of an internal high-resolution ' *projection screen'* , so as to guide the spatial trajectory of the drawing-hand with the requisite precision. It thus closes the full processing 'loop' from perception through memory to precisely controlled motor action (Likova, 2012a).

We suggest that the classic model of working memory provides a framework for understanding the memory processes involved in the drawing task. In this model, working memory (WM) is the "ability to retain information for several seconds to guide goal-directed behaviors" (Baddeley and Hitch, 1974; Baddeley, 1986, 2000, 2003). The WM model has provided major insights into functional neuroimaging on memory, and conversely, has been in turn updated based on neuroimaging data. Recently, for example, it has been suggested that WM processes are not restricted to short-term memory but also reflect activation of long-term memory (LTM) representations (e.g., Ranganath, 2009; Buchsbaum and D'Esposito, 2009; Ishai, 2009). Our treatment of WM is consistent with this recently expanded interpretation.

Baddeley's model consists of four major components, the one we find of interest here being the visuo-spatial 'sketchpad', which conveys the idea that memory is 'drawing' or generating a mental sketch of the memorized object, an internal representation that can be further spatially manipulated. Thus, this 'sketchpad' concept provides much of the functionality of the internal 'projection screen' introspectively needed for drawing.

However, where in the brain the WM 'sketchpad' might be implemented? The neural substrate required to serve such 'sketchpad' function has to provide a large, high-resolution topographic 'screen' or 'map'. Although the full neural implementation of the sketchpad concept is still a puzzle, these requirements point out to the primary visual cortex, area V1, as the best candidate. A few theoretical and neurophysiological studies in non-human primates (e.g., Mumford, 1992; Super et al., 2001a,b; Lee and Mumford, 2003; Super, 2003) had already suggested that V1 may provide the high-resolution visuo-spatial 'sketchpad' function, but there has been little supporting evidence in human. Traditionally, all regions of the early visual cortex have been considered predominantly bottom-up, purely sensory, regions, specifically devoted to the visual modality. However, it is now known that this is not the case, as many of these regions are also subject to *top-down visual* processes such as visual imagery (Ishai and Sagi, 1995; Kastner et al. 1998; Ishai et al., 2000; Kosslyn et al., 1996, 1997, 1999; Kosslyn and Thompson 2003; Kreiman et al., 2000; Lambert et al., 2004; Mechelli et al., 2004; O'Craven and Kanwisher, 2000; Ganis et al., 2004; 2005; Amedi et al., 2005; Slotnick et al. 2005), and - most recently – to short-term visual memory (e.g., William at al., 2008; Harrison and Tong, 2009). Beyond visual top-down effects, different regions of the visual cortex have been also activated cross-modally in a number of auditory and tactile *sensation* tasks (e.g., Sadato et al., 1996; Cohen et al., 1997; Zangaladze et al., 1999; Pascual-Leone and Hamilton, 2001; Block, N., 2003). Moreover, two recent studies have found V1 activation during verbal and episodic memory tasks (Amedi et al., 2003; Raz et all, 2005). No investigation has been done, however, on cross-modal *tactile memory* involvement in these regions.

1.3. Can blind drawing help in solving the puzzle? If there is working memory sketchpad, may it be amodal?

Recently, I hypothesized that the early visual areas, and V1, in particular, can support *modality-independent (i.e., amodal)* 'sketchpad' in human (Likova, 2010b; 2012a; 2013). This hypothesis, which is of importance for models of memory and functional brain architecture, is investigated under our novel drawing-based paradigm. To critically test the amodal hypothesis, the studies in this chapter focus on groups of participants with different forms of total ocular visual deprivation – congenitally blind, late-onset blind and blindfolded – of brain reorganization is studied by fMRI before and after C-K training. To our knowledge, there are no previous studies on the *learning* to draw in the blind and on the *corresponding dynamic phases* of adult brain reorganization. The data showed strong, well-structured V1 activation in a *tactilely-acquired memory* task. These results are consistent with V1 implementing the memory sketchpad concept, however, as no vision is involved, they imply a reconceptualization of the sketchpad from being 'visuo-spatial' to being ' *'amodal-spatial'*.

2. General methods

2.1. Innovative experimental platform

As there are no preceding neuroimaging studies of such training, we had to develop a unique experimental platform integrating a number of innovations, such as: (i) the *Cognitive-Kinesthetic Method* , (ii) a *multisensory MRI-Compatible Drawing Tablet (for both tactile and visual drawing)* , incorporating a motion-capture stylus, (iii) a *Method for Estimating Topographic Maps in the Blind,* (iv) as well as the first implementation of *Visual Probabilistic Maps* in blind individuals.

2.2. Experimental design

A battery of raised-line models of faces and objects was developed as the drawing targets, and a three-task block fMRI paradigm, with task duration being 20 s, interleaved with a 20 s null intervals (Fig. 4 A). The tasks were as follows: *Explore/Memorize, E/M—* perceptual exploration and memorization of the model to be drawn; *MemoryDraw, MD—* a memory-guided non-visual drawing task; and *Scribble, S—* a motor-control and 'negative' memory-control task. Importantly, as opposed to the traditional null intervals, the subjects not only rested motionless during these intervals *(NullInterval, NI)* but were instructed (and practiced) to clear any memory or image structures from awareness ('mind blank'). The start of each task or null interval was prompted by an auditory cue. The whole three-task sequence with interleaved null intervals (*NI, E/M, NI, MD, NI, S, NI)* was repeated 12 times in each 1-hour fMRI session, using a new drawing model for each repeat.

In *Explore/Memorize,* using the left hand only, the subjects had to explore tactually a raised-line drawing model on the left slot of the drawing tablet continuously for 20 s, and to develop a full memory representation of the image in preparation for the *MemoryDraw* task. Then the model was removed and the subjects rested motionless for 20 s with no image in mind (*NullInterval*). In the following *MemoryDraw* phase, the fiber-optic stylus was used to draw the image (from tactile memory) on the right slot of the tablet using the right hand only. In the control task *Scribble* , the subjects moved the stylus with the right hand in a random trajectory matching the extent and rate of the drawing movements but with 'mind-blank'.

This design ensures that the drawing was performed exclusively by the right hand while keeping the left hand motionless during *MemoryDraw* ; moreover, because the virtual stylus was used to draw on the plastic surface of the tablet slot, there was no tactually perceivable trace and no possibility for tactile tracing with the left hand during drawing in the scanner. The lack of left hand movement during drawing was also confirmed by the lack of BOLD activation in the left hand motor area. These restrictions thus enforce the encoding of robust *memory* representations in order to guide the drawing trajectory.

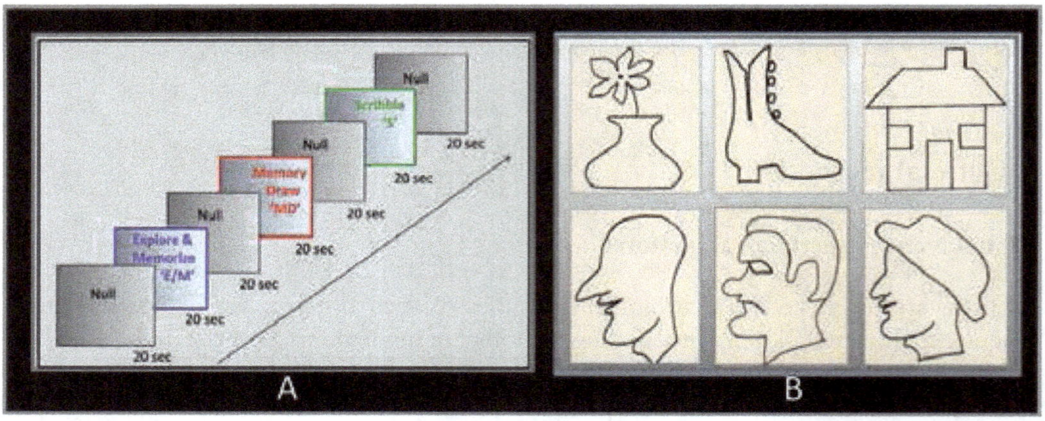

Figure 4. Experimental design. (A) Drawing was investigated in a three-phase paradigm consisting of a memory-guided drawing task, abbreviated as "MemoryDraw" *(MD)*, plus two control tasks: a motor and "negative" memory control task "Scribble" *(S)*, and a task of perceptual exploration and memorization of the model to be drawn "Explore/Memorize" *(E/M)*. Each task's duration was 20 s, with 20 s null intervals interposed between the tasks, the whole 140 s trial sequence being repeated 12 times in each of the 1-hour pre- and post-training fMRI sessions using a new image for each repeat. (B) Raised-line drawings of realistic faces and objects were presented as templates to be explored by the subject using her left hand in the *E/M* phase. Two repetitions of each stimulus were run. The quality of the reproductions was assessed by a masked rating procedure, based on recognition and similarity to the templates. Eexamples of reproduction are shown in in Figs. 3 & 6B.

2.3. Tactile stimulus presentation and hand-movement control

A custom-built, multisensory MRI-compatible drawing system. To run drawing studies within the scanner is not a conventional protocol and faced a lot of challenging technological problems. The special-purpose drawing system (Fig. 5) that we have developed (1) is MRI-compatible, (2) is ergonomically adaptable to the small space available inside the scanner bore, (3) allows multiple tactile models to be presented sequentially in the scanner, (4) captures and records the drawing trajectory with high precision, and (5) can provide real-time visual feedback of the drawn trajectory (when appropriate in *visual* drawing). It incorporates a dual-slot drawing tablet that is height/distance adjustable for the subject's arm length and a specially-adapted version of a fiber-optic motion-capture system for on-line recording of the drawing movements. This multisensory system supports fMRI investigations of *tactually-* guided drawing by providing for the presentation of multiple raised-line models in the scanner without the need of any operator assistance. It also allows us to record relevant behavioral events and to correlate them to the brain activation for full off-line analysis.

Auditory cue presentation. The auditory stimuli were presented through Resonance Technologies Serene Sound earphones (Resonance Technologies, Salem, MA). To reduce scanner noise, this equipment employs external ear protectors with perforated earplugs that conduct the auditory cues directly into the auditory passage while blocking much of the scanner noise.

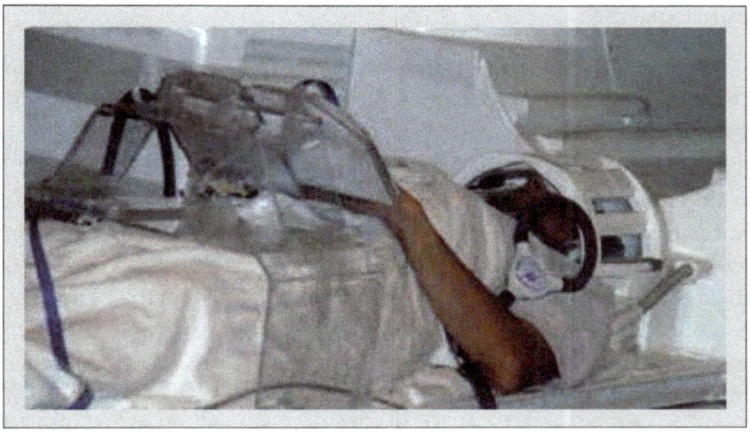

Figure 5. A subject on the scanner bed operating our novel multimodal MRI-compatible drawing device. The plexiglass gantry supports a drawing tablet while a fiber-optic drawing stylus captures and records the drawing movements with high precision. The motion capture information synchronized with the fMRI allows the effect of behavioral events to be analyzed to high precision.

2.4. Computerized Recognizability Index (CR Index)

The C-K training results in dramatic drawing improvements (e.g., Fig. 3B, top row; Fig. 7B) in all forms of visual deprivation, but to be able to quantify that improvement we developed the CR Index, which is based on an optimized spatial-correlation fit across the full spectrum of affine transformations (translation, rotation, scaling and shear). It is applied to each recorded drawing with respect to the set of template images to be drawn, cumulating the proportion of the image that contains matching contours (with sparse-matrix correction for incomplete drawings). The total CR Index of the drawings can then be compared before and after training, to quantify the improvement in the quality of the drawing skill that has been achieved. The CR Index was validated by a masked rating procedure for the quality of the drawing reproductions based on perceptual similarity to the templates.

2.5. MRI data collection, analysis, and visualization

FMRI acquisition

MR data were collected on a Siemens Trio 3T scanner equipped with 8-channel EXCITE capability, a visual stimulus presentation system and response buttons. A high-resolution anatomical (T1-weighted) volume scan of the entire brain was obtained for each observer (0.8 × 0.8 × 0.8 mm voxels). The fMRI blood-oxygenation-level-dependent (BOLD) responses were collected with EPI acquisition from the whole head coil. There were 34 axial slices at 2 s TR, with TE of 28 ms and flip angle of 80°, providing 3.0 × 3.0 × 3.5 mm voxels throughout the brain. The functional activations were processed for slice-time correction and motion correction. An anatomical segmentation algorithm (mrGray, part of the VISTA software package specified below) was applied to the T1 scan, ensuring localization of the signal within the cortical gray matter close to the activated neurons.

FMRI time course analyses

The analysis software was Stanford Vision and Imaging Science and Technology (VISTA, Stanford University) software. The data were analyzed to estimate the effective neural activation amplitudes (e.g., Friston et al., 1994) for each task across the 12 repeats of the 3-task sequence in the one-hour scan by the following procedure. A General Linear Model (GLM) consisting of a (3+1)-parameter boxcar neural activation model convolved with an estimated hemodynamic response function (HRF) was fitted to the BOLD responses for each 3-task sequence, combined with a 1-parameter boxcar model of the 8 auditory cue presentations and an additive 4th-order polynomial to capture low-frequency drift in the BOLD signal. (The HRF was determined once per session by optimizing it to a subset of gray matter voxels identified as those whose average modulation (as a result of the task alternation sequence across the E/M, MD and S tasks) exceeded the statistical level of $z = 3$ in each voxel ($p < 0.001$).) Thus, the parameters of the activation model consisted of the boxcar activation amplitudes for the three task periods, relative to the remainder of the 140 s scan duration.

Voxel-wise parametric maps

For each task, statistical parametric maps were generated, based on the estimated activation amplitudes from the above GLM in each voxel. As is standard for GLM, the boxcar neural activation model for each 20 s task period was contrasted with the entire remainder of the 140 s scan duration. All three task-models were optimized jointly to the detrended BOLD waveform. These maps could be viewed in the 3D volume or projected onto 3D views of the inflated cortex or on flatmaps of cortical regions of particular interest.

ROI activation analysis

The effective neural activation amplitudes (bar graphs) for each condition in each region of interest (ROI) were estimated by the same GLM procedure but now applied to the average signal across all voxels within the ROI. This procedure also provided high-quality time courses for evaluation of the response dynamics and its comparison across tasks and stages of training.

The confidence intervals and error bars were defined by the amplitude variability of the 12 repeats of the 3-task sequence in each one-hour scan. The dashed lines represent the 99% "zero" confidence interval within which the activation amplitudes are not significantly different from zero (at $p < 0.05$, corrected for multiple applications within each figure). The error bars are "difference" confidence intervals designed to illustrate the t-test for the significance of differences between any two activation levels.

In the text, the significance of all ROI-comparisons are specified by the t-test using a statistical criterion threshold of $p < 0.05$ corrected for multiple comparisons.

Retinotopic maps and motion localizer in the sighted

There is a topographic 'projection' or 'mapping' of the visual input information to the retinal surface, and from the retinal surface to corresponding points on the surface of the visual cortex of the brain, thus forming what are known as retinotopic cortical maps. The boundaries of the retinotopic projection areas in the occipital cortex V1, V2d, V2v, V3d and V3v were established as described in Sereno et al. (1995); Tootell et al. (1996) and Engel, Glover and Wandell (1997).

Retinotopic projection areas V3A, V3B, hV4 and V7 were specified in accordance with Tyler et al. (2005) and Schira et al (2010). The hMT+ motion complex was identified using the standard stimuli of an expanding and contracting motion vector field of low-contrast random dots, alternating with a field of static dots as previously implemented in Likova and Tyler, 2007.

Topographic maps in the blind

On the one hand, no informed analysis of the visual cortex could be done without knowledge of its retinotopic and functional organization; on the other hand, no retinotopic mapping is possible in the blind (other than cerebral blindness, which does not apply to any of our participants), so it is a challenge to localize any specific visual area. To resolve this issue and determine the borders of different 'visual' areas in the blind participants, we combined three different approaches. First, we used an innovative 14-step procedure (Likova, 2010a) to warp the brains of sighted and blind subjects to the same MNI brain coordinates. Second, for the primary visual cortex in particular, the location of the V1 ROI was confirmed by its intersection with its anatomical markers (the calcarine sulcus). Additionally, we also compared the result with the Freesurfer probability map of V1, which aligned sufficiently accurately (within 87% overlap of the voxels) with those from the other methods.

3. Where may the amodal spatial memory be implemented? Blindfolded studies and reconceptualization of the WM sketchpad

3.1. Beyond the traditional view of modality-specific cortices specialized for sensory processing

According to the traditional view of brain architecture, the so-called 'sensory' cortical areas are modality-specific and specialized for sensory processing only. Although this view is still prevalent in textbooks, increasing evidence suggests that the function of these areas is not restricted to sensory processing, but (as discussed in the Introduction) is also subject to a number of top-down processes such as modality-specific imagery; furthermore, many of these 'sensory' areas are activated in cross-modal tasks. A body of experimental data shows that in blind individuals, brain areas commonly associated with the processing of visual information can undergo reorganization and be recruited in tasks such as Braille reading, naming, tactile object perception or tactile motion (e.g., Sedato et al., 1996; Uhl et al., 1991, 1993; Cohen et al., 1997; DeVolder et al., 1997; Buechel et al., 1998; Hamilton et al., 2000; Burton et al., 2002, 2003, 2004; Gizewski et al. 2003; Theoret et al., 2004; Merabet et al., 2005; Merabet, 2008; Pascual-Leone et al., 2005; Amedi et al., 2003, 2004, 2008; Goyal et al., 2006; Borowsky et al., 2007 ; Ptito et al., 2008; Deibert et al. 1999; Pietrini et al.; Cohen et al., 2004; Hagen et al., 2002; Matteau et al., 2010) and during drawing in blind individuals (Amedi et al., 2008; Likova, 2010a,b; 2012a,b). Transcranial magnetic stimulation (TMS) of the visual cortex has been found to disrupt Braille reading or verb-generation in the blind (Cohen et al., 1997; Hamilton & Pascual-Leone, 1998; Amedi et al., 2004).

This section probes deeper levels of cross-modal interactions that are of importance for advanced models of functional architecture of the brain.

3.2. Subjects and methods

A group of six subjects with normal vision were blindfolded throughout the experimental procedures. The subjects ranged in age from 25 to 59 and were 4 females and 2 males, right-handed with no formal training in visual art and with no cognitive disorders. All subjects gave informed consent for the experimental protocol approved by the local research ethics committee. Each subject underwent training in blindfolded drawing (1 to 1.5 hour/day for a week with our Cognitive-Kinesthetic Method.)

3.3. Results

Functional MRI, run before and after the blindfolded training, revealed strong activation in the primary visual cortex (area V1) for the tactile memory-guided drawing task (Memory-Draw, Fig. 6A), while, by contrast, no significant V1 activation was recorded for the non-memory drawing task (Scribble, Fig. 6B).

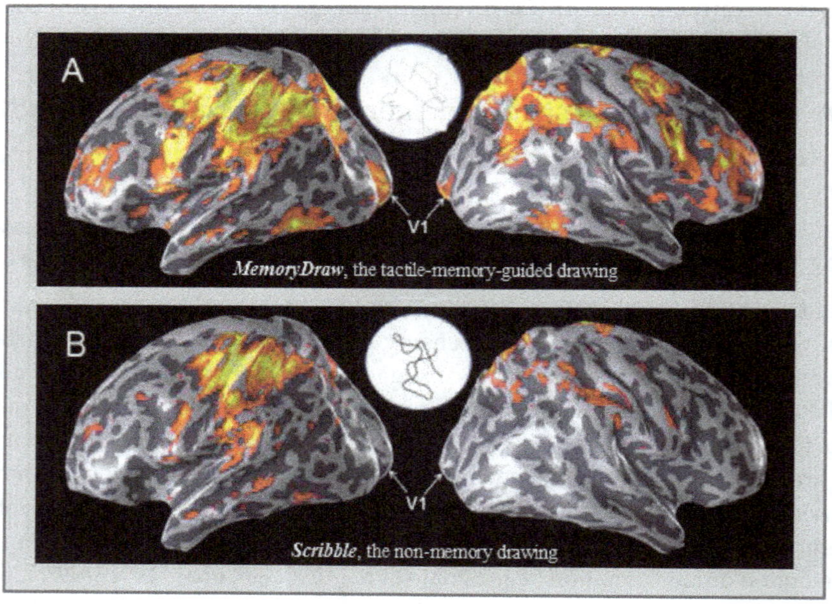

Figure 6. Comparison of the activation networks in the two types of drawing:(A) MemoryDraw (the tactile memory-guided drawing): Successful recall from memory of the specific tactile template explored 20 s earlier during E/M is critical for guiding the detailed movements of the drawing hand. (B) Scribble (the tactile non-memory, 'mindless'drawing) was used as motor control and 'negative memory' control condition. Note the dramatic difference between the two types of drawing activity (Avs B): The memory-guided drawing activates an expanded bilateral network; remarkably, there is a well-localized activation in the primary visual cortex, V1. In contrast, the non-memory drawing predominantly activates the left hemisphere within the right hand region; most importantly, it does not activate the visual cortex at all.

Remarkably, without any visual involvement at any stage of the learning or drawing process, the C-K training enable the blindfolded participants to memorize and draw well complex images in only 20 s, guided solely by memory acquired during haptic exploration! Note how well coordinated and recognizable these drawings are (see Fig. 7 B).

3.3.1. Retinotopic maps for memory-guided drawing in the blindfolded

The best way to look in detail at the puzzling activation in the visual cortex is to present the data in a flatmap format with the retinotopic maps delineated (Fig. 7 A).

MemoryDraw in the blindfolded produced an unexpected, unique occipital response. Despite the lack of any visual (or even tactile) stimulation, there was extensive activation of the primary retinotopic area, V1, while the rest of the visual hierarchy showed a pronounced suppression of the BOLD response relative to the baseline level.

The other two activated regions seen on the flat map are the caudal intraparietal sulcus (cIPS) and an additional locus at the temporo-occipital border in LOtv. The latter site, although in close proximity and often partially overlapping with the ventro-anterior visual LOC, is shifted anteriorly towards the temporal lobe. These two non-occipital loci have been previously reported to be involved in tactile perception (Prather & Sathian, 2002; Amedi et al., 2001, 2002; James et al., 2002; Stoesz et al., 2003; Pietrini et al., 2004; Reed et al., 2004; Merabet et al., 2005; Van Boven et al., 2005; Weisser et al., 2005; Zhang et al., 2005).

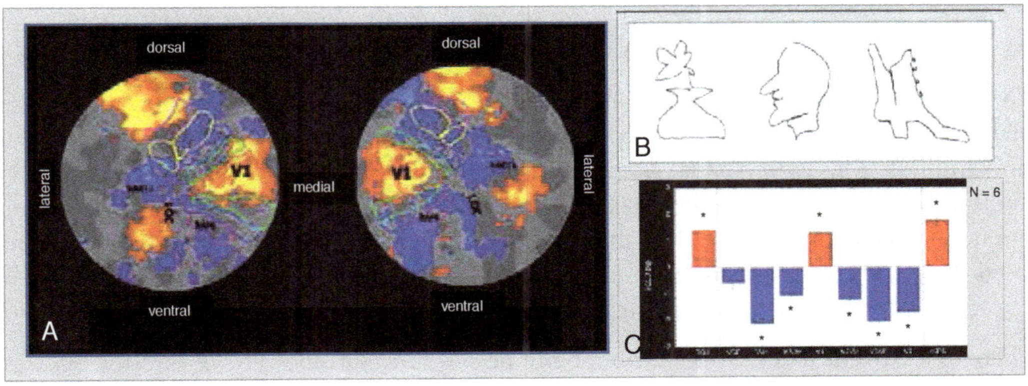

Figure 7. A. MD flat maps centered on the occipital pole. ROIs for the retinotopic hierarchy are indicated by colored outlines. The post-training MD map shows a unique 'triad' of three activation regions (orange-yellow coloration). Note in particular that the (non-visually-stimulated) primary visual cortex, V1, forms an isolated 'island' of activation surrounded by a 'sea' of suppression in the adjacent retinotopic areas. The other two activated regions seen on the flat map are the caudal intraparietal sulcus (cIPS) dorsally and an additional locus at the temporo-occipital border (LOtv). B.Post-training examples of blindfolded drawings demonstrating the level of detail the participants became able to complete in 20 s in the MRI scanner. Note that no vision was involved at any stage of the learning or drawing process! Recorded by the virtual stylus in the scanner are drawings of a vase with a flower, a face profile and a boot, each of which is easy to recognize (the corresponding templates are the 1st and the 2nd on the top row, and the 1st on the bottom row in Fig. 4B). C. Average response amplitude with standard errors for blindfolded memory-guided drawing in a group of 6 subjects, showing positive signal in the triad of areas – primary visual area V1, cIPS and LOtv; these three 'islands' of positive activation are separated by strong deactivation throughout boththe ventral and the dorsal extrastriate areas. Error bars represent 1 standard error of the means. Asterisks indicate activations significant at $p < 0.01$. [After Likova, 2013].

3.4. Discussion

3.4.1. Reconceptualization of the memory sketchpad

Tactile memory processing in the primary visual cortex?

Employing a pioneering memory paradigm based on non-visual drawing demonstrated that V1 can be strongly activated in a non-visual working memory task in the blindfolded. The V1 activation we have found is remarkable in many respects: i) the retinotopic analysis shows that the activation is rather well localized within V1, ceasing rapidly at a specific eccentricity; ii) surprisingly, its extension of about 10 deg (in terms of the retinotopic mapping) corresponds approximately to the angular subtense at the face that the drawings would have if projected optically; and iii) most remarkably – there is a massive deactivation surrounding V1, thus effectively 'cutting-off' any signal propagation from or through the extrastriate cortex. These results have major implications as discussed below.

To our knowledge, this study is the first evidence of involvement of the primary visual cortex in a tactile-memory task. We also know no other neuroimaging study either on the learning to draw, or on the effect of training on tactile-memory under visual deprivation. In MemoryDraw, the tactile template under the fingers of the left hand is memorized and then removed, so the drawing movements of the right hand are guided solely by that tactilely-acquired memory with no concurent tactile input from the drawn template (Penfield & Boldrey, 1937; Penfield & Rasmussen, 1950).

Amodal spatial memory vs visual imagery interpretation: Distinct patterns

To put the present results in a neurobiological perspective, we need a relevant concept about memory encoding and retrieval for the kinds of detailed spatial images used in the drawing task. The visuo-spatial sketchpad component of the classic WM model (Baddeley and Hitch, 1974; Baddeley, 1986, 2000, 2003) conveys the idea that working memory incorporates a detailed mental sketch of the retrieved object that can be further spatially manipulated (Fig. 8). This model provided us with a basis to generating specific hypothesis about the activation components in the drawing task.

There is a current tendency to attribute any new result that does not fit into the classical feedforward model of brain architecture, to a narrow number of top-down processes and - most recently - to 'visual imagery'. However, the pattern that we found of strong V1 activation surrounded by deactivation in the higher extrastriate areas (Fig. 7 A,B) is distinct, essentially the inverse of the known visual imagery pattern. In direct contrast to our results, the known neural substrate for visual imagery has been found to exhibit a gradient of activation decreasing from the higher visual areas toward V1, where the activation is much weaker or even lacking entirely. Although a weak level of V1 activation has sometimes been reported during imagery (Kosslyn et al., 1993; Le Bihan et al., 1993; Sabbah et al., 1995; Chen et al., 1998; Thompson et al., 2001; Ishai, Haxby, and Ungerleider, 2002; Lambert, Sampaio, Scheiber, and Mauss, 2002 ; Ganis et al., 2004), a larger number of other studies did not find any V1 activation at all (Goldenberg et al., 1991; Charlot et al., 1992; D'Esposito et al., 1997; Mazard et al., 2004; Mellet et al., 1995, 1998a, 1998b; Ishai, et al., 2000; Knauff et al., 2000;

Trojano et al., 2000; Wheeler et al., 2000; Formisano et al., 2002; Sack et al., 2002; Kaas et al., 2010). This decreasing gradient of activation implies that the imagery signal propagates from higher cortical regions in a top-down manner through the visual hierarchy towards V1.

In summary, while substantial imagery activation in the higher occipital areas has been consistently found across studies, this has not been the case with V1; furthermore, imagery does not produce any significant negative signal in the occipital cortex (Ganis et al., 2004; also see that paper for an overview of the imagery areas throughout the brain).

Our approach allows for testing between the following hypotheses: Hypothesis I: If the memory-based activation is due to the visual imagery mechanism, the predicted response-profile in the visual cortex would have the top-down 'imagery signature' of activation significantly decreasing from the higher extrastriate areas toward V1 (as reviewed above). Hypothesis II: If V1 was being employed as a WM sketchpad independently from the visual imagery process, it would be activated by a separate pathway external to the visual hierarchy, together with activation of WM-related sites beyond the occipital lobe.

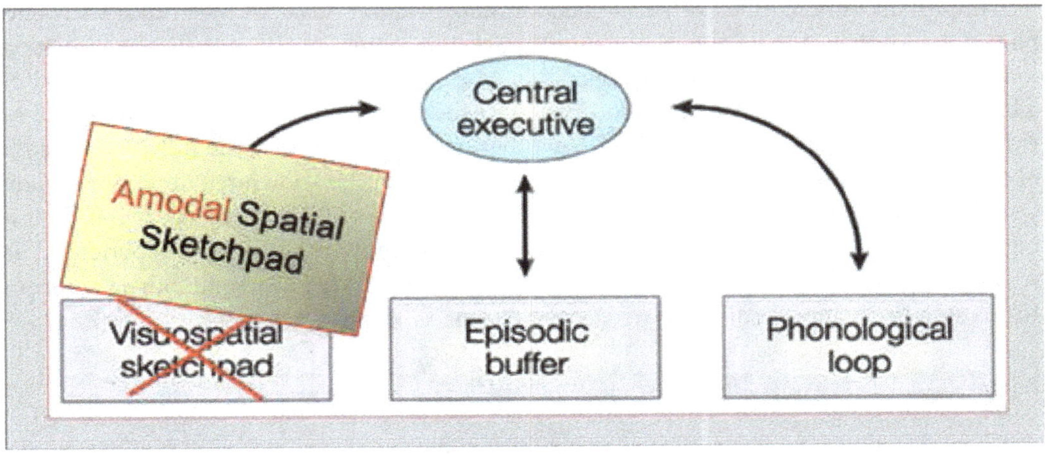

Figure 8. Our proposal for a re-conceptualization of the visuo-spatial sketchpad as an amodal-spatial sketchpad. Modified schematic of the main modules of Baddeley's classic model of working memory including the visuo-spatial sketchpad [after Baddeley, 2003], where the added "Amodal Spatial Sketchpad" block depicts our re-conceptualization of the visuo-spatial sketchpad as being accessible to any sensory modality. [From Likova, 2012a]

The imagery hypothesis seems not to be supported by the data because we find the inverse gradient of strong activation in the iconic visual area V1, and not only decreased but negative response in the higher occipital areas. The deactivation means that it is implausible the signal to be 'delivered' through the visual hierarchy, because this hierarchy is suppressed, i.e., V1 is 'cut-off' from the higher-level cortical regions that could generate and propagate imagery signals. Thus, this activation pattern is incompatible with the main principle of visual imagery as a top-down process propagating through the visual pathway towards V1. Instead, this pattern seems to be more consistent with Hypothesis II that V1 is operating as a working memory component, such as the hypothetical spatial memory buffer/sketchpad of the composite working memory model.

Re-conceptualization of the visuo-spatial sketchpad as an amodal-spatial sketchpad

The overall pattern of our results suggests that, even under complete visual deprivation, the high-resolution, topographically organized early visual cortex can operate as the conscious 'projection screen' for working memory, even when evoked by non-visual tasks. The spatiotopic organization and inherently parallel processing of the largest cortical map, V1, and most importantly, the small receptive fields providing the high-spatial resolution of the V1 map (e.g., Hubel & Wiesel, 1968; van Essen & Maunsell, 1980; van Essen et al., 1984; Mumford, 1992), makes it a very attractive candidate for precise spatial and spatial-memory processing, in particular, once it is freed up from visual processing, as in blindfolding or blindness (see sections 4 & 5). The data described in this chapter provide a direct evidence supporting such an implementation of a spatial sketchpad in human V1; most notably, our results make another step forward implying for a first time a generalization of the 'visuo-spatial' sketchpad concept beyond the visual modality, into a modality-independent or amodal spatial sketchpad.

It is important to note, however, that such an interpretation does not mean that V1 is employed for long-term storage of the memory trace, but merely for its operational activation in working memory to meet the task demands. Moreover, in contrast to the usual format of a baseline condition, we instructed and practiced the subjects to eliminate any rehearsal of either the just-explored templates or of any other memory images for the full 20 s duration of each null interval, which was also too long to account for the known retention time of any visual or iconic image of the memory trace, which is of the order of a second or less (Sperling, 1963; Di Lollo, 1980; Loftus et al., 1992). Since the drawings were not experienced as spatial images during the null interval, they were evidently held in some other, non-conscious storage location until it was needed for the subsequent drawing task.

3.4.2. Why is V1 surrounded by extrastriate suppression?

The current analysis was not designed to directly answer the question of the role of the extrastriate suppression (Fig. 7), but it allows several general considerations to be drawn. For instance, our results demonstrate a unique activation/suppression pattern produced without either visual or tactile stimulation in the occipital cortex. This fact eliminates potential sensory mechanisms, such as a direct drive of the primary visual cortex through direct connections from the primary somatosensory cortex.

Why is this suppression needed? One possible explanation is the existence of a mechanism homologous to what we have found previously in a figure/ground paradigm: a topographically precise, suppressive top-down feedback to the ground projection in V1 (Likova and Tyler, 2008). We suggested that such suppression of the less relevant information (that of the ground) makes strong computational sense. Such an interpretation is also consistent with theoretical predictions in Tsotsos et al. (1995). It seems logical that a similar principle of active suppression of the task-irrelevant regions (i.e., of the extrastriate visual pathways) may operate in our non-visual memory task but on a much larger scale, i.e., on a cross-modal instead of intramodal scale. This principle allows task-irrelevant or conflicting pathways to be excluded or 'cut-off' from functional involvement. Thus, the extrastriate suppression surrounding V1 prevents any potential propagation of the entirely non-visual V1 signal through the visual hierarchy pathway, which would be an inappropriate pathway in this case.

4. How does the learning-based reorganization develop? Insights from a congenitally blind case

4.1. Introduction

A congenitally blind novice with no experience with drawing or writing provides an ideal paradigm for investigating the earliest stages of V1 reorganization, and also provides for a critical probe of our amodal sketchpad idea, because congenital blindness eliminates the possibility of any visual mechanisms influencing the neural processing. Specifically, it abolishes not only the bottom-up visual input but also any potential top-down visual processing, such as visual imagery (since congenital blindness eliminates any visual experience on which to base such processing). We were lucky to find such an absolute novice. This individual was well-adapted to operating in the spatial world, including longstanding familiarity with complex tactile manipulations and Braille reading, but had no drawing, writing or even pen-holding experience. Functional MRI was run before and after a week's C-K training in order to test our hypothesis that V1 uses an amodal spatial representation in its operation as the putative memory buffer and to investigate the evolution of brain reorganization as a function of learning to draw.

4.2. Methods: The methods were as described in the general methods section

4.2.1. Subject and training

The congenitally blind subject was a 61-year-old right-handed female, totally blind with no light perception, who lost her vision shortly after birth as a result of rubella (German measles) in her expectant mother, severely and permanently damaging the fetal optic nerves, and also degrading her hearing to some degree. She had not been previously studied by fMRI or behavioral methods of any kind. She is a sophisticated intellect and a fluent Braille reader, with a graduate education and lifetime employment including the professional use of a computer keyboard, and was highly motivated to participate in the study. Nevertheless, despite her Braille fluency, the subject had no experience with writing or drawing, so her training to draw had to start with the basics, such as the proper holding of the pen and key spatial concepts of the representation of 3D structure on a 2D plane. She had relied heavily on active tactile exploration for her whole life, so it was quite surprising that she did not have clear idea of elementary geometric concepts such as a straight line vs a curve, right angles, etc.; she also was unable to reproduce any simple geometric figure or object by drawing. These issues were manifested at all levels of the experimental process – the tactile recognition and memorization phase, the memory recall in drawing, the understanding of spatial relationships, and even the kinesthetic feedback and self-evaluation of her own performance. For example, she could think she had just drawn a straight line when she had actually drawn an almost-closed curve, and so on.

It became clear, however, that these 'negatives' could be turned into significant 'positives' that would allow better tracking of the full evolution of the process of learning to draw. Another advantage was the fact that this subject was an intelligent adult, able both to readily follow instructions and to express back her introspections.

The special C-K technique allowed our subject to learn to draw without using any tactile feedback from the non-drawing (left) hand. As specified in 3.4.1. by eliminating the tactile feedback during drawing, this approach enforces the use of memory signals for guiding the drawing trajectory.

The training procedure was able to inspire and motivate this blind subject to acquire the exciting drawing skill. After only a week, she significantly advanced relative to her starting level, although her capability was still not satisfactory to her. Two months later she came back for two 'refresher' training sessions which she felt brought her up to an adequate skill level. To study the dynamics of the learning process, we ran fMRI before training, as well as after the prolonged period of consolidation.

4.3. Results

4.3.1. Comparative pre/post-training analysis: Increased activation and development of memory specialization

Training-induced enhancement of V1 activation for the memory-guided drawing

The focus of analysis is the occipital region along the calcarine sulcus corresponding to the location of the primary visual cortex, area V1. Comparison of the voxelwise parametric maps in the primary visual cortex during the MemoryDraw task (Fig. 9) reveals dramatic enhancement of the activation (orange coloration) in V1 (green outline) from negligible patchy activation before training (Fig. 9 A) to a massive task-specific activation after training (Fig. 9 B). Remarkably, the extension of post-training activation in V1 approximately corresponds to the spatial extent of that in the blindfolded (normally-sighted) subjects.

Lack of task-specificity before training, but development of MemoryDraw dominance after training

Bar-graphs for the estimated activation in V1 in each hemisphere before training (Fig. 9 C) indicate a lack of task specificity, i.e., similar activation levels for the MD (red) and both control tasks in the left hemisphere, with negligible responses to E/M and MD in the right hemisphere.

In contrast, after training (Fig. 9 D), the MD response (red bars) dominates in both left and right V1. As indicated by the confidence intervals, the following relationships are statistically significant post-training ($p < 0.01$): MD > E/M and MD > S in both hemispheres, and E/M >

S in the left hemisphere. Thus, MD is the task that most powerfully activates V1 bilaterally, showing highly significant % BOLD responses at a low noise level; the E/M task gives much weaker, left-dominant responses; while the motor-control scribbling task, S (which lacks any memory component), is suppressed even in the left hemisphere.

Pre/post comparison of the pattern of response in V1 across tasks shows significant reorganization in this response pattern as a result of training

Pre/post comparison of the pattern of V1 response across three tasks after training (Fig. 9 D) to that before training (Fig. 9 C) shows the following statistically significant ($p < 0.01$) relationships: $E/M_{post} \equiv E/M_{pre}$, $DM_{post} > DM_{pre}$ and $S_{post} < S_{pre}$ in both the left and the right hemispheres. This analysis implies a significant reorganization in the V1 response pattern as a result of training. Importantly, the V1 response in the memory-guided drawing task (MD) was substantially increased, while the response of the non-memory motor-control task (S) became insignificant. Note that no such increase was present in the area of the left motor cortex (controlling the drawing right hand), which even showed a reduction in response after training, as may be expected when a motor task becomes familiar (e.g., Jenkins et al., 1994). The E/M condition, which used the left hand (controlled by contralateral right motor cortex), developed the expected suppression in the ipsilateral (unused) cortex after training, manifesting the known cross-hemispheric competition in motor cortices (e.g., Nowak et al., 2009).

Bar-graphs show the estimated average activation in each hemisphere (left – LH, right – RH) for Explore/Memorize (E/M, blue), MemoryDraw (MD, red), non-memory drawing Scribble (S, green). The dashed lines indicate 99% confidence interval for the significance of the activation relative to zero. Error bars represent the 99% confidence intervals for assessing significant differences between pairs of activation levels. Pairs of activations are significantly different if they exceed the 99% confidence intervals for both activations. Time-courses show the average time courses of BOLD activity (black lines) for the sequence of three task intervals (white bars). The four dark-grey bars indicate the 20 s rest intervals separating E/M, MD and S tasks.

Top row (A, B): No significant V1 activation before training (in A), but massive, spatiotopic recruitment of V1 in the MemoryDraw task as a result of the CK-training (in B). Second row (C, D): Pre/post training comparison of response amplitudes across all three tasks reveals the development of a clear functional specialization for the MD task after training (in D). Third row (E, F): Response waveform analysis reveals how the immature and non-specific transient 'bursts' before the CK-training (in E) are transformed into a well-developed response waveforms for the memory-drawing MD (in F), but any significant response is lacking for the non-memory drawing S. Bottom row (G, H): In contrast to V1, the left motor area M1 produced well-formed responses for the two right-hand tasks (MD and S) both before (in G), and after training (in H) (but did not respond, and became significant suppressed for the left-hand task E/M).

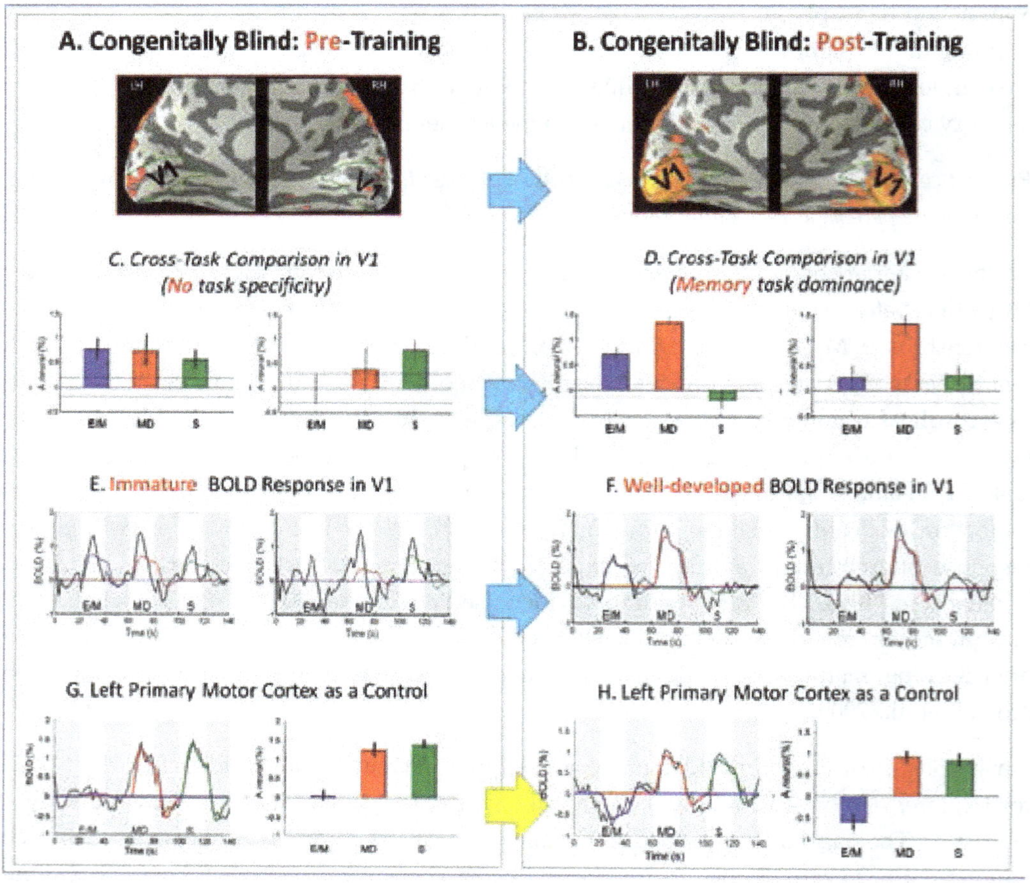

Figure 9. The first three rows present a comparative pre/post-training analysis of the primary visual cortex V1 (green outline), revealing its dramatic training-based functional reorganization, specific to the memory task. The fourth row is a control to show that nonvisual areas, such as the area of the left primary motor cortex that controls the right (drawing) hand, does not significantly change their response characteristics (as opposed to the dramatic pre/post reorganization in V1).

4.3.2. Time course of the BOLD response in V1: Dramatic post-training changes

Before Training: Immature BOLD Response Wave forms in V1 (Fig. 9 E)

The advantage of training a total novice was also manifested by allowing us to capture the very early stages of functional reorganization as expressed in the changes of the time course of the BOLD responses. As seen in Fig. 8 E the average time courses for the sequence of the three task intervals (white bars) have substantial deviations of the waveforms (black lines) from the model prediction fits (color curves). The model takes into account both the task duration and the estimated HRF (see General Methods). The pre-training response waveforms are rudimentary, poorly-developed and noisy, with a prominent transient nature and early offsets long before the end of the 20 s task periods, in spite of the continuous hand movements during the full task period (these continuous hand movements are evident from both the motion-capture records and also from the fully-fledged time course in the motor hand area, Fig. 8 G). Such early offset in V1 implies that the neural response was essentially a brief transient pulse that was immediately withdrawn, suggesting an unsuccessful attempt to activate this area. The subject's self-report and drawing performance were consistent with such undeveloped utilization.

After Training: Well-Developed BOLD Response Waveform in V1 (Fig. 9 F)

Notably, as a result of training, the temporal waveform of the V1 response regularized to become a good match to the linear model prediction (colored curves in Fig. 9 F), with maximum strength for the MemoryDraw task bilaterally. We no longer see the transient early-offset signals. Importantly, however, Scribble, which has no memory involvement, is lacking any significant response.

4.4. Discussion

4.4.1. Support of the amodal spatial 'sketchpad' and its implementation in the primary visual cortex

This study is the first to investigate the temporal evolution of functional reorganization of V1 as a result of a non-visual memory training task. Working with an adult who was an absolute novice has the advantage that such a subject can provide full introspection and produce complex behavioral measures (as opposed to working with difficult-to-communicate-with infants). This investigation thus opens a window to research the developmental evolution of both neural and behavioral changes, benefiting by effectiveness of the Cognitive-Kinesthetic training.

Except for her blindness and reduced hearing, this congenitally blind subject was in a very good physical and mental health, with robust BOLD responses in right-hand motor cortex, M1 (Fig. 9 G, H), so there were no reasons to expect abnormal BOLD responses in V1. Thus, a primary explanation of her V1 response patterns of undifferentiated, transient activation across all the tasks (Fig. 9 C, E) implies the lack of memory-specific role for V1 at that early stage. In particular, the poor response pattern may mean that, despite her lifetime of tactile experience including the professional use of a computer keyboard, the primary visual cortex was not able to serve as an effective 'amodal memory sketchpad' before training. The immature, early-offset waveforms suggest a rudimentary and unsuccessful attempt to activate V1, showing that the six decades of reliance on tactile perception in everyday tasks was evidently insufficient for the development of V1 functionality as demanded by the challenging memory-drawing task.

The rapid, learning-based recruitment of V1 in the MemoryDraw task after blind training (Fig. 9D, F), supports our reconceptualization of the memory 'sketchpad' as an amodal-spatial sketchpad, implemented in the primary visual cortex. Importantly, several parallel measures, such as subject's self-reports on the quality of the memory recall and the objective memory readout (the drawings recorded by our motion-capture system) with the concurrently recorded fMRI activation, all converged in supporting this hypothesis. Importantly, the learning paradigm itself provides causal inferences about the cross-modal changes in V1.

4.4.2. General considerations

Although a mature adult, this congenitally blind individual showed rapid functional reorganization of her brain in the process of learning to draw. It seems particularly surprising to find such reorganization in the primary visual cortex, whose main role is considered to be the early processing modality-specific information from visual input. The implication is that, although this cortical region had never been visually stimulated during the six decades of this blind subject's life, it is still retained sufficient plasticity to be accessible for use when the need arose. Thus, the drawing task was sufficiently demanding to activate functional reorganization that was not instigated by any other task during her life (despite the intensive use of other forms of detailed spatial information such as Braille characters for reading). Further studies are needed to investigate the specific cross-modal mechanisms mediating the V1 reorganization; in general, there is a wide range of theoretical possibilities, such as unmasking of pre-existing connections, synaptic weight changes, or a combination of a number of different mechanisms (e.g., Florence and Kaas, 1995; Jones, 2000; Raineteau and Schwab, 2001; Merabet, 2008; Van Brussel at al., 2011; Likova, 2012a).

Furthermore, the MemoryDraw post-training response map extended to an eccentricity of ~ 10 deg, which is in accordance with that in the blindfolded subjects. Such multidimensional consistency between the congenitally blind and the blindfolded responses is likely not to be accidental but to reflect common mechanisms operating under both short- and long-term visual deprivation. To further explore this finding, a comparative analysis of groups of congenitally and late blind individuals is described in the next section.

5. Is there a universal 'language' of modality-independent space?

5.1. Introduction

The eccentricity overlap of the post-training MD activation in V1 for the congenitally blind (Fig. 9 B) and the blindfolded (Fig. 7 A) appears even more remarkable knowing that what they had in common was that they all memorized the same battery of tactile images, with all images being of the same overall size. Thus, the consistent extent of V1 activation raises a number of fundamental questions, as it is suggestive of i) preservation of the form of topographic organization in V1 despite complete visual deprivation, and moreover, ii) utilization of this topography by cross-modal memory.

Does a topographic operation of the amodal memory sketchpad reflect a universal (i.e., modality-independent) 'language' of spatial representation? This section does not aim to provide complete answers but to raise questions and show their legitimacy based on our results in two additional groups of totally blind people.

5.2. Subjects and methods

A group of 6 congenitally blind and 7 late-onset blind individuals were studied before and after C-K training. All methods were as described in the General Methods section, with delineation of the normal retinotopic and functional organization in the whole-brain averaging by means of the novel training method we have developed. The late-onset blind group had blindness onsets ranging from 3 to 39 years of age. Only patients with total ocular blindness, but not cerebral blindness, were included. (Human vision is well-established to be close to adult level by the age of 3, so the primary requirements for visually processing would have been well developed before the onset of blindness in this late-onset group.)

5.3. Results and discussion

Consistent with the findings from sections 3 and 4, MemoryDraw strongly activated V1 along the calcarine in both blind groups, and remarkably, the activation did not fill in the whole of V1 but extended only about half way posteriorly, covering what in the sighted would be approximately the central 10 deg retinotopic representation. The dashed white lines in Fig. 10 A, B show the 10 deg eccentricity contour, on the basis of our approach to enabling retinotopic mapping in the blind (see Methods). Both the late-onset blind (Fig. 10A) who had full visual experience during early development, and the congenitally blind (Fig. 10B) who did not, show activation extending from the foveal representation all along 10 deg eccentricity contour but not beyond it (to an accuracy of ± 10% of its cortical extent). Thus, despite their total lack of visual experience, even the congenitally blind group adheres to a similar mapping principle as for those with some sighted development.

The fact that eccentricity-robust V1 post-training activation was systematically obtained in all visually-deprived populations is suggestive of topographically organized non-visual processing, and raises an array of questions. How would a topographic organization developin the congenitally blind despite the absence of visual experience to drive it? Is its development entirely genetically predetermined and independent from visual stimulation? How is an already developed retinotopy preserved after the total loss of visual input, as in the case of the late-onset blind subjects? How is a still functioning retinotopy, such as in the blindfolded, rapidly recruited by cross-modal memory? Does it develop by a nature or nurture mechanism, or by an interplay between the two? What is the frame of reference for the implemented metrics?

The current studies leave open questions for future research. A basis for some answers is already emerging. Interestingly, a recent 7-T high-resolution structural MRI study in congenitally blind individuals has established the presence of the stria of Gennari in the human cortex, which is another organizational landmark of V1 (Trampel et al., 2011), indicating that neither the development nor the preservation of this V1 landmark depends on the existence of visual input. Moreover, Cang et al. (2008) demonstrated for the first time that the development of the topographic axes of V1 is genetically controlled. The same group has also shown, however, strong experience-based plasticity in V1 (reviewed in Espinosa and Stryker, 2012). Thus, the plasticity mechanisms in V1 appear to be a complex interplay between genetic and environmental factors, which further tune-up and refine the genetically-determined layout (for a recent review see Maya-Vetencourt and Origlia, 2012).

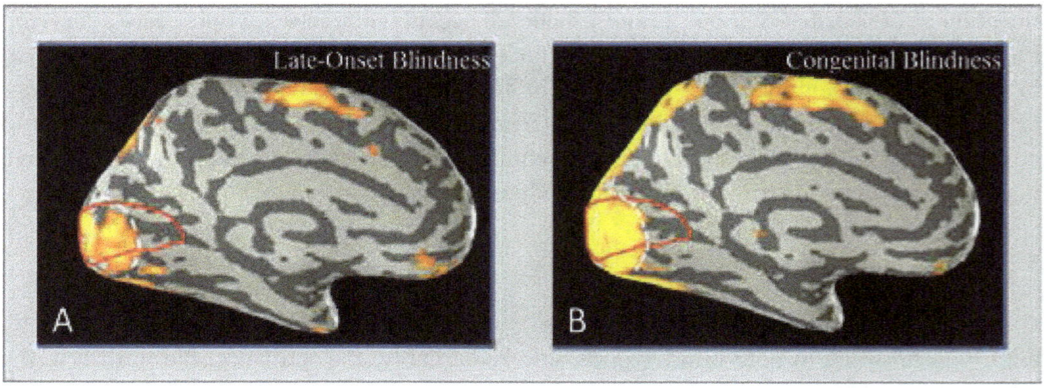

Figure 10. Group data in the blind. (A) The post-training group activation in V1 for the MemoryDraw task in the late-onset blind group expanded to approximately 10 deg eccentricity (dashed white line), similarly to the results in previous sections. (B) Remarkably, even the group data of congenitally blind individuals with no visual experience throughout their life manifested similar eccentricity (dashed white line).

6. Concluding comments

Detailed discussions are included in each of the experimental sections. Here, to sum up, the analyses of the fMRI data from our novel drawing-based memory paradigm and the Cognitive-Kinesthetic training led us to discover a unique pattern of V1 response, cut-off from propagation throughout the visual hierarchy by surrounding deactivation. Consideration of these results, in turn, excludes the most expected hypotheses and suggested a novel straightforward interpretation: That V1 in human implements the visuo-spatial working memory sketchpad concept but does so in an amodal form that transcends the sensory-modality specialization of the visual hierarchy. Based on this reasoning, we generated the prediction that, under the same memory paradigm, V1 will be activated even in the congenitally blind, who had never had any visual stimulation. This prediction was tested in a subsequent experiment, which replicated the freehand memory-drawing paradigm in a congenitally-blind novice. The data from this unique case study confirmed our initial interpretations of i) an amodal working memory role of V1, and ii) a spatiotopic character of the amodal memory representation. Furthermore, they also revealed for the first time the temporal evolution of the BOLD response during this learning-based cross-modal reorganization in the primary visual cortex. The large-scale study in groups of both congenitally and late-onset totally blind participants provided further strong evidence of these discoveries, and also contributed to the formulation of new research questions. The strong training effect implies causal or functionally relevant reorganization of the (non-visual) processing in area

V1. It is also particularly noteworthy that effectiveness of the Cognitive-Kinesthetic training was felt as transformative by the blind individuals in opening a new domain of experience.

Our findings of unusual immature BOLD waveforms in V1 before training might be taken as a warning for neuroimaging studies on plasticity, indicating that finding some unspecified activation is not sufficient as an indicator of functional employment. Additional criteria considering the time-course characteristics of the response have to be analyzed as well. The training-based evolution of cortical response to becoming task-specific and developing fully-fledged BOLD waveforms, eliminates epiphenomenon-based explanations such as those related to excess of excitability or a generic lack of synaptic pruning.

The research reviewed here exemplifies how an innovative learning method, integrated with a complex memory paradigm employing art, can further empower functional neuroimaging to shed light on long-standing puzzles concerning memory and cross-modal plasticity, and lead to re-conceptualization of organizational principles of the brain.

7. Acknowledgements

This research was supported by NSF/SLC Grant to Lora T. Likova. The author thanks Spero Nicholas for his help in data pre-processing and analysis tools, and Christopher W. Tyler for helpful discussions.

Author details

Lora Likova

The Smith-Kettlewell Eye Research Institute, San Francisco, CA, USA

References

[1] Amedi, A., Malach R., Hendler T., Peled S., Zohary E. (2001) Visuo-haptic object-related activation in the ventral visual pathway. Nat Neurosci 4:324–330.

[2] Amedi, A., Jacobson G., Hendler T., Malach R., Zohary E. (2002) Convergence of visual and tactile shape processing in the human lateral occipital complex. Cereb Cortex 12:1202–1212.

[3] Amedi, A., Raz, N., Pianka, P., Malach, R., and Zohary, E. (2003) Early 'visual' cortex activation correlates with superior verbal memory performance in the blind. Nature Neuroscience 6:758–766.

[4] Amedi, A., Floel, A., Knecht, S., Zohary, E., and Cohen, L.G. (2004) Transcranial magnetic stimulation of the occipital pole interferes with verbal processing in blind subjects. Nature Neuroscience 7:1266–1270.

[5] Amedi A., Malach, R., and Pascual-Leone, A. (2005) Negative BOLD Differentiates Visual Imagery and Perception. Neuron, Dec 8 Vol. 48, 859–872.

[6] Amedi, A., Merabet, L.B., Camprodon, J., Bermpohl, F., Fox, S., Ronen, I., Kim, D.S., and Pascual-Leone, A. (2008) Neural and behavioral correlates of drawing in an early blind painter: a case study. Brain Res. 25 1242:252-62.

[7] Baddeley, A.D. (1986) Working Memory. Oxford University Press: New York.

[8] Baddeley, A.D. (2000) The episodic buffer: a new component of working memory? Trends Cognit Sci 4 (11): 417–23.

[9] Baddeley, A.D., and Hitch, G.J. (1974). Working memory. In G Bower (Ed.), The Psychology of Learning and Motivation, Vol. 8, pp. 47-90. San Diego, CA: Academic Press.

[10] Baddeley, A.D. (2003) Working memory: looking back and looking forward. Nature Reviews Neuroscience 4: 829-839.

[11] Block, N. (2003) Tactile sensation via spatial perception. Trends Cogn. Sci. 7, 285-286.

[12] Borowsky, R., Esopenko, C., Cummine, J., and Sarty, G.E. (2007) Neural representations of visual words and objects: a functional MRI study on the modularity of reading and object processing. Brain Topogr. 20:89-96.

[13] Buchsboum, B.R., and D'Esposito, M., (2009) Is there anything special about working memory? In Neuroimaging of Human Memory. Rosler, F., Ranganath, C., Roder, B., Kluwe, R., (Eds.) Oxford Univ. Press: Oxford.

[14] Buechel, C., Price, C., Frackowiak, R.S., and Friston, K. (1998) Different activation patterns in the visual cortex of late and congenitally blind subjects. Brain 121:409–419.

[15] Burton, H., Snyder, A.Z., Conturo, T.E., Akbudak, E., Ollinger, J.M., and Raichle M.E. (2002) Adaptive changes in early and late blind: a fMRI stud of Braille reading. J Neurophysiol 87:589–607.

[16] Burton, H. (2003) Visual cortex activity in early and late blind people. J Neurosci, 23(10):4005–4011.

[17] Burton, H., Sincler, R.J., MacLaren, D.C. (2004) Cortical activity to vibrotactile stimulation: an fMRI study in blind and sighed individuals. Hum Brain Mapp 23:210–228.

[18] Cohen, L.G., Celnik, P., Pascual-Leone, A., Corwell, B., Falz, L., and Dambrosia, J. (1997) Functional relevance of cross-modal plasticity in blind humans. Nature 389:180e–183.

[19] Deibert, E., Kraut M., Kremen S., Hart J.Jr. (1999) Neural pathways in tactil eobject recognition. Neurology. 52:1413–1417.

[20] DeVolder, A.G., Bol, A., Blin, J., Robert, A., Arno, P., and Grandin, C. (1997) Brain energy metabolism in early blind subjects: neural activity in the visual cortex. Brain Res 750:235–244.

[21] Engel, S.A., Glover, G.H., and Wandell, B.A. (1997). Retinotopic organization in human visual cortex and the spatial precision of functional MRI. Cereb. Cortex 7, 181–192.

[22] Florence, S.L., and Kaas, J.H. (1995) Large-scale reorganization at multiple levels of the somatosensory pathway follows therapeutic amputation of the hand in monkeys. 15(12): 8083-95.

[23] Friston, K. J., Jezzard, P., and Turner, R. 1994. Analysis of functional MRI time-series. *Hum.* Brain Map. 1:153–171.

[24] Ganis, G., Thompson, W. L., & Kosslyn, S. M. (2004). Brain areas underlying visual mental imagery and visual perception: An fMRI study. Cognitive Brain Research, 20, 226-241.

[25] Gizewski, E.R., Gasser, T., de Greiff, A., Boehm, A., and Forsting, M. (2003) Cross-modal plasticity for sensory and motor activation patterns in blind subjects. Neuroimage 19(3):968-75.

[26] Goyal, M.S., Hansen, P.J., and Blakemore, C.B. (2006) Tactile perception recruits functionally related visual areas in the late-blind. Neuroreport 17(13):1381-4.

[27] Grossi D and Trojano L. (1999) Constructional apraxia. In Denes G, and Pizzamiglio L (Eds), Handbook of Clinical and Experimental Neuropsychology. Hove: Psychology Press.

[28] Hagen, M.C., Franzen, O., McGlone, F., Essick, G., Dancer, C., Pardo, J.V. (2002) Tactile motion activates the human middle temporal /V5(MT/V5) complex. Eur J Neurosci. 16:957–964.

[29] Hamilton, R.H., Pascual-Leone, A., (1998) Cortical plasticity associated with Braille learning. Trends in Cognitive Sciences, Elsevier, 2(5), 168-174..

[30] Hamilton, R.H, Keenan, J.P., Catala, M., and Pascual-Leone, A. (2000) Alexia for Braille following bilateral occipital stroke in an early blind woman. NeuroReport 11:237–240.

[31] Harrison, S.A., Tong, F. (2009) Decoding reveals the content of visual working memory in early visual cortex. Nature 458:632-5.

[32] Hubel DH, Wiesel TN (1968) Receptive fields and functional architecture of monkey striate cortex. J Physiol. 195:215-43.

[33] Ishai, A., and Sagi, D. (1995) Common mechanisms of visual imagery and perception. Science 268, 1772–1774.

[34] Ishai, A., Ungerleider, L.G., and Haxby, J.V. (2000). Distributed neural systems for the generation of visual images. Neuron 28, 979–990.

[35] Ishai, A., Haxby, J.V., and Ungerleider, L.G. (2002) Visual imagery of famous faces: effects of memory and attention revealed by fMRI. Neuroimage 17, 1729–1741.

[36] Ishai, A. (2009) Retrieving pictures from long-term memory. In Neuroimaging of Human Memory. Rosler, F., Ranganath, C., Roder, B., Kluwe, R., (Eds.) Oxford Univ. Press: New York.

[37] James, T.W., Humphrey, G.K., Gati, J.S., Servos, P., Menon, R.S., and Goodale, M. A. (2002) Haptic study of three-dimensional objects activates extrastriate visual areas. Neuropsychologia 40:1706-1714.

[38] Jenkins, I. H., Brooks, D. J., Nixon, P. D., Frackowiak, R.S.J., Passingham, R. E. (1994) Motor sequence learning: a study with positron emission tomography. J. Neurosci. 14:3775–3790.

[39] Kastner, S., De Weerd, P., Desimone, R., Ungerleider, L.G. (1998) Mechanisms of directed attention in the human extrastriate cortex as revealed by functional MRI. Science 282: 108–111.

[40] Kennedy, J. M. (1993) Drawing and the Blind. New Haven, CT: Yale University Press.

[41] Kennedy, J.M. (2000) Recognizing outline pictures via touch: Alignment theory. In M.A. Heller (Ed.) Touch, Representation and Blindness. Oxford University Press: Oxford (pp. 67-98).

[42] Kennedy, J.M., and Igor, J. (2003) Haptics and projection: Drawings by Tracy, a blind adult. Perception 32(9):1059 –1071.

[43] Kennedy, J.M., and Juricevic, I. (2006) Foreshortening, convergence and drawings from a blind adult. Perception 35(6):847 851.

[44] Kosslyn, S.M., Thompson, W.L., & Alpert, N.M. (1997). Neural systems shared by visual imagery and visual perception: A positron emission tomography study. NeuroImage, 6, 320-334.

[45] Kosslyn, S. M., Thompson, W. L., Kim, I. J., Rauch, S. L., & Alpert, N. M. (1996). Individual differences in cerebral blood flow in area 17 predict the time to evaluate visualized letters. J Cognit Neurosci, 8, 78-82.

[46] Kosslyn, S.M., Pascual-Leone, A., Felician, O., Camposano, S., Keenan, J.P., Thompson, W.L., Ganis, G., Sukel, K.E., and Alpert, N.M. (1999) The role of area 17 in visual imagery: convergent evidence from PET and rTMS. Science 284, 167–170.

[47] Kosslyn, S.M., Thompson, W.L. (2003) When is early visual cortex activated during visual mental imagery? Psychol Bull 129: 723–746, 2003.

[48] Kreiman, G., Koch, C., and Fried, I. (2000) Imagery neurons in the human brain. Nature 408, 357–361.

[49] Lambert, S., Sampaio, E., Mauss, Y., and Scheiber, C. (2004) Blindness and brain plasticity: contribution of mental imagery? An fMRI study. Brain Res. Cogn. Brain Res. 20, 1–11.

[50] Lee, T.S., and Mumford, D. (2003) Hierarchical Bayesian inference in the visual cortex. J Opt Soci Amer, A. 20: 1434-1448.

[51] Likova, L.T., Tyler, C.W., (2008) Occipital network for figure/ground organization. Experimental Brain Research, 2008, 189: 258-67.

[52] Likova, L.T. and Tyler C.W. (2007). Stereomotion processing in the human occipital cortex. NeuroImage 38:293-304.

[53] Likova, L.T. (2010a) Drawing in the blind and the sighted as a probe of cortical reorganization. Human Vision and Electronic Imaging XV. Edited by Rogowitz, Bernice E.; Pappas, Thrasyvoulos N. Proceedings of the SPIE, Volume 7527, 8-14.

[54] Likova, L.T. (2010b) The primary visual cortex as a modality-independent 'screen' for working memory. J Vision, 10(7): 776,

[55] http://www.journalofvision.org/content/10/7/776.

[56] Likova L.T. (2012a) Drawing enhances cross-modal memory plasticity in the human brain: A case study in a totally blind adult. Frontiers in Human Neuroscience.6:44. doi: 10.3389/fnhum.00044.

[57] Likova L.T. (2012b) The spatiotopic 'visual' cortex of the blind. Proc. SPIE 8291, Human Vision and Electronic Imaging XVII, 8291-10L doi:10.1117/12.912257.

[58] Likova L.T. (2013) A cross-modal perspective on the relationships between imagery and working memory. Front. Psychology, 3:561. doi: 10.3389/fpsyg.00561.

[59] Loomis, K.M., and Klatzky R. (2008) Functional equivalence of spatial representations from vision, touch, and hearing: Relevance for sensory substitutions. In M.A. Heller (Ed.) Touch, Representation and Blindness (pp. 67-98), Oxford University Press: New York.

[60] Matteau, I., Kupers, R., Ricciardi, E., Pietrini, P., Ptito, M. (2010) Beyond visual, aural and haptic movement perception: hMT+ is activated by electrotactile motion stimulation of the tongue in sighted and in congenitally blind individuals. Brain Res Bull. Jul 30;82(5-6):264-70.

[61] Mechelli, A., Price, C.J., Friston, K.J., and Ishai, A. (2004) Where bottom-up meets top-down: neuronal interactions during perception and imagery. Cereb. Cortex 14, 1256–1265.

[62] Merabet, L., Rizzo, J., Amedi, A., Somers, D., and Pascual-Leone, A. (2005) What blindness can tell us about seeing again: Merging neuroplasticity and neuroprostheses. Nature Rev. Neurosci 6:71–77.

[63] Merabet, L. (2008) The plastic brain in blind individuals: The cause of disability and the opportunity for rehabilitation. In, Blindness and Brain Plasticity in Navigation and Object Perception. Lawrence Erlbaum Associates, London.

[64] Mumford, D. (1992) On the computational architecture of the neocortex II Biol. Cybern. 66, 241–251.

[65] Nowak DA, Grefkes C, Ameli M, Fink GR (2009) Interhemispheric competition after stroke: brain stimulation to enhance recovery of function of the affected hand. Neurorehabil Neural Repair. 23:641-56.

[66] O'Craven, K.M., and Kanwisher, N. (2000) Mental imagery of faces and places activates corresponding stimulus-specific brain regions. J Cogn Neurosci 12, 1013–1023.

[67] Pascual-Leone, A., Hamilton, R., 2001. The metamodal organization of the brain. Prog. Brain Res. 134, 427-445.

[68] Pascual-Leone, A., Amedi, A., Fregni, F., Merabet, L. (2005) The plastic human brain. Annual Review of Neuroscience, 28: 377-401.

[69] Penfield W, Boldrey E (1937) Somatic motor and sensory representation in the cerebral cortex of man as studied by electrical stimulation. Brain 60:389–443.

[70] Penfield W, Rasmussen T. (1950) The Cerebral Cortex of Man. Macmillan: New York.

[71] Perkel, D.J., Bullier, J., Kennedy, H. (1986) Topography of the afferent connectivity of area 17 in the macaque monkey: a double-labelling study. J Comp Neurol 253:374–402.

[72] Piercy, M., Hecaen H., and Ajuriaguerra, J. (1960) Constructional apraxia associated with unilateral cerebral lesion—Left and right-sided cases compared. Brain 83: 225–242.

[73] Pietrini, P., Furey, M.L., Ricciardi, E., Gobbini, M.I., Wu, W.H., Cohen, L., Guazzelli, M., Haxby, J.V. (2004) Beyond sensory images: Object-based representation in the human ventral pathway. Proc Natl Acad Sci USA 101:5658–5663.

[74] Ponchilla, P. E. (2008) Non-visual sports and Arts: fertile substrates for the growth of knowledge about brain plasticity in people who are blind or have low vision. In Blindness and Brain Plasticity in Navigation and Object Perception. Lawrence Erlbaum Associates, London.

[75] Prather, S.C., Sathian, K. (2002) Mental rotation of tactile stimuli. Brain Res Cogn Brain Res 14: 91–98.

[76] Ptito, M., Fumal A., de Noordhout A.M., Schoenen J., Gjedde A., and Kupers R. (2008) TMS of the occipital cortex induces tactile sensations in the fingers of blind Braille readers. Exp Brain Res. Jan; 184(2):193-200.

[77] Raineteau, O., and Schwab, M.E., (2001) Plasticity of motor systems after incomplete spinal cord injury. Nat Rev Neurosci. 2(4):263-73.

[78] Ranganath, H., (2009) Interrelationships between working memory and long-term memory. In Neuroimaging of Human Memory. Rosler, F., Ranganath, C., Roder, B., Kluwe, R., (Eds.) Oxford Univ. Press: Oxford.

[79] Raz, N., Amedi, A., and Zohary, E. (2005). V1 activation in congenitally blind V1 activation in congenitally blind humans is associated with episodic retrieval. Cereb. Cortex 15, 1459–1468.

[80] Reed, C.L., Shoham, S., Halgren, E. (2004) Neural substrates of tactile object recognition: an fMRI study. Hum Brain Mapp 21:236–246.

[81] Sadato, N., Pascual-Leone, A., Grafman, J., Ibanez, V., Deiber, M.P., Dold, G., Hallett, M. (1996) Activation of the primary visual cortex by Braille reading in blind subjects. Nature 380:526–528.

[82] Schira, M.M., Breakspear, M., Spehar, B., Tyler, C.W., (2010) Modeling magnification and anisotropy in the primate foveal confluence. PLoS, Computational Biology, 6(1):e1000651.

[83] Sereno, M.I., Dale, A.M., Reppas, J.B., Kwong, K.K., Belliveau, J.W., Brady, T.J., Rosen, B.R., and Tootell, R.B. (1995). Borders of multiple visual areas in humans revealed by functional magnetic resonance imaging. Science 26, 889–893.

[84] Slotnick, S.D., Thompson, W.L., Kosslyn, S.M. (2005) Visual mental imagery induces retinotopically organized activation of early visual areas. Cereb Cortex 15:1570–1583.

[85] Sperling G (1963) A model for visual memory tasks. Human Factors, 5: 19-31.

[86] Stoesz, M.R., Zhang, M., Weisser,V.D., Prather, S.C., Mao, H., Sathian, K. (2003) Neural networks active during tactile form perception: common and differential activity during macrospatial and microspatial tasks. Int J Psychophysiol 50: 41–49.

[87] Theoret, H., Merabet, L., Pascual-Leone A. (2004) Behavioral and neuroplastic changes in the blind: Evidence for functionally relevant cross-modal interactions. J Physiol, Paris 98(1-3): 221–233.

[88] Tootell, R.B., Reppas, J.B., Kwong, K.K., Malach, R., Born, R.T., Brady, T.J., Rosen, B.R., Belliveau, J.W. (1995) Functional analysis of human MT and related visual cortical areas using magnetic resonance imaging. J Neurosci 15: 3215–3230.

[89] Trampel, R., Derek, V. M., Ott, R.T. (2011). Do the Congenitally Blind Have a Stria of Gennari? First Intracortical Insights in Vivo. Cereb Cortex, 21(9): 2075-2081.

[90] Trojano L., Grossi D, Flash T. (2009) Cognitive neuroscience of drawing: Contributions of neuropsychological, experimental and neurofunctional studies. *Cortex* , 45(3): 269-277.

[91] Tsotsos, J.K., Culhane, S.M., Kei Wai, W.Y., Lai, Y., Davis, N., NuXo, F. (1995) Modeling visual attention via selective tuning. Artif Intell, 78:507–545.

[92] Tyler, C.W., Likova. L.T., Kontsevich, L.L., Schira, M.M., Wade, A.R. (2005) Enhanced concept of ocipital retinotopy. Current Medical Imaging Reviews 1: 319-329.

[93] Van Boven, R.W., Ingeholm, J.E., Beauchamp, M.S., Bikle, P.C., Ungerleider, L.G. (2005) Tactile form and location processing in the human brain. Proc Natl Acad Sci USA 102:12601–12605.

[94] Uhl, F., Franzen, P., Lindinger, G., Lang, W., Deecke, L. (1991) On the functionality of the visually deprived occipital cortex in early blind persons. Neurosci Lett 124: 256–9.

[95] Uhl, F., Franzen, P., Podreka, I., Steiner, M., Deecke, L. (1993) Increased regional cerebral blood flow in inferior occipital cortex and cerebellum of early blind humans. Neurosci Lett 150: 162–4.

[96] Van Brussel, L., Gerits, A., Arckens, L. (2011) Evidence for cross-modal plasticity in adult mouse visual cortex following monocular enucleation. Cereb. Cortex 21(9): 2133-2146.

[97] Van Essen DC, Maunsell JH (1980) Two-dimensional maps of the cerebral cortex. J Comp Neurol. 191:255-81.

[98] Van Essen DC, Newsome WT, Maunsell JH (1984) The visual field representation in striate cortex of the macaque monkey: asymmetries, anisotropies, and individual variability. Vision Res. 24:429-48.

[99] Weisser, V., Stilla, R., Peltier, S., Hu, X., Sathian, K. (2005) Short-term visual deprivation alters neural processing of tactile form. Exp Brain Res 166:572–582.

[100] Williams, M., Baker, C. I., Op de Beeck, H. P., Shim, W. M. Dang, S., Triantafyllou, C., and Kanwisher, N. (2008) Feedback of visual object information to foveal retinotopic cortex. Nature Neuroscience. 11:1439-45.

[101] Zangaladze, A., Epstein, C.M., Grafton, S.T., Sathian, K (1999). Involvement of visual cortex in tactile discrimination of orientation. Nature 401, 587-590.

[102] Zhang, M., Mariola, E., Stilla, R., Stoesz, M., Mao, H., Hu, X., Sathian, K. (2005) Tactile Discrimination of grating orientation: fMRI activation patterns. Hum Brain Mapp 25:370–377.

9

The Contribution of fMRI in the Study of Visual Categorization and Expertise

Natasha Sigala

1. Introduction

We recognize and categorize objects around us within a fraction of a second and in a number of different ways, depending on context, our experience with them, and the purpose of the categorization. For example the same animal can be *a dog, a bow wow* or *a bulldog, a mammal or a Canis lupus familiaris.* We are also able to recognize it in a variety of lighting conditions, orientations and positions, despite the large number of two dimensional images that every three dimensional object generates. It is therefore not surprising that our extraordinary ability to recognize objects has fascinated philosophers for a very long time. In *Categories* Aristotle made an attempt to categorize everything, mainly by analysing patterns of language and speech, answering questions like "τί ἐστί", "what is it?", "what like is it?" (Cross, 1959), and by describing the defining qualities that all instances of a particular category share, e.g. all soft things share the quality of softness.

Real progress in describing and understanding such qualities (features) was made by Fred Attneave in experiments of visual perception during his Ph.D. research at Stanford University (Attneave, 1957). Specifically his results showed that subjective ratings of the perceived dissimilarities between stimuli (letter stings and shapes) and the frequency of errors while learning those stimuli, could both be explained in terms of distances between stimuli represented as points in a "psychological space". The idea of describing subjective psychological experiences with geometry influenced Roger Shepard, who applied and extended multidimensional scaling (MDS), the representation of objects (e.g. shapes, words, faces) as points in space, so that the distances between the points represent the perceived similarities between the objects (Richardson, 1938), (Torgerson, 1952), (Shepard, 1958), (Shepard, 1962a), (Shepard, 1962b), (Shepard, 1987).

The exact ways in which similarity of a perceived object and its mental representation is measured have been the focus of research for over half a century. According to the theory of prototypes, we categorize new objects by comparing them to abstracted representations that are the central tendency of all the examples of the categories that we have experienced (Posner and Keele, 1968), e.g. a prototypical triangle or square. According to exemplar theories, the perceived objects are compared with stored representations of exemplars, grouped by category (Medin and Schaffer, 1978), e.g. memories of actual triangles and squares we have experienced. Although the early exemplar models postulated equal weights for all stimulus features, later contributions included an attention-optimisation hypothesis, allowing the perceived distance (similarity) between objects to vary with context and task demands (Generalised Context model, (Nosofsky, 1986)). For example this implies that for a layperson the representations of a trout and bass may be close together (similar), but for an ichthyologist or fisherman those representations are further apart (less similar) because they can identify a number of features that make the two types of fish different.

Eleanor Rosch analyzed language patterns and visual perception across cultures and did the experiments that I suspect Aristotle would have liked to perform himself (Heider, 1972, Rosch et al., 1976a). She showed that the categorizations we make rely on features of high validity (e.g. feathers and wings for birds) which form prototypes that aid cognitive economy and reflect perceived world structure (Boden, 2006), pp. 520-521. In other words "robin" is a more typical bird example, than "ostrich", and this helps us recognise and make decisions about objects faster, and also reflects the likelihood to encounter such objects in our environment. Rosch named the hierarchical level where category prototypes are found as the basic level of categorization (e.g. bird, fish, tree), which is the one that provides the most useful information, the first to be named by children, and the most necessary in language (Rosch, 1976, Rosch et al., 1976b). The level below (subordinate) contains more specific information (e.g. robin, sparrow), while the level above (superordinate) (e.g. animal, plant) less specific information. These results explained how we structure information about the world around us, to a large extent in a universal, rather than arbitrary or culture-dependent way. The opposite conclusion would render the following "ancient Chinese" animal taxonomy, presented by Jorge Luis Borges (1966) (in (Boden, 2006), p. 519) entirely possible:

"[Animals] are divided into (a) those that belong to the Emperor, (b) embalmed ones, (c) those that are trained, (d) suckling pigs, (e) mermaids, (f) fabulous ones, (g) stray dogs, (h) those that are included in this classification, (i) those that tremble as if they were mad, (j) innumerable ones, (k) those drawn with a very fine camel's hair brush, (l) others, (m) those that have just broken a flower vase, (n) those that resemble flies from a distance".

Crucially for the question of expertise, Rosch's basic level of categorization, can be and is modified by experience. Based on their observation that an airplane mechanic answered questions about airplanes differently to other (non-expert) participants, Rosch and colleagues suggested that one way to study what part a person's previous knowledge plays in categorization, would be a systematic variation of the participants' level of expertise and the object categories (Rosch et al., 1976a). They also speculated that an ichthyologist would use as a basic level, what a novice would consider a more specific, subordinate one (e.g. trout or salmon, instead of fish). Tanaka and Taylor performed such an experiment, and compared the categorization performance of dog and bird experts in listing distinctive features, as well as speed and level of categorizing animals in and out of their area of expertise. They found that the most informative category for the experts was the more specific, subordinate level, rather than the basic one (Tanaka and Taylor, 1991), e.g. crow or robin, rather than bird for the bird experts, and beagle or collie, rather than dog for the dog experts.

Despite long-running debates about the usefulness of the concept of similarity in explaining categorization (e.g. Goodman, 1972), and the merits of prototype, exemplar or other theories, most researchers agree that categorization is based on an expanded notion of similarity, an overall similarity, which encompasses physical, functional and overall features, reflecting a person's theoretical understanding of the world, e.g. (Murphy and Medin, 1985) in (Ahn and Dennis, 2001). The concept of similarity has furthermore inspired computational theories of vision, where "the representation of similarity is taken to be the goal of the visual system" (Edelman, 1998), modern extensions of which are particularly appropriate for relating neural data, behaviour and models across species and neuroscientific methods (Kriegeskorte, 2009).

In this chapter I will first review some background work that sets the context for the subsequent discussion of a subset of fMRI studies that have shed light on the questions of perceptual and cognitive categorization and expertise over the last 15 years.

2. Computational and experimental work

During the end of the 20th and the beginning of the 21st century, the idea that neuronal populations code representations which reflect both physical stimulus similarity and perceived stimulus similarity, as shaped by task demands, received significant experimental support. In order to bridge the species gap between human and non-human primates, and study meaningfully the neuronal representations in the macaque brain, it was first necessary to test if the categorizations that monkeys make can also be explained with MDS, and prototype and/or exemplar theories. This involved the creation of novel, parametrically designed stimuli with a known number of varying dimensions (features). The premise here was inspired by computational theories of vision that called for representations that were two-dimensional viewpoint-dependent snapshots of three-dimensional objects (Poggio and Edelman, 1990) that preserved the geometry of similarity amongst the objects (Edelman, 1998) (as opposed to stored three-dimensional representations of the objects themselves (Marr and Nishihara, 1978) (Biederman, 1987)). The first study to show that MDS was a useful tool for understanding object categorization in the monkey was described in (Sands et al., 1982). Crucially, they did not provide categorization training to the animals, and they explored how macaques perceived and represented pictures of various natural categories (faces, fruit, colours). They reached the conclusion that macaques treat pictorial stimuli categorically cf. (Sigala, 2009). Several years later (Sugihara et al., 1998) employed novel stimuli (computer-generated 3D animals) to test the usefulness of MDS in the study of object recognition, following a previous demonstration with the human visual system (Cutzu and Edelman, 1996). After systematic training of the monkeys to report their perception of the stimuli, Sugihara et al. showed that the psychophysical representation of the novel stimuli, as revealed by MDS, captured the similarities built in the stimulus space. This means that the monkey visual system could successfully recover a two-dimensional configuration of the stimuli that were originally built in a high-dimensional space (set of 56 variables), and reliably capture their relative similarities. This was the first piece of evidence for the non-human primate visual system that representations of the stimuli might be representations of the similarities of the stimuli.

Following this psychophysical experiment, Sigala and colleagues also created two parametrically designed stimulus sets (schematic faces and fish) with four varying dimensions (Sigala et al., 2002). The participants (both humans and non-human primates) first had to report how similar the stimuli were to them, then were trained to categorize them at the subordinate level based on the combination of two features, and then reported how similar the stimuli were to them a second time. By collecting similarity ratings before and after the categorization training, it was possible to show that the perceptual similarity of the stimuli changed, particularly for the macaques, after they had learnt to categorize the stimuli based on two features (ignoring the other two equally varying features) (Fig. 1). The initial MDS solution of the similarity ratings showed that the stimulus features were not consistently used when comparing the stimuli (Fig. 1a).

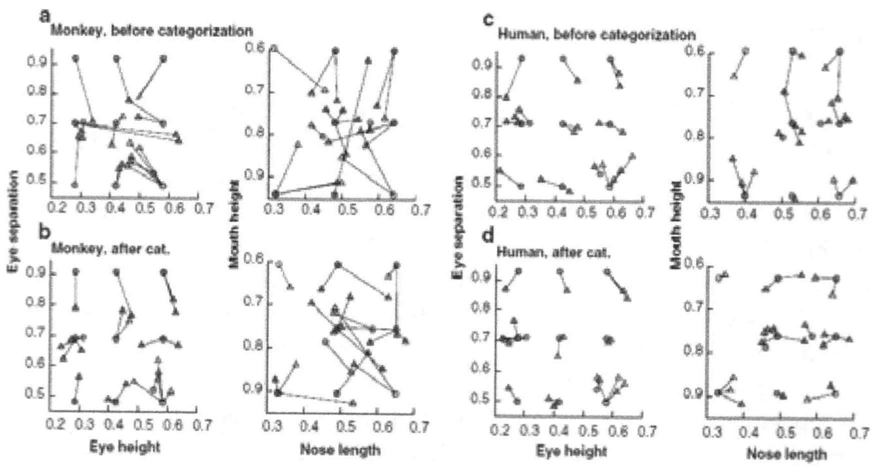

Figure 1. Psychophysical representation of schematic faces in a non-human (a, b) and a human (c, d) participant, as revealed by Multi Dimensional Scaling (MDS) on similarity ratings of the stimuli before and after categorization training. (Triangles: psychophysical representation based on similarity ratings; circles: physical stimulus values). 20 schematic faces are represented by: red and yellow circles, for category 1 and 2 exemplars used in training respectively; blue circles for the test exemplars used in the transfer phase of categorization; purple circles: prototypes for categories 1 and 2. The two categories were linearly separable along the Eye Height, Eye Separation dimensions, but not along the Nose Length, Mouth Height. Lines connect matching physical stimulus representations. When several patterns share the same combination of physical dimension values, multiple triangles are connected to the same circle. Longer lines correspond to less faithful psychophysical representation of corresponding physical stimulus values. Reproduced from (Sigala et al., 2002) with permission.

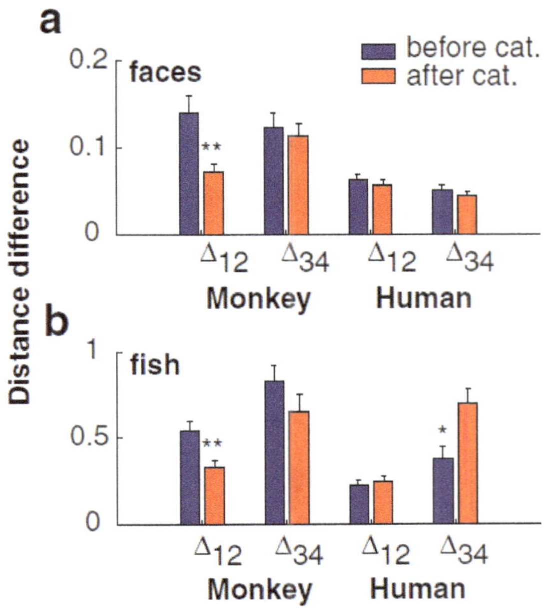

Figure 2. a) Mean distance difference between psychophysical and physical stimuli along the dimensions that were diagnostic for the categorization task (Δ12) and the dimensions that also varied, but were not diagnostic for the categorization task (Δ34), before and after training, averaged over 20 schematic faces (error bars are standard error of mean). b) Average distance difference along the non-diagnostic and diagnostic dimensions before and after categorization for schematic fish stimuli. Data before and after categorization taken from two different monkeys and a single human subject. Signif cance levels (t-test): (∗∗) corresponds to P<0.005 and (∗) to P<0.01. Reproduced from (Sigala et al., 2002) with permission.

However training to categorize the stimuli based on a subset of their features, changed the way they perceived and represented them, even in the context of a different task (similarity ratings vs. categorization) (Fig. 1b, Fig. 2, Fig. 3). Looking for the neuronal underpinnings that supported this perceptual change (Sigala and Logothetis, 2002) found that cells in the anterior inferior temporal cortex selectively represented the values of the features that were important (diagnostic) for the categorization task, over the values of the features that were not (Fig. 4). This was clear evidence that perceptual expertise correlated with selective tuning of cells in the temporal cortex, which presumably developed over the course of training, since the stimuli were unlike anything the animals encountered in their normal environment. It was also evidence in favour of the Generalised Context Model (Nosofsky, 1986), according to which selective attention processes make the perceptual multidimensional stimulus space to shrink or expand reflecting the importance of the most relevant stimulus dimensions (Fig. 5) (Gauthier and Palmeri, 2002). It is clear that if one input the firing rates of the recorded cells in an MDS analysis, the result would resemble the solution recovered for the behavioural data after training (Fig. 1b), where the diagnostic feature values (that separate the categories) are perceived as dissimilar and end up further away from each other, while the non-diagnostic feature values (that don't separate the categories) are perceived as similar and end up close together in space. A similar finding was reported in a single-unit study of inferior temporal neurons, where the stimulus space of parametrically designed shapes was recovered both by psychophysical and neurophysiological measurements (Op de Beeck et al., 2001).

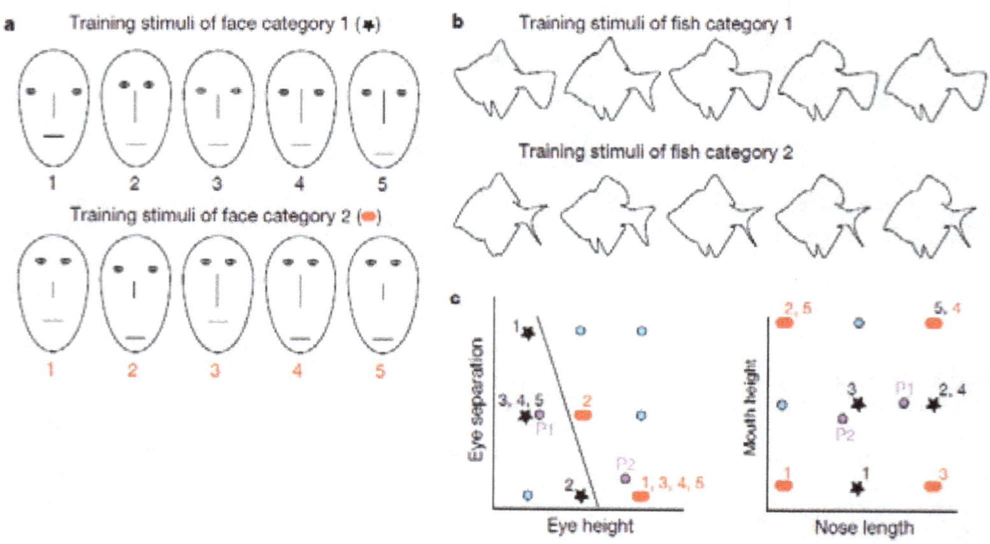

Figure 3. Stimuli and category structure used by (Sigala et al., 2002) and (Sigala and Logothetis, 2002). a. The first stimulus set consisted of line drawings of faces with four varying features: eye height, eye separation, nose length and mouth height. b, The second stimulus set consisted of fish outlines with four varying features: the shape of the dorsal fin, tail, ventral fins and mouth. In both stimulus sets, each feature could take one of three discrete values. The categories were separable along two of the four stimulus features, but information about only one of the diagnostic features was insufficient for optimal performance. The monkeys were presented with one stimulus at a time. c, Two-dimensional representation of the stimulus space. Black stars represent the stimuli of the first category and red ovals represent the stimuli of the second category. Each number indicates the position of one corresponding stimulus from a. As the stimuli differ along four dimensions, the two-dimensional representations in this figure result in overlap of stimuli that are distinct. The purple circles (P1 and P2) represent the prototypes. Cyan circles represent test exemplars that did not belong to a fixed category. The two categories were linearly separable along the eye height, eye separation (EH, ES) dimensions (solid line) but not along the nose length, mouth height (NL, MH) dimensions. Reproduced from (Sigala and Logothetis, 2002) with permission.

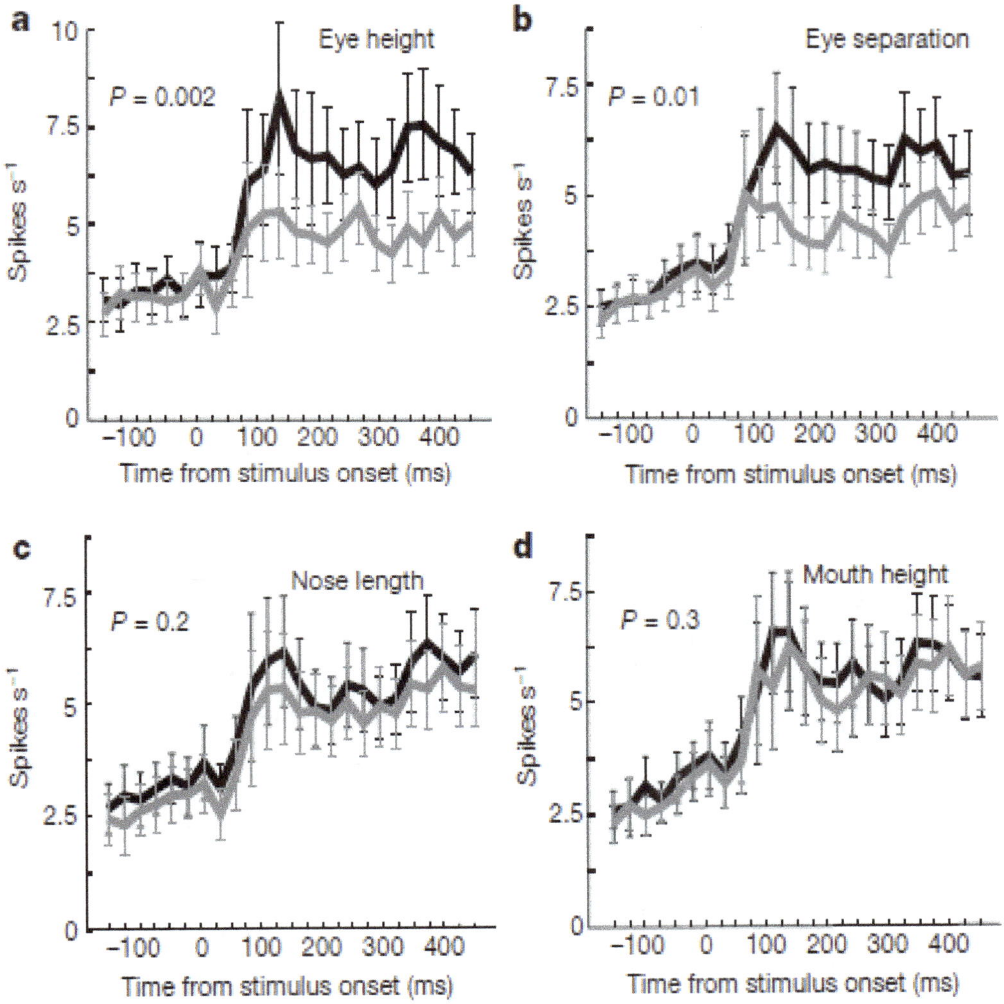

Figure 4. Population average of neuronal tuning to the features that were diagnostic for the categorization task in (Sigala and Logothetis, 2002) (reproduced with permission). The average activity is sorted by stimulus feature (eye height (a), eye separation (b), nose length (c) and mouth height (d)). Black traces indicate average responses to the best feature value; grey traces indicate average responses to the worst feature value. The bars indicate standard error of the mean. For each feature (a–d) a t-test was performed for the time window 100–475 ms after stimulus presentation, testing the hypothesis that the mean firing rate to the best feature was higher than the mean firing rate to the worst feature. The hypothesis could not be rejected in the case of the diagnostic features (eye height (a) and eye separation (b)).

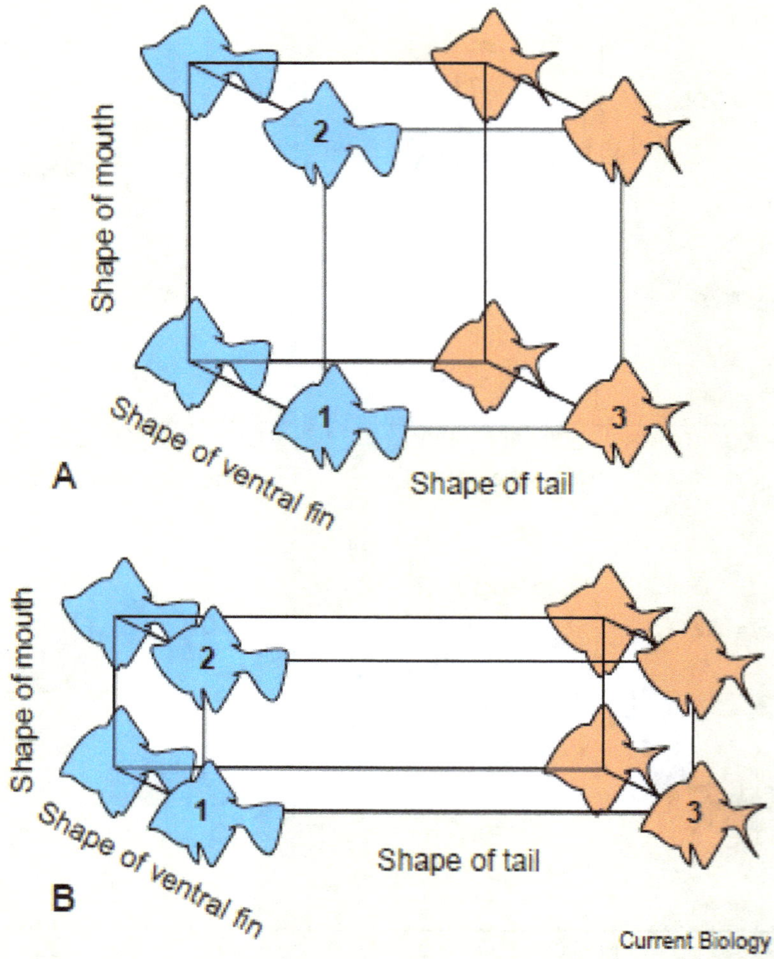

Figure 5. Stretching and compression of the stimulus space by selective attention according to the task demands. As the subjects learn to categorize fish into two groups the multidimensional space becomes relatively stretched along a diagnostic dimension (here shape of the tail) relative to the non-diagnostic dimensions. Before categorization (A), object 1 is equally similar to objects 2 and 3. During categorization (B), object 1 becomes more similar to object 2 than to object 3 through selective attention to the shape of the tail. Reproduced from (Gauthier and Palmeri, 2002) with permission.

3. The brave new era of fMRI

Until the nineties the study of the neural substrates of object recognition in the human brain relied mainly on patients with brain damage, e.g. (Farah, 1992). However behavioural and event-related potential studies of normal subjects, as well as behavioural, lesion and single-unit recording studies in macaque monkeys, had provided a wealth of evidence for the functional organisation of the primate visual system, and of object recognition in particular. With the advent of functional imaging (initially PET, but mainly of fMRI) it became possible to see the normal human brain in action for the first time. Two of the very first questions people wanted to ask concerned the localisation and functional organisation of object recognition: where does recognition happen in the brain, and are there specialized cortical modules for different object categories. These were really important question to ask because a) single-unit recordings (Desimone et al., 1984) and cortical field recordings in human patients (Allison et al., 1994) did not have the global coverage necessary to show the extent of clusters of inferior temporal neurons tuned to faces or other trained object classes e.g. paperclips (Logothetis and Pauls, 1995), and to assess hemispheric laterality; b) structural models of vision and object recognition (Marr and Nishihara, 1978), (Biederman, 1987) did not suggest different representations for different types of objects, or multiple levels of recognition; but c) neuropsychological studies had provided evidence for at least three different brain modules, specific for faces, common objects and words, see (Farah, 1992) for a review.

In this chapter, I present some experimental and theoretical progress that has followed from the literature of perceptual similarity, and will review contributions of the fMRI literature.

(Sergent et al., 1992) provided the first neuroimaging evidence for category-selective responses for face stimuli, with PET imaging of normal subjects. They showed a dissociation between face processing in the right ventromedial hemisphere, and object processing in the left occipito-temporal cortex. The first study to employ fMRI to address the localisation question was by (Puce et al., 1995). They compared faces vs. scrambled faces and reported a number of bilateral activations, with the strongest in the right fusiform gyrus. But it was the study by (Kanwisher et al., 1997) (see (Kanwisher et al., 1996) for preliminary results) that thoroughly tested the response specificity of a proposed face module for the first time, and coined the acronym, the Fusiform Face Area (FFA) that has been with us for almost 15 years now (Fig. 6).

Nancy Kanwisher and her colleagues first localised the area that was significantly more active for faces than objects, then tested if the activity of the area could be explained by a number of variables: low level features; the fact that all faces belonged in the same level category, while the objects were from different categories, by comparing with houses; the fact that faces were compared with inanimate objects, by comparing with hands; attentional factors, by comparing passive fixation with a one-back task. That study was important for several reasons: a) because it showed a clear selectivity for faces over other object categories; b) it pointed to the need for different theories of computation for object and face recognition; c) brought the discussion about whether faces were special, or this specificity could be expected to develop for every class of objects that one was expert in (Diamond and Carey, 1986), in the neuroimaging field.

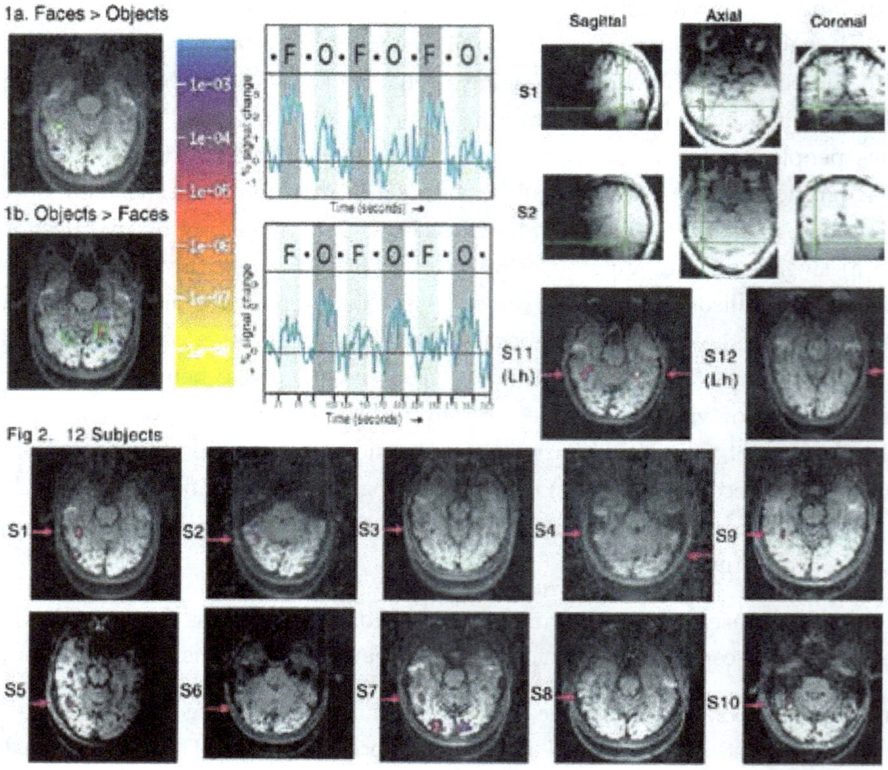

Figure 6. The Fusiform Face Area first reported in (Kanwisher et al., 1997) (reproduced with permission). Results from one subject. The right hemisphere appears on the left. The brain images at the left show in colour the voxels that produced a significantly higher MR signal intensity during the epochs containing faces than during those containing objects (1a) and vice versa (1b) for 1 of the 12 slices scanned. These significance images are overlaid on a T1-weighted anatomical image of the same slice. In each image, an ROI (Region Of Interest) is shown outlined in green, and the time course of raw percentage signal change over the 5 min 20 sec scan (based on unsmoothed data and averaged across the voxels in this ROI) is shown at the right. Epochs in which faces were presented are indicated by the vertical gray bars marked with an "F"; gray bars with an "O" indicate epochs during which assorted objects were presented; white bars indicate fixation epochs.

4. Car, bird and greeble experts

Gauthier and her colleagues had also been working on the question of functional specialization using fMRI (Gauthier et al., 1996a) (Gauthier et al., 1996b), and had preliminary evidence that FFA may also be recruited in subordinate categorizations (e.g. for the basic level "bird", the subordinate level –requiring additional perceptual processing-could be "skylark" or "blackbird") (Gauthier et al., 1997). Their fMRI work with greebles, novel objects created to provide a control set equivalent for faces (Fig. 7), indicated that the FFA may be an area involved in visual expertise in general and not just for faces (Gauthier et al., 1999). This proposal has become known as the expertise hypothesis.

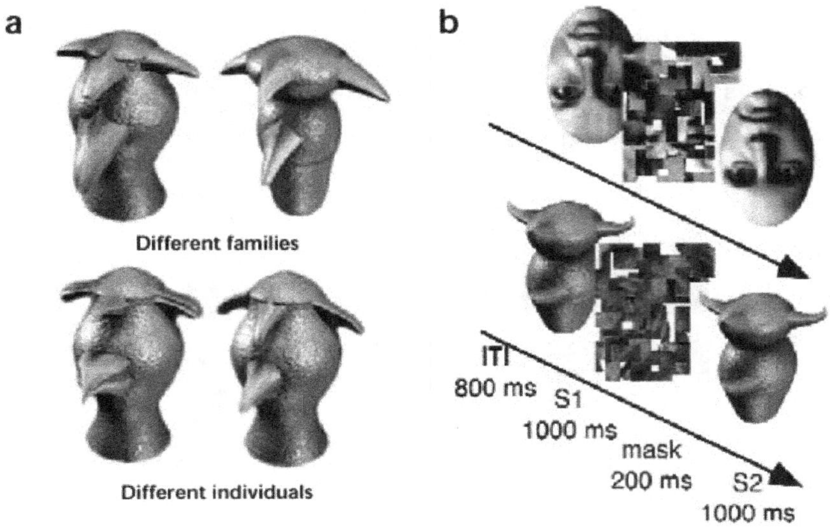

Figure 7. Meet the Greebles. Two greebles from different 'families', as defined by the shape of the large central part, as well as two individual greebles from the same family, differing only in the shape of the smaller parts. Adapted from (Gauthier et al., 1999) with permission

The greebles however have been criticised as being too similar to faces (in terms of symmetry, features, configural processing), which would make them less than ideal controls for the face specificity hypothesis of FFA (see below for neuro-imaging evidence). In a different experiment, Gauthier and her colleagues, recruited car and bird experts in order to test whether FFA was recruited during categorization of objects in their domain of expertise (Gauthier et al., 2000). The results showed that while the FFA response was still greater for faces, rather than other objects, it was nonetheless involved in processing the objects in the participants' area of expertise as well (e.g. birds for bird experts). This finding has been subsequently replicated by other laboratories (Xu, 2005), as well as in different domains of expertise (e.g. with moths and butterflies) (Rhodes et al., 2004). The BOLD signal intensity of the FFA in these studies is greater for faces than other stimuli, so there is specificity, but not exclusivity, for face stimuli, a domain of expertise that most humans share.

Another way to test the expertise hypothesis, instead of recruiting real world experts, is to effectuate expertise in the lab following intense training until a certain discrimination criterion has been reached, and/or a certain number of training hours (e.g. 10) have been completed. These paradigms, not only allow to test the responses of FFA or any other brain area, but also to study other changes as a result of training. For example (Op de Beeck et al., 2006) tested changes in cortical activations before and after 10 hours of training to discriminate novel 3D shapes at a subordinate level in a match-to-sample task. The authors used three novel shape categories, which they named "smoothies", "spikies" and "cubies" based on the type of protrusions they had (Fig. 8).

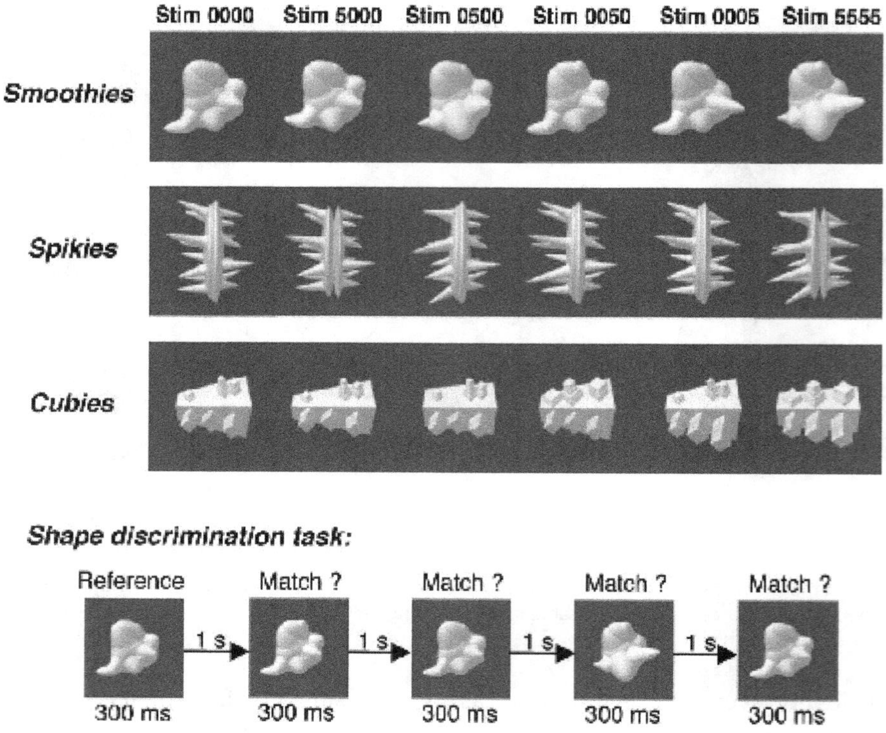

Figure 8. Stimuli and task used in (Op de Beeck et al., 2006), reproduced with permission. For each of the three classes (smoothies, spikies, and cubies), exemplars were constructed from a four-dimensional object space. Each exemplar had a value from 0 to 5 on each of four shape dimensions. The top three rows show exemplars from each class: value 0 on each dimension (far left), value 5 on one dimension and value 0 on the other dimensions (middle four exemplars), and value 5 on each dimension (far right). The bottom half of the figure shows the task used to train subjects in shape discrimination.

The approach of using artificial stimuli avoids confounds of prior, uncontrolled experience of the participants with the stimuli, and should lead to new cortical representations that are formed during the course of training. The participants were scanned before and after the training sessions, and while performing an orthogonal task to shape discrimination (colour change detection task), so any observed changes in the cortical activations could not be attributed to changes in task performance or differences of other cognitive factors e.g. attention, task difficulty etc. This study showed that the behavioural improvement in shape discrimination (one trained class for each participant) was accompanied by the following changes in cortical activations: 1) more voxels, therefore more groups of neurons, responded to the trained rather untrained stimuli in the post-training scan; 2) these voxels did not form a large cluster, but multiple small clusters in the extrastriate visual cortex (Fig. 9); 3) the Lateral Occipital Cortex (LOC) showed more activity to the trained stimuli compared to the FFA and early retinotopic visual areas, but also showed more activity to the stimuli before the training had taken place, especially in the right hemisphere; 4) the right FFA did not show increased responsiveness to the trained stimuli, except in one participant trained with "smoothies", who

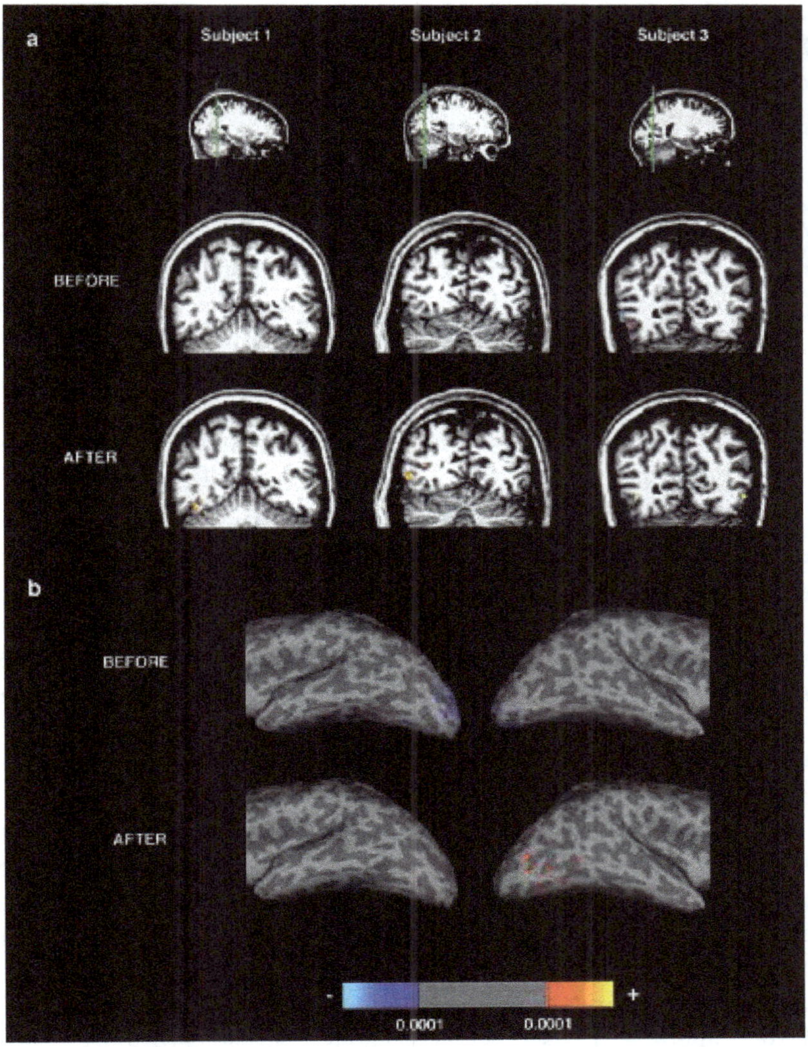

Figure 9. fMRI evidence that categorization training changes object representations in human extrastriate cortex, reproduced from (Op de Beeck et al., 2006) with permission. Activations (significance maps thresholded at $p < 0.0001$, uncorrected) are shown for the contrast [trained > untrained], with red/yellow indicating positive contrast and blue indicating negative contrast. a, Functional activation overlaid on a coronal anatomical slice for three subjects. The left, middle, and right subjects were trained with the smoothies, spikies, and cubies, respectively. These subjects were representative in the size of training effects seen across the population. Slices are shown with right hemisphere at the left. b, Functional activation overlaid on a ventrolateral view of the inflated brain of a fourth subject (trained with the smoothies).

during debriefing reported interpreting the stimuli as "women wearing hats", in other words face-like (Fig. 9).

This last observation shed light as to what could be driving the FFA responses in the studies with greebles, which are also face-like stimuli. This was further tested in a recent study by

(Brants et al., 2011) which replicated the design of the original greeble fMRI study (Gauthier et al., 1999) and extended it by scanning the participants both before and after training with the greebles. The main finding of this experiment is that even before training the participants showed an inversion effect[1] with the Greebles (that did not increase after training), indicating that these objects are interpreted as living entities with faces, and the cortical activations elicited by them may not be due to expertise.

Two more studies that contrasted the effect of mere exposure vs. categorization training (van der Linden et al., 2008) and a categorization vs. individuation task (Wong et al., 2009) with computer-generated, parametrically designed stimuli also showed increased cortical activations after training in areas near and somewhat overlapping with the right FFA.

5. The extent of the brain areas involved in categorization revealed with fMRI

Lack of increased right FFA response to trained stimuli (morphed cars) within a subordinate category was also reported by (Jiang et al., 2007) in a study of categorization training that revealed a large number of areas, including prefrontal, insular, parietal and inferior temporal cortices, as well as the thalamus that responded to the trained stimuli vs. a fixation baseline (Table 1). A similar network of cortical and subcortical areas, including the striatum, was also revealed by a study of categorization of dynamic moving patterns (Li et al., 2007), contrasted with a rotation detection task of the same stimuli. This study indicated a different role for temporal and parietal areas, and for prefrontal and striatal areas. For the former areas, the selectivity to diagnostic visual features was tuned according to task demands. Prefrontal and striatal areas are thought to provide top-down control by shaping the neural representations in the cortical areas involved in the relevant stimulus feature processing (e.g. inferior temporal cortex for shape). This study replicated and extended a number of key finding from separate single unit studies in the macaque, partly because of the global brain coverage that fMRI affords, but also thanks to careful parametric design of the stimulus space, and the sensitivity of Multi Voxel Pattern Analysis (MVPA) methods that capitalize on differences across distributed patterns of activity in the brain, e.g. (Cox and Savoy, 2003), (Norman et al., 2006) (Fig. 10).

MVPA, an approach that uses a variety of powerful pattern classification algorithms to decode the information in multi-voxel patters of activity, is particularly well suited for the study of distributed cortical representations. Although single unit studies had already pointed to the distributed nature of information coding e.g. (Young and Yamane, 1992), it is the excellent spatial coverage and non-invasive nature of fMRI that can provide information about where categories are represented in the human brain. The advantages of MVPA include: a) the

1 n fMRI experiments the inversion effect is associated with higher activity in FFA for upright than for inverted stimuli. The inversion effect is a hallmark of holistic processing (the integration of the stimulus parts into a whole representation), which may be specific to faces, as opposed to part-based processing for other types of stimuli, like animals or artifacts.

Region	mm^3	T	MNI Corrrdinates X	Y	Z
Stimuli > baseline					
Left Visual Cortex	26912	10.53	-44	-88	-8
		9.26	-22	-102	-2
		7.13	-26	-92	-14
Right Visual Cortex	33024	9.06	26	-105	4
		8.70	32	-100	8
		8.55	20	-100	-6
Left Inf/Sup Parietal	12280	8.25	-30	-60	50
		7.80	-38	-42	44
		7.00	-24	-68	48
R/L Sup Mot	7504	7.45	4	6	52
		7.12	-6	2	56
		6.94	-2	12	48
R Cerebelum	544	5.12	18	-64	-46
R Sup Parietal	1232	5.12	28	-66	54
		4.35	26	-52	48
L Brainstem	1584	4.93	-16	-18	12
		4.48	-14	-16	2
L Thalamus	216	4.85	-10	-26	-12
R Thalamus	728	4.78	16	-18	8
L Cerebelum	528	4.76	-16	-54	-20
L Precentral	656	4.65	-48	6	32
		3.87	-50	0	42
R Mid/Sup Frontal	408	4.65	32	-2	58
L Mid Frontal	240	4.60	-50	32	32
R Inf Parietal/Supramarginal	328	4.59	44	-36	46
L Sup/Mid Frontal	1008	4.57	-22	-8	44
		4.07	-26	-4	54
L Insula	568	4.49	-32	20	2
L Cerebum	280	4.46	-6	-28	26
		3.94	-8	-20	28
L Cerebelum	368	4.45	-16	-64	-50
R Cerebelum	480	4.43	36	-18	54
L Cerebelum	472	4.43	-8	-74	-20
L Rolandic	264	4.40	-46	-6	10
R Postcentral	208	4.34	62	-18	50
R Sup/Mid Occipital	760	4.33	28	-74	32

Table 1. Table of brain areas that are activated by the trained stimuli (cars) in (Jiang et al.,2007) (Supplementary Table 1, reproduced with permission).

sensitivity to signals that can be ignored in univariate approaches, where each voxel is treated independently and its activity modulation must reach a statistical significance threshold; b), brain activity and behaviour can be related on a trial-by-trial basis (as in single unit studies) rather than hundreds of averaged trials; and c) most importantly, it allows to characterize the structure of neural representations in individual subjects with or without the use of pattern classifiers (Norman et al., 2006). The earliest attempt to examine and relate the entire distributed pattern of voxel activations in object-related cortical areas to object categories was pioneered by Edelman and colleagues (Edelman et al., 1998), and showed promising results in recovering stimulus spaces with MDS. Pictures of natural stimuli, human and animal faces (Figure 11), and computer-generated stimuli resembling fighter planes, human bodies, sharks, four-legged animals, cars and vans (Figure 12), separated in meaningful categories based on the fMRI activity patterns. This study pioneered the multivariate analysis approach with fMRI

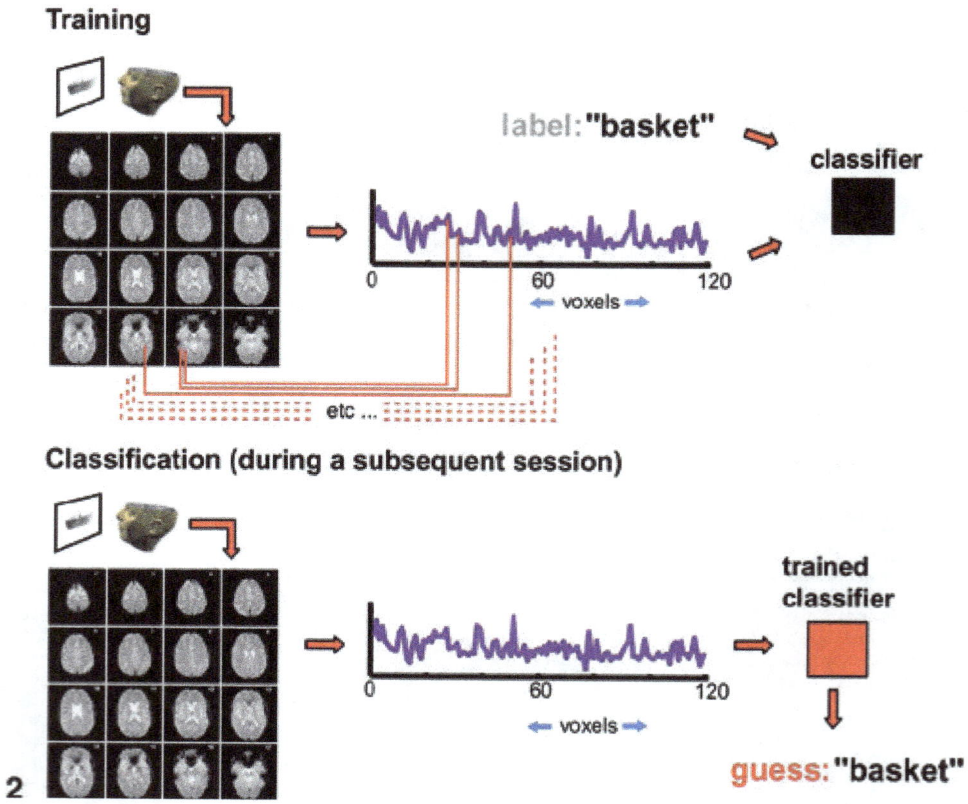

Figure 10. Basic classification scheme in MVPA (adapted from (Cox and Savoy, 2003) with permission). Each participant viewed block of images belonging to 1 of 10 categories. The pattern of activity over a previously selected subset of voxels, based on a feature selection procedure, is treated as a high-dimensional vector, shown here as a profile plot (the mapping between the voxels in the brain and points in the profile plot is symbolized by red lines). These vectors, along with labels corresponding to the category, are given to a classifier, which learns statistical regularities in the patterns, and maps between brain patterns and experimental conditions. In a subsequent session (separated in time by as much as a month), the same subject is shown the same category of objects. fMRI data are collected with the same spatial sampling, and the pattern over the same voxel subset is extracted. This pattern is given to the trained classifier that infers the category the subject was viewing, based on the decision boundary it extracted. The same steps can be followed with data collected in a single session, where half the data is used to train the classifier, and half is used in the testing phase.

data, and further suggested that both perceptual and cortical representations may be representations of similarity, which can vary according to the importance of the stimulus features and level of experience with the stimuli, e.g. (Schyns and Rodet, 1997), (Op de Beeck H, 2000), (Sigala, 2004).

The finding of distributed, rather than category-specific clusters of activation in the cortex, was later confirmed with a now seminal study by (Haxby et al., 2001) who showed that despite a small number of areas specialized for specific categories (see section: Other specific modules: Bodies, Places, Words), the representations of objects in the ventral temporal cortex are very distributed and overlapping. This means that the representation of a particular object, or object

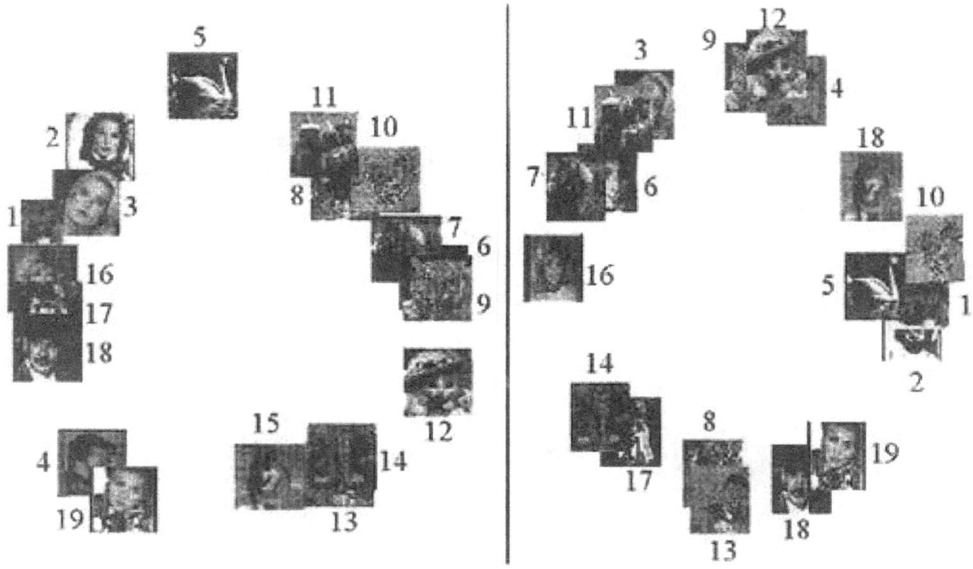

Figure 11. The left panel illustrates the stimulus space configuration, as it was derived with MDS from seven participants' most significant voxels that responded preferentially to whole objects, but not to their scrambled versions. Those voxels were bilaterally in the Lateral Occipital Complex (area LO).The number labels indicate the serial number of the picture in the epoch. The main result is the separation of faces and animals in two linearly separable clusters. The panel on the right shows the result of a bootstrap procedure, where MDS was applied to randomly permuted time courses. This result shows no clustering that corresponds to specific stimulus categories. (Figure from Edelman et al. 1998, reproduced with the permission of the Psychonomic Society.)

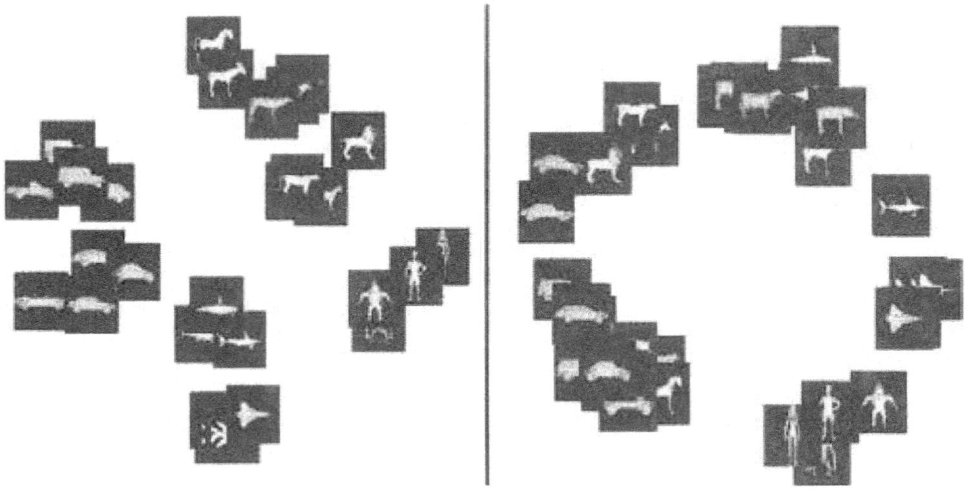

Figure 12. Comparison of the stimulus space derived with MDS applied on perceptual judgments of similarities (left panel) and fMRI activation patterns (right panel). (Figure from Edelman et al. 1998, reproduced with the permission of the Psychonomic Society.)

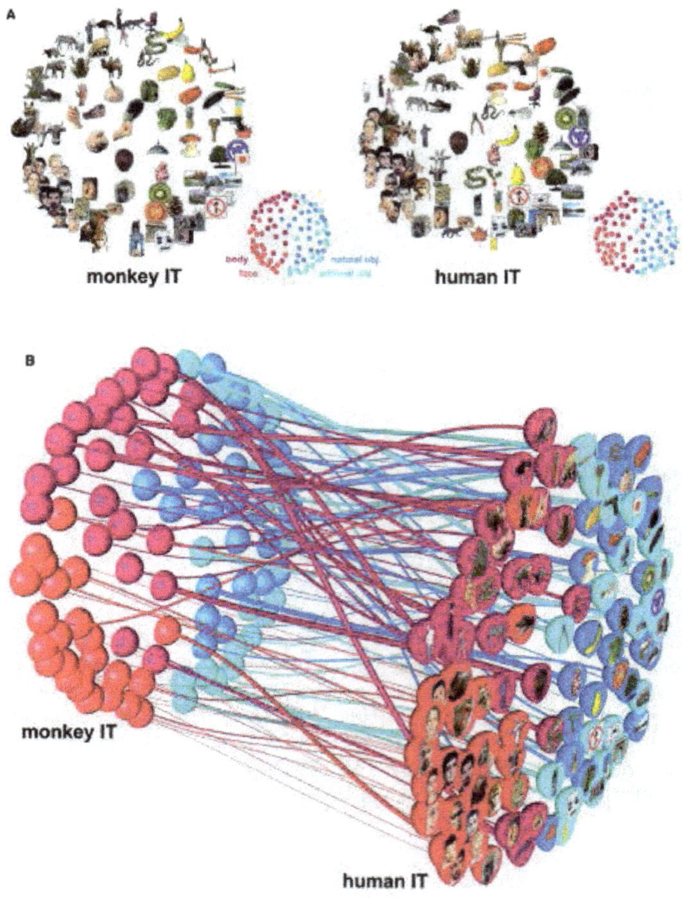

Figure 13. Similarity of representations in human and monkey Inferior Temporal Cortex (IT). Reproduced from (Kriegeskorte et al., 2008b) with permission. (A) Stimulus space reflecting the similarity of responses in IT. The stimuli have been arranged such that their pairwise distances approximately reflect response-pattern similarity (MDS, dissimilarity: 1 – Pearson r, criterion: metric stress). In each arrangement, images placed close together elicited similar response patterns. Images placed far apart elicited dissimilar response patterns. The arrangement is unsupervised: it does not presuppose any categorical structure. (B) Fiber-flow visualization emphasizing the interspecies differences. This visualization combines all the information from (A) and links each pair of dots representing a stimulus in monkey and human IT by a "fiber." The thickness of each fiber reflects to what extent the corresponding stimulus is inconsistently represented in monkey and human IT. The interspecies consistency ri of stimulus i is defined as the Pearson correlation between vectors of its 91 dissimilarities to the other stimuli in monkey and human IT. The thickness of the fiber for stimulus i is proportional to (1 – ri)2, emphasizing the most inconsistently represented stimuli.

category, is encoded in the activity pattern created by a large number of neurons, and each of these neurons takes part in instantiating multiple object representations.

In the most recent and visually compelling demonstrations of the power of combining the notion of similarity with multivariate analyses, (Kriegeskorte et al., 2008b) demonstrated the close correspondence of the activity patterns in human and non-human IT cortex, and revealed a mostly orderly representation of object super-ordinate categories (e.g. animate, inanimate),

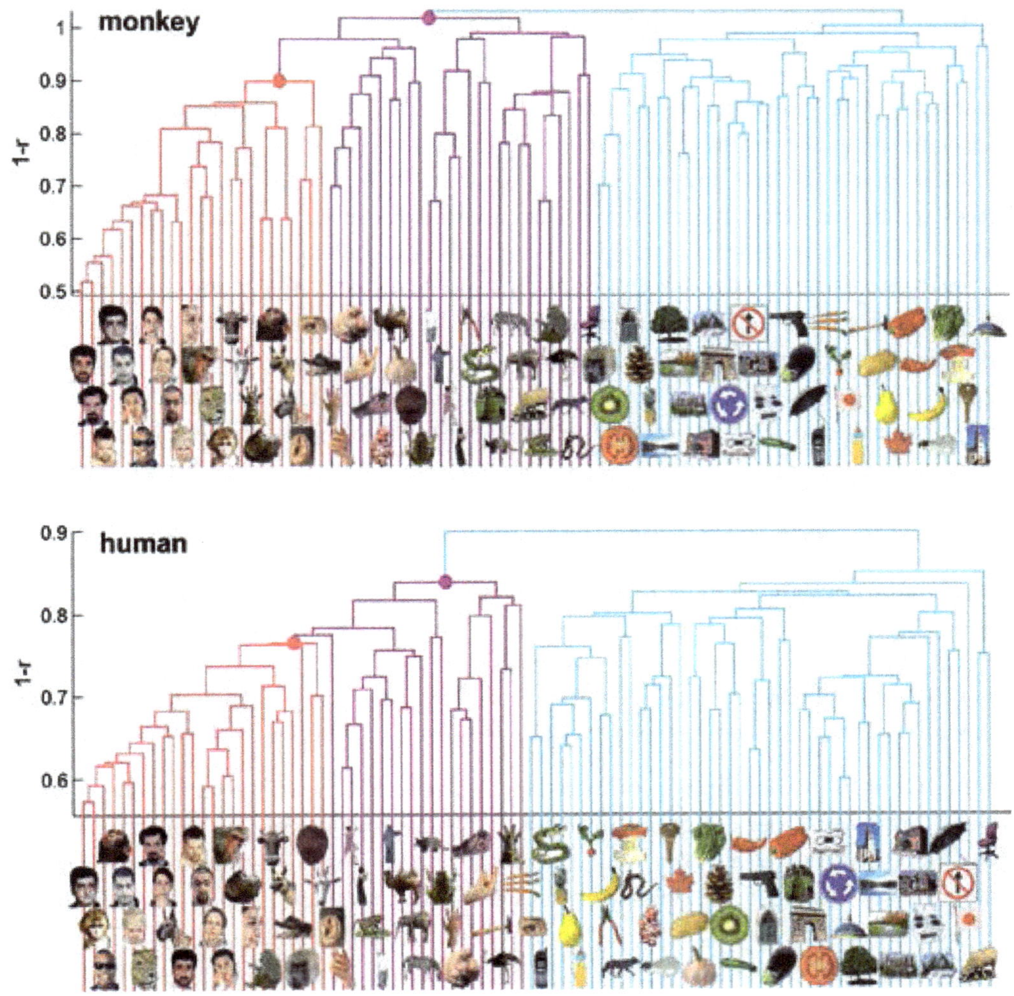

Figure 14. Hierarchical clustering of Inferior Temporal Cortex (IT) response patterns. Reproduced from (Kriegeskorte et al., 2008b) with permission. This analysis proceeds from single-image clusters (bottom of each panel) and successively combines the two clusters closest to each other in terms of the average response-pattern dissimilarity, so as to form a hierarchy of clusters (tree structure in each panel). The vertical height of each horizontal link indicates the average response-pattern dissimilarity (the clustering criterion) between the stimuli of the two linked subclusters (dissimilarity: 1 − r). The cluster trees for monkey and human are the result of completely independent experiments and analysis pipelines. This data-driven technique reveals natural-category clusters that are consistent between monkey and human. For easier comparison, subcluster trees were colored (faces, red; bodies, magenta; inanimate objects, light blue).

as well as a continuous representations of categories and exemplars (Fig.13, 14). This approach promises to help bridge the gap of relating the different approaches (computational, imaging, electrophysiological and psychophysical) and species (mainly human and non-human primates) that have figured in the field of object recognition and categorization over the decades (Kriegeskorte et al., 2008a).

6. Other selective modules: Bodies, places, words

The answer to the question "are faces special" is probably yes – the question refers to visual processing mechanisms that may be unique to faces. The case study of a boy who sustained brain damage on the first day he was born, resulting in an inability to recognise individual faces (while his object recognition is largely intact) even after acquired experience and plasticity, as he was tested at the age of 16 (Farah et al., 2000), indicates that the brain is equipped to cope with face recognition at birth and this core ability may not be restored with experience. The FFA therefore may be the result of natural selection for copying with a common and important stimulus for survival, which occupies a dense stimulus/similarity space. This is because all faces look largely similar in terms of number and configuration of features, and multiple categorizations need to be applied on them in a very short time (e.g. identity, sex, emotion). This does not mean however that experience is not important, since the fine tuning of face recognition ability also depends on experience, as seen e.g. in the other-race effect[2] (Lindsay et al., 1991), (Feng et al.).

Other modules selective for processing certain categories of stimuli that have been revealed with fMRI are the Parahippocampal Place Area (PPA), which is selective for the geometry of the local environment including pictures of houses (Epstein R, 1998), the Extrastriate Body Area (EBA) selective to human body parts (Downing et al., 2001), as well as the letter string area, which has been elegantly shown to form as a result of experience (Baker et al., 2007).

Imaging work in the non-human primate has also revealed the full extent of the representation of faces and other categories in the brain. The equivalent of the human FFA, seems to be still elusive (Ku et al., 2011), but a network of areas that respond more to faces than to other objects has been repeatedly shown with fMRI in the macaque brain including the temporal and prefrontal cortex, and the amygdala (Logothetis et al., 1999), (Tsao et al., 2003), (Hoffman et al., 2007), (Tsao et al., 2008b), (Tsao et al., 2008a), (Ku et al., 2011). The exact role of each face patch is not clear, but what we do know is that it only takes a small amount of micro-stimulation of a small group of face selective neurons to affect the perception of a macaque categorizing face vs. non-face stimuli and bias the response towards the face category (Afraz et al., 2006). A direct comparison of the reported locations of these face patches from different groups, reveals such a dense network of selective cell groups, which clearly points to a very distributed representation of faces in the non-human primate brain (Fig. 15). However, it should be noted that the majority of these face patches are also active in the anaesthetised preparation (Logothetis et al., 1999), (Ku et al., 2011), complicating the interpretation of the findings and the role of these activations in conscious perception.

---

2 he other race effect (or own-race bias): the phenomenon describes the fact that, despite our impressive ability to effortlessly recognize and remember faces, we make more errors when we remember and recognize faces from another, less familiar race (O'Toole et al., 1994).

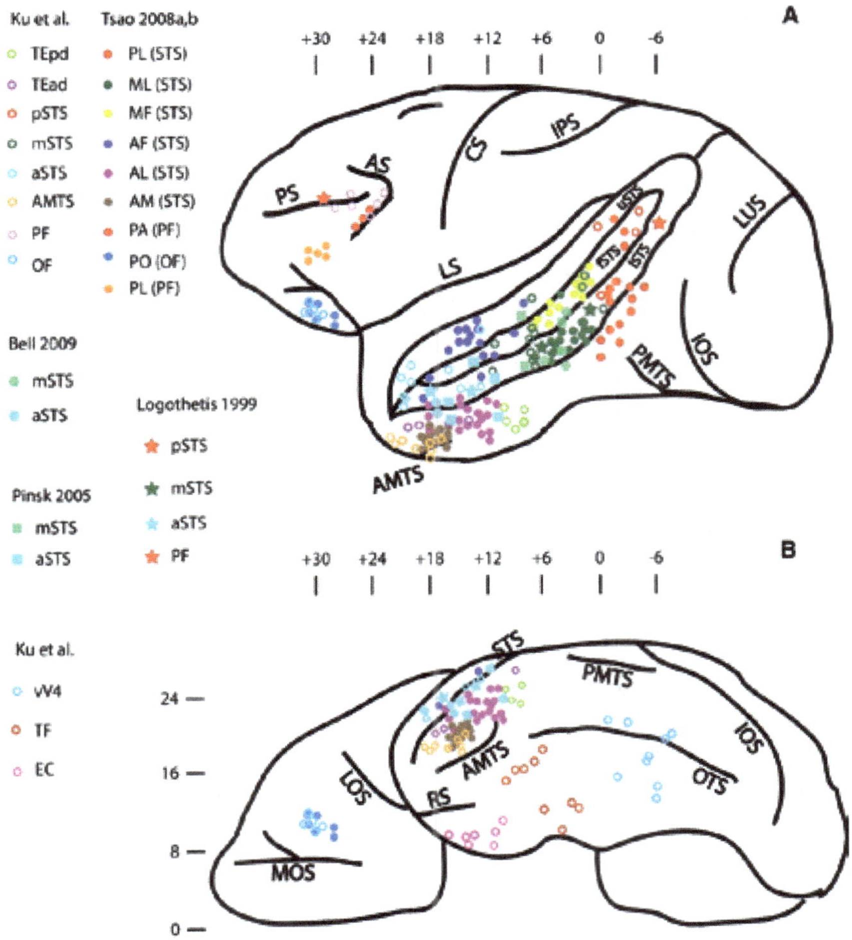

Figure 15. Comparison of Face-Selective Activation Found in the Current Study with Face-Selective Activation Described in the Literature Superimposed on a Side and Ventral View of the Brain. (A) Side view of the brain. The locations of face-selective patches found in the literature ((Bell et al., 2009), (Logothetis et al., 1999), (Pinsk et al., 2005), (Tsao et al., 2008a) and (Tsao et al., 2008b) are marked by closed symbols and locations found in the current study are indicated by the open circles. For the activated areas described by (Tsao et al., 2008a) and (Tsao et al., 2008b), naming conventions used by the authors were retained with the locations in parentheses. Locations were estimated based on AP positions when given; otherwise positions were estimated by comparing the coronal slices to the atlas by (Saleem and Logothetis, 2006). In cases where activation extended over multiple slices the average position was taken. The locations shown are after normalization to the macaque template (McLaren et al., 2009). Note that not all studies (including the present one) make a distinction between STS patches located on the lip and the fundus. (B) Ventral view of face-selective activation in this study (open circles) and the literature (closed symbols). Abbreviations: LOS: lateral orbital sulcus; MOS: medial orbital sulcus; OTS: occipitotemporal sulcus; PMTS: posterior middle temporal sulcus; RS: rhinal sulcus. Figure reproduced from (Ku et al., 2011) with permission.

7. Conclusion

It would be unfortunate if the reader was left with the impression that fMRI has only revealed locations and representations of stimuli that are compatible with certain computational and theoretical accounts of visual perception and long term memory. Other important contributions of fMRI in the literature of expertise relate to evidence for the improvement of working memory abilities in experts (Moore et al., 2006), as well as the demands of encoding strategies (e.g. chunking) that can make certain tasks easier (Bor et al., 2003), and the possibility that a frontoparietal cortical network may be a general purpose expertise-based network, e.g. (Bor and Owen, 2007).

Despite its relatively young age, the fMRI community has engaged with and made important contributions to most of the questions that had been keeping single-unit electrophysiologists busy for decades, regarding for example functional specialisation, local vs. distributed processing, hierarchical representations and the malleability of those representations. The emphasis in the field has slowly but surely shifted from where functions are taking place to how the underlying computations are achieved.

The unprecedented ability to see the whole human brain in action has reassured us about its similarities with non-human primate brains, e.g. (Orban et al., 2004), but also pinpointed differences, e.g. (Petit et al., 1997), and has revealed the extent to which the brain operates as a functional network, e.g. (Vogel et al., 2010, Van Dijk KR et al., 2010).

In the field of visual categorization and expertise, fMRI has revealed a number of specialised areas for processing biologically and culturally important categories of stimuli, like faces and letter strings. At the same time fMRI has revealed how distributed the representations of most object categories are, and how these may be organised in a hierarchical way that breaks up the complexity of the world in manageable chunks, governed by perceptually and cognitively defined similarity rules, that take into account task demands.

Author details

Natasha Sigala*

Clinical Imaging Sciences Centre, Brighton and Sussex Medical School, University of Sussex, United Kingdom

References

[1] Afraz, S. R., Kiani, R. & Esteky, H. (2006). Microstimulation of inferotemporal cortex influences face categorization. *Nature* 442, 692-695.

[2] Ahn, W. & Dennis, M. J. (2001) Dissociation between categorization and similiarity judgement: differential effect of causal status on feature weights. In: *Similarity and Categorization*, (eds.) U. Hahn & M. Ramscar, pp. 87-107. Oxford: Oxford University Press.

[3] Allison, T., Ginter, H., McCarthy, G., Nobre, A. C., Puce, A., Luby, M. & Spencer, D. D. (1994). Face recognition in human extrastriate cortex. *J Neurophysiol* 71, 821-825.

[4] Attneave, F. (1957). Transfer of experience with a class-schema to identification-learning of patterns and shapes. *Journal of experimental psychology* 54, 81-88.

[5] Baker, C. I., Liu, J., Wald, L. L., Kwong, K. K., Benner, T. & Kanwisher, N. (2007). Visual word processing and experiential origins of functional selectivity in human extrastriate cortex. *Proc Natl Acad Sci U S A* 104, 9087-9092. doi:0703300104 [pii] 10.1073/pnas.0703300104.

[6] Bell, A. H., Hadj-Bouziane, F., Frihauf, J. B., Tootell, R. B. & Ungerleider, L. G. (2009). Object representations in the temporal cortex of monkeys and humans as revealed by functional magnetic resonance imaging. *J Neurophysiol* 101, 688-700. doi:90657.2008 [pii] 10.1152/jn.90657.2008.

[7] Biederman, I. (1987). Recognition-by-Components: a theory of human image understanding. *Psychological review* 94, 115-147.

[8] Boden, M. A. (2006) *Mind as machine: a history of cognitive science*. Oxford: Oxford University Press.

[9] Bor, D., Duncan, J., Wiseman, R. & Owen, A. M. (2003). Encoding strategies dissociate prefrontal activity from working memory demand. *Neuron* 37, 361-367.

[10] Bor, D. & Owen, A. M. (2007). Cognitive training: neural correlates of expert skills. *Curr Biol* 17, R95-97. doi:S0960-9822(07)00821-4 [pii] 10.1016/j.cub.2007.01.019.

[11] Brants, M., Wagemans, J. & Op de Beeck, H. P. (2011). Activation of Fusiform Face Area by Greebles is Related to Face Similarity but Not Expertise. *Journal of Cognitive Neuroscience*. doi:doi:10.1162/jocn_a_00072.

[12] Cox, D. D. & Savoy, R. L. (2003). Functional magnetic resonance imaging (fMRI) "brain reading": detecting and classifying distributed patterns of fMRI activity in human visual cortex. *Neuroimage* 19, 261-270.

[13] Cross, R. C. (1959). Category DIfferences. *Proceedings of the Aristotelian Society* 59, 255-270.

[14] Cutzu, F. & Edelman, S. (1996). Faithful representation of similarities among three-dimensional shapes in human vision. *Proc. Natl. Acad. Sci. USA* 93, 12046-12050.

[15] Desimone, R., Albright, T. D., Gross, C. G. & Bruce, C. (1984). Stimulus-selective properties of IT neurons in the macaque. *The Journal of Neuroscience* 4, 2051-2062.

[16] Diamond, R. & Carey, S. (1986). Why faces are and are not special: an effect of expertise. *Journal of Experimental Psychology: General* 115, 107-117.

[17] Downing, P. E., Jiang, Y., Shuman, M. & Kanwisher, N. (2001). A cortical area selective for visual processing of the human body. *Science* 293, 2470-2473. doi:10.1126/science.1063414, 293/5539/2470 [pii].

[18] Edelman, S. (1998). Representation is representation of similarities. *Behavioral & Brain Sciences* 21, 449-467.

[19] Edelman, S., Grill-Spector, K., Kushnir, T. & Malach, R. (1998). Towards direct visualization of the internal shape representation space by fMRI. *Psychobiology* 26, 309-321.

[20] Epstein R, K. N. (1998). A cortical representation of the local visual environment. *Nature* 392, 598-601.

[21] Farah, M. J. (1992). Is an object an object an object? Cognitive and neuropsychological investigations of domain-specificity in visual object recognition. *Current Directions in Psychological Science* 1, 164-169.

[22] Farah, M. J., Rabinowitz, C., Quinn, G. E. & Liu, G. T. (2000). Early commitment of neural substrates for face recognition. *Cogn Neuropsychol* 17, 117-123. doi:713751844 [pii], 10.1080/026432900380526.

[23] Feng, L., Liu, J., Wang, Z., Li, J., Li, L., Ge, L., Tian, J. & Lee, K. The other face of the other-race effect: An fMRI investigation of the other-race face categorization advantage. *Neuropsychologia.* doi:S0028-3932(11)00438-6 [pii], 10.1016/j.neuropsychologia.2011.09.031.

[24] Gauthier, I., Anderson, A. W., Tarr, M. J. & Gore, J. C. (1996a) Levels of categorization in visual object recognition studied with fMRI. In: *3rd Annual Meeting of the Cognitive Neuroscience Society*. San Fransisco.

[25] Gauthier, I., Anderson, A. W., Tarr, M. J., Skudlarski, P. & Gore, J. C. (1997). Levels of categorization in visual recognition studied using functional magnetic resonance imaging. *Current Biology* 7, 645-651.

[26] Gauthier, I., Behrmann, M., Tarr, M. J., Anderson, A. W., Gore, J. C. & McClelland, J. L. (1996b) Subordinate-level categorization in human inferior temporal cortex: Converging evidence from neuropsychology and brain imaging. In: *Society for Neuroscience Abstracts.*

[27] Gauthier, I. & Palmeri, T. J. (2002). Visual Neurons: Categorization-Based Selectivity. *Current Biology* 12, 282-284.

[28] Gauthier, I., Skudlarski, P., Gore, J. C. & Anderson, A. W. (2000). Expertise for cars and birds recruits brain areas involved in face recognition. *Nat Neurosci* 3, 191-197.

[29] Gauthier, I., Tarr, M. J., Anderson, A. W., Skudlarski, P. & Gore, J. C. (1999). Activation of the middle fusiform 'face area' increases with expertise in recognizing novel objects. *Nat Neurosci* 2, 568-573. doi:10.1038/9224.

[30] Haxby, J., Gobbini, M., Furey, M., Ishai, A., Schouten, J. & Pietrini, P. (2001). Distributed and overlapping representations of faces and objects in ventral temporal cortex. *Science* 293, 2425-2430.

[31] Heider, E. R. (1972). Universals in color naming and memory. *J Exp Psychol* 93, 10-20.

[32] Hoffman, K. L., Gothard, K. M., Schmid, M. C. & Logothetis, N. K. (2007). Facial-expression and gaze-selective responses in the monkey amygdala. *Curr Biol* 17, 766-772. doi:S0960-9822(07)01144-X [pii], 10.1016/j.cub.2007.03.040.

[33] Jiang, X., Bradley, E., Rini, R. A., Zeffiro, T., Vanmeter, J. & Riesenhuber, M. (2007). Categorization training results in shape- and category-selective human neural plasticity. *Neuron* 53, 891-903. doi:S0896-6273(07)00114-6 [pii], 10.1016/j.neuron.2007.02.015.

[34] Kanwisher, N., Chun, M. M., McDermott, J. & Ledden, P. J. (1996). Functional imaging of human visual recognition. *Brain Res Cogn Brain Res* 5, 55-67.

[35] Kanwisher, N., McDermott, J. & Chun, M. M. (1997). The fusiform face area: a module in human extrastriate cortex specialized for face perception. *Journal of Neuroscience* 17, 4302-4311.

[36] Kriegeskorte, N. (2009). Relating Population-Code Representations between Man, Monkey, and Computational Models. *Front Neurosci* 3, 363-373.

[37] Kriegeskorte, N., Mur, M. & Bandettini, P. (2008a). Representational similarity analysis - connecting the branches of systems neuroscience. *Front Syst Neurosci* 2, 4. doi: 10.3389/neuro.06.004.2008.

[38] Kriegeskorte, N., Mur, M., Ruff, D. A., Kiani, R., Bodurka, J., Esteky, H., Tanaka, K. & Bandettini, P. A. (2008b). Matching categorical object representations in inferior temporal cortex of man and monkey. *Neuron* 60, 1126-1141. doi:S0896-6273(08)00943-4 [pii], 10.1016/j.neuron.2008.10.043.

[39] Ku, S. P., Tolias, A. S., Logothetis, N. K. & Goense, J. (2011). fMRI of the face-processing network in the ventral temporal lobe of awake and anesthetized macaques. *Neuron* 70, 352-362. doi:S0896-6273(11)00205-4 [pii], 10.1016/j.neuron.2011.02.048.

[40] Li, S., Ostwald, D., Giese, M. & Kourtzi, Z. (2007). Flexible coding for categorical decisions in the human brain. *J Neurosci* 27, 12321-12330.

[41] Lindsay, D. S., Jack, P. C., Jr. & Christian, M. A. (1991). Other-race face perception. *J Appl Psychol* 76, 587-589.

[42] Logothetis, N. K., Guggenberger, H., Peled, S. & Pauls, J. (1999). Functional imaging of the monkey brain. *Nat Neurosci* 2, 555-562.

[43] Logothetis, N. K. & Pauls, J. (1995). Psychophysical and physiological evidence for viewer-centered object representations in the primate. *Cereb Cortex* 5, 270-288.

[44] Marr, D. & Nishihara, H. K. (1978). Representation and recognition of the spatial organization of three-dimensional shapes. *Proc R Soc Lond B Biol Sci* 200, 269-294.

[45] McLaren, D. G., Kosmatka, K. J., Oakes, T. R., Kroenke, C. D., Kohama, S. G., Matochik, J. A., Ingram, D. K. & Johnson, S. C. (2009). A population-average MRI-based atlas collection of the rhesus macaque. *Neuroimage* 45, 52-59. doi:S1053-8119(08)01176-2 [pii], 10.1016/j.neuroimage.2008.10.058.

[46] Medin, D. L. & Schaffer, M. M. (1978). Context theory of classification learning. *Psychological Review* 85, 207-238.

[47] Moore, C. D., Cohen, M. X. & Ranganath, C. (2006). Neural mechanisms of expert skills in visual working memory. *J Neurosci* 26, 11187-11196.

[48] Murphy, G. L. & Medin, D. L. (1985). The role of theories in conceptual coherence. *Psychol Rev* 92, 289-316.

[49] Norman, K. A., Polyn, S. M., Detre, G. J. & Haxby, J. V. (2006). Beyond mind-reading: multi-voxel pattern analysis of fMRI data. *Trends Cogn Sci* 10, 424-430.

[50] Nosofsky, R. (1986). Attention, similarity, and the identification-categorization relationship. *J of experimental psychology: general* 115, 39-57.

[51] Op de Beeck H, B. E., Wagemans J, Sunaert S, Van Hecke P (2000). The representation of shape in the context of visual object categorization tasks. *Neuroimage* 12, 28-40.

[52] Op de Beeck, H., Wagemans, J. & Vogels, R. (2001). Inferotemporal neurons represent low-dimensional configurations of parameterized shapes. *Nat Neurosci* 4, 1244-1252. doi:10.1038/nn767, nn767 [pii].

[53] Op de Beeck, H. P., Baker, C. I., DiCarlo, J. J. & Kanwisher, N. G. (2006). Discrimination training alters object representations in human extrastriate cortex. *J Neurosci* 26, 13025-13036. doi:26/50/13025 [pii], 10.1523/JNEUROSCI.2481-06.2006.

[54] Orban, G. A., Van Essen, D. & Vanduffel, W. (2004). Comparative mapping of higher visual areas in monkeys and humans. *Trends Cogn Sci* 8, 315-324.

[55] O'Toole, A. J., Deffenbacher, K. A., Valentin, D. & Abdi, H. (1994). Structural aspects of face recognition and the other-race effect. *Mem Cognit* 22, 208-224.

[56] Petit, L., Clark, V. P., Ingeholm, J. & Haxby, J. V. (1997). Dissociation of saccade-related and pursuit-related activation in human frontal eye fields as revealed by fMRI. *J Neurophysiol* 77, 3386-3390.

[57] Pinsk, M. A., DeSimone, K., Moore, T., Gross, C. G. & Kastner, S. (2005). Representations of faces and body parts in macaque temporal cortex: a functional MRI study.

Proc Natl Acad Sci U S A 102, 6996-7001. doi:0502605102 [pii], 10.1073/pnas.0502605102.

[58] Poggio, T. & Edelman, S. (1990). A network that learns to recognize three-dimensional objects. *Nature* 343, 263-266.

[59] Posner, M. I. & Keele, S. W. (1968). On the genesis of abstract ideas. *Journal of Experimental Psychology* 77, 353-363.

[60] Puce, A., Allison, T., Gore, J. C. & McCarthy, G. (1995). Face-sensitive regions in human extrastriate cortex studied by functional MRI. *J Neurophysiol* 74, 1192-1199.

[61] Rhodes, G., Byatt, G., Michie, P. T. & Puce, A. (2004). Is the fusiform face area specialized for faces, individuation, or expert individuation? *J Cogn Neurosci* 16, 189-203. doi:10.1162/089892904322984508.

[62] Richardson, M. W. (1938) Multidimensional Psychophysics. In: *46th annual meeting of the American Psychological Association*, pp. 659. Colombus, Ohio: Psychological Bulletin.

[63] Rosch, E. (1976) Classification of real-world objects: origins and representations in cognition. In: *Thinking: readings in cognitive science*, (eds.) P. N. Johnson-Laird & P. C. Wason, pp. 212-277. Cambridge University Press.

[64] Rosch, E., Mervis, C. B., Gray, W. D., Johnson, D. M. & Boyes-Braem, P. (1976a). Basic objects in natural categories. *Cognitive Psychology* 8, 382-439.

[65] Rosch, E., Simpson, C. & Miller, R. S. (1976b). Structural bases of typicality effects. *J Exp Psychol: Hum Perception Performance* 2, 491-502.

[66] Saleem, K. S. & Logothetis, N. K. (2006) A Combined MRI and Histology Atlas of the Rhesus Monkey Brain. Academic Press.

[67] Sands, S. F., Lincoln, C. E. & Wright, A. A. (1982). Pictorial similarity judgments and the organization of visual memory in the rhesus monkey. *Journal of Experimental Psychology: General* 111, 369-389.

[68] Schyns, P. G. & Rodet, L. (1997). Categorization creates functional features. *Journal of Experimental Psychology: Learning, Memory & Cognition* 23, 681-696.

[69] Sergent, J., Ohta, S. & MacDonald, B. (1992). Functional neuroanatomy of face and object processing. A positron emission tomography study. *Brain* 115 Pt 1, 15-36.

[70] Shepard, R. (1958). Stimulus and response generalisation: tests of a model relating ganeralization to distance in psychological space. *Journal of Experimental Psychology* 55, 509.

[71] Shepard, R. (1962a). The analysis of proximities: Multidimensional scaling with an unknown distance function. Part I. *Psychometrika* 27, 125-140.

[72] Shepard, R. (1962b). The analysis of proximities: Multidimensional scaling with an unknown distance function. Part II. *Psychometrika* 27, 219-246.

[73] Shepard, R. (1987). Toward a universal law of generalization for psychological science. *Science* 237, 1317-1323.

[74] Sigala, N. (2004). Visual categorization and the inferior temporal cortex. *Behav Brain Res* 149, 1-7. doi:S0166432803002249 [pii].

[75] Sigala, N. (2009). Natural images: a lingua franca for primates? *The Open Neuroscience Journal* 3, 48-51. doi:10.2174/1874082000903010048.

[76] Sigala, N., Gabbiani, F. & Logothetis, N. K. (2002). Visual categorization and object representation in monkeys and humans. *J Cogn Neurosci* 14, 187-198. doi: 10.1162/089892902317236830.

[77] Sigala, N. & Logothetis, N. K. (2002). Visual categorization shapes feature selectivity in the primate temporal cortex. *Nature* 415, 318-320. doi:10.1038/415318a, 415318a [pii].

[78] Sugihara, T., Edelman, S. & Tanaka, K. (1998). Representation of objective similarity among 3D shapes in the monkey. *Biological Cybernetics* 78, 1-7.

[79] Tanaka, J. W. & Taylor, M. (1991). Object categories and expertise: is the basic level in the eye of the beholder? *Cognitive Psychology* 23, 457-482.

[80] Torgerson, W. (1952). Multidimensional scaling: I. Theory and method. *Psychometrica* 17, 401-419.

[81] Tsao, D. Y., Freiwald, W. A., Knutsen, T. A., Mandeville, J. B. & Tootell, R. B. (2003). Faces and objects in macaque cerebral cortex. *Nat Neurosci* 6, 989-995.

[82] Tsao, D. Y., Moeller, S. & Freiwald, W. A. (2008a). Comparing face patch systems in macaques and humans. *Proc Natl Acad Sci U S A* 105, 19514-19519. doi:0809662105 [pii], 10.1073/pnas.0809662105.

[83] Tsao, D. Y., Schweers, N., Moeller, S. & Freiwald, W. A. (2008b). Patches of face-selective cortex in the macaque frontal lobe. *Nat Neurosci* 11, 877-879. doi:nn.2158 [pii], 10.1038/nn.2158.

[84] van der Linden, M., Murre, J. M. & van Turennout, M. (2008). Birds of a feather flock together: experience-driven formation of visual object categories in human ventral temporal cortex. *PLoS One* 3, e3995. doi:10.1371/journal.pone.0003995.

[85] Van Dijk KR, Hedden T, Venkataraman A, Evans KC, Lazar SW & RL., B. (2010). Intrinsic functional connectivity as a tool for human connectomics: theory, properties, and optimization. *J Neurophysiol.* 103, 297-321.

[86] Vogel, A. C., Power, J. D., Petersen, S. E. & Schlaggar, B. L. (2010). Development of the brain's functional network architecture. *Neuropsychol Rev* 20, 362-375. doi:10.1007/s11065-010-9145-7.

[87] Wong, A. C., Palmeri, T. J., Rogers, B. P., Gore, J. C. & Gauthier, I. (2009). Beyond shape: how you learn about objects affects how they are represented in visual cortex. *PLoS One* 4, e8405. doi:10.1371/journal.pone.0008405.

[88] Xu, Y. (2005). Revisiting the role of the fusiform face area in visual expertise. *Cereb Cortex* 15, 1234-1242. doi:bhi006 [pii], 10.1093/cercor/bhi006.

[89] Young, M. P. & Yamane, S. (1992). Sparse Population Coding of Faces in the Inferotemporal Cortex. Science 256, 1327.

Permissions

All chapters in this book were first published by InTech Open; hereby published with permission under the Creative Commons Attribution License or equivalent. Every chapter published in this book has been scrutinized by our experts. Their significance has been extensively debated. The topics covered herein carry significant findings which will fuel the growth of the discipline. They may even be implemented as practical applications or may be referred to as a beginning point for another development.

The contributors of this book come from diverse backgrounds, making this book a truly international effort. This book will bring forth new frontiers with its revolutionizing research information and detailed analysis of the nascent developments around the world.

We would like to thank all the contributing authors for lending their expertise to make the book truly unique. They have played a crucial role in the development of this book. Without their invaluable contributions this book wouldn't have been possible. They have made vital efforts to compile up to date information on the varied aspects of this subject to make this book a valuable addition to the collection of many professionals and students.

This book was conceptualized with the vision of imparting up-to-date information and advanced data in this field. To ensure the same, a matchless editorial board was set up. Every individual on the board went through rigorous rounds of assessment to prove their worth. After which they invested a large part of their time researching and compiling the most relevant data for our readers.

The editorial board has been involved in producing this book since its inception. They have spent rigorous hours researching and exploring the diverse topics which have resulted in the successful publishing of this book. They have passed on their knowledge of decades through this book. To expedite this challenging task, the publisher supported the team at every step. A small team of assistant editors was also appointed to further simplify the editing procedure and attain best results for the readers.

Apart from the editorial board, the designing team has also invested a significant amount of their time in understanding the subject and creating the most relevant covers. They scrutinized every image to scout for the most suitable representation of the subject and create an appropriate cover for the book.

The publishing team has been an ardent support to the editorial, designing and production team. Their endless efforts to recruit the best for this project, has resulted in the accomplishment of this book. They are a veteran in the field of academics and their pool of knowledge is as vast as their experience in printing. Their expertise and guidance has proved useful at every step. Their uncompromising quality standards have made this book an exceptional effort. Their encouragement from time to time has been an inspiration for everyone.

The publisher and the editorial board hope that this book will prove to be a valuable piece of knowledge for researchers, students, practitioners and scholars across the globe.

List of Contributors

Julia Kivistö
Department of Neurology, Kuopio University Hospital, Kuopio, Finland

Hilkka Soininen and Maija Pihlajamäki
Department of Neurology, Kuopio University Hospital, Kuopio, Finland
Unit of Neurology, Institute of Clinical Medicine, School of Medicine, University of Eastern Finland, Kuopio, Finland

Aymeric Guillot, Franck Di Rienzo and Christian Collet
Centre de Recherche et d'Innovation sur le Sport, Performance Motrice, Mentale et du Matériel (P3M), Université de Lyon, Université Claude Bernard Lyon 1, France

Deborah A. Hall
NIHR National Biomedical Research Unit in Hearing, Nottingham, UK

Cornelis P. Lanting
MRC Institute of Hearing Research, Nottingham, UK

Douglas E.H. Hartley
Department of Otorhinolaryngology, Nottingham University, UK

Alyssa A. Brewer and Brian Barton
Center for Cognitive Neuroscience and Department of Cognitive Sciences, University of California, Irvine, CA, USA

Aaron J. Suminski
Biomedical Engineering, Marquette University, Milwaukee, WI, USA
Organismal Biology and Anatomy, University of Chicago, Chicago, IL, USA

Tessa M. van Leeuwen and Mark Rijpkema
Donders Institute for Brain, Cognition and Behaviour, Radboud University Nijmegen, The Netherlands

Robert A. Scheidt
Biomedical Engineering, Marquette University, Milwaukee, WI, USA
Neurology, Medical College of Wisconsin, Milwaukee, WI, USA
Physical Medicine and Rehabilitation, Feinberg School of Medicine, Northwestern University, Chicago, IL, USA

Karl Magnus Petersson and Peter Hagoort
Donders Institute for Brain, Cognition and Behaviour, Radboud University Nijmegen, The Netherlands
Max Planck Institute for Psycholinguistics, Nijmegen, The Netherlands

Oliver Langner
Donders Institute for Brain, Cognition and Behaviour, Radboud University Nijmegen, The Netherlands
Behavioural Science Institute, Radboud University Nijmegen, The Netherlands

T. Dorina Papageorgiou
Departments of Neuroscience and Neurology, Baylor College of Medicine, Houston, Texas, USA

Amalia Papanikolaou
Departments of MaxPlanck Institute for Biological Cybernetics, Tuebingen, Germany

Stelios M. Smirnakis
Departments of Neuroscience and Neurology, Baylor College of Medicine, Houston, Texas, USA
Departments of MaxPlanck Institute for Biological Cybernetics, Tuebingen, Germany

Lora Likova
The Smith-Kettlewell Eye Research Institute, San Francisco, CA, USA

Natasha Sigala
Clinical Imaging Sciences Centre, Brighton and Sussex Medical School, University of Sussex, United Kingdom

Index

www.ingramcontent.com/pod-product-compliance
Lightning Source LLC
LaVergne TN
LVHW062231200926
848484LV00006B/1518